THE ORGANIC CHEMISTRY

OF

MEDICINAL AGENTS

THE ORGANIC CHEMISTRY

OF

MEDICINAL AGENTS

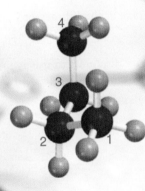

ADAM RENSLO, PHD

Associate Professor
Department of Pharmaceutical Chemistry
School of Pharmacy
University of California, San Francisco

Mc
Graw
Hill
Education | Medical

New York Chicago San Francisco Athens London Madrid Mexico City
Milan New Delhi Singapore Sydney Toronto

The Organic Chemistry of Medicinal Agents

1 2 3 4 5 6 7 8 9 0   CTP/CTP   20 19 18 17 16 15

ISBN 978-0-07-179421-3
MHID 0-07-179421-2

This book was set in Sabon LT Std by MPS Limited.
The editors were Michael Weitz and Peter J. Boyle.
The production supervisor was Richard Ruzycka.
Project management was provided by Ruchika Abrol, MPS Limited.
The designer was Eve Siegel.
China Translation & Printing Services, Ltd., was printer and binder.

This book was printed on acid-free paper.

Cataloging-in-publication data for this book is on file at the Library of Congress.

McGraw-Hill books are available at special quantity discounts to use as premiums and sales promotions, or for use in corporate training programs. To contact a representative please e-mail us at bulksales@mcgraw-hill.com.

Contents

Contributors   ix

Preface   xi

1. The Nature of Bonding in Organic Molecules   1
Adam Renslo & Dmitry Koltun

Introduction   1

The Nature of Covalent and
   Ionic Bonds   2

Box 1.1—Drawing organic molecules   4

Polarization of Covalent Bonds   4

Atomic Orbitals and Valence Bond
   Theory   5

Hybridization of Orbitals and Tetrahedral
   Carbon   8

Hybrid Orbitals of Oxygen and Nitrogen
   and Common Functional Groups   11

Box 1.2—Functional groups containing
   phosphorus or sulfur   12

Aromaticity   14

Heteroaromatic Ring Systems in
   Drug Structures   17

Summary   19

Exercises   20

2. Non-Covalent Interactions   23
Adam Renslo

Introduction   23

Enthalpic and Entropic Contributions
   to Ligand/Drug Binding   25

The Strength of Non-Covalent
   Interactions   27

Desolvation and the
   Hydrophobic Effect   27

Ionic Interactions   29

Box 2.1—Ionic interactions in a proton
   channel from influenza virus   29

Hydrogen Bonds   29

C–H Bonds as Hydrogen Bond
   Donors   32

Aryl Rings as Hydrogen
   Bond Acceptors   33

Box 2.2—A π-hydrogen bond in
   glutathione S-transferase   33

Aryl-Aryl Interactions   34

Cation-π Interactions   34

Box 2.3—Hydrophobic and cation-π
   interactions in the binding of
   neurotransmitters and drugs   35

Halogen Bonds   35

Box 2.4—C–F bonds as hydrogen
   bond acceptors and in orthogonal
   interactions with carbonyl groups   36

Summary   37

Case Study—Inhibitors of Factor Xa as
   Anticoagulants   38

Exercises   40

3. Stereochemistry   41
Adam Renslo

Introduction   41

Chirality and the Shape of Molecules   42

Stereoisomers—Some Important
   Definitions   42

Box 3.1—Determining isomeric and stereochemical relationships between molecules   *43*

Avoiding Confusion   *43*

Stereoisomers of 1,3-Dimethylcyclohexane   *43*

Chirality Centers   *44*

Assigning the Configuration of Chirality Centers   *44*

Box 3.2—Cahn–Ingold–Prelog rules in brief   *46*

Configurational Assignment and Stereochemical Relationships   *46*

Meso Compounds   *46*

Chirality Centers at Non-Carbon Atoms   *48*

Other Sources of Chirality and Stereoisomerism   *48*

Box 3.3—Atropisomerism   *49*

Summary   *49*

Case Study—Racemic and Non-Racemic Drugs   *51*

Exercises   *53*

4. Conformations of Organic Molecules   *57*
Adam Renslo

Introduction   *57*

Newman Projections and Dihedral Angles   *58*

Conformations and Energies of Ethane—Torsional Strain   *58*

Conformations and Energies of Larger Acyclic Molecules—Steric Strain   *60*

Conformations of Small Rings   *62*

Box 4.1—The three major types of strain in organic molecules   *63*

Conformations of Cyclohexane and Related Six-Membered Rings   *64*

Estimating the Conformational Preferences of Substituted Cyclohexanes   *66*

Box 4.2—Drawing chair conformations   *68*

Conformationally Constrained Ring Systems   *69*

Box 4.3—Conformational constraint in opiate analgesics   *70*

Summary   *71*

Case Study—Neuraminidase Inhibitors and the Influenza Virus   *72*

Exercises   *74*

5. Acid-Base Chemistry of Organic Molecules   *77*
Susan Miller

Introduction   *77*

Three Theories of Acids and Bases   *77*

Self-Ionization of Water and the pH Scale   *79*

Avoiding Confusion—Use of "Acid" and "Base" and Related Terms   *79*

The Acid Dissociation Constant K_a and pK_a as a Measure of Acid Strength   *80*

Electronegativity and Size of Atoms and Acid/Base Strength   *82*

Atom Hybridization and Acid/Base Strength   *85*

Resonance Electronic Effects on Acid/Base Strength   *86*

Inductive Electronic Effects of Substituents on Acid/Base Strength   *89*

Combined Inductive and Resonance Effects on Acid/Base Strength   *92*

Proximity and Through-Space Effects on Acid/Base Strength   *95*

The Henderson–Hasselbalch Relationship and Acid/Base Equilibria as a Function of pH   *96*

Summary   *97*

Case Study—Discovery of Tagamet   *99*

Exercises   *101*

6. Nucleophilic Substitution, Addition, and Elimination Reactions   *105*
Jie Jack Li & Adam Renslo

Introduction   *105*

Nucleophiles   *106*

Electrophiles   *108*

Box 6.1—Electrophiles in cancer drugs   *109*

Leaving Groups   *109*

Nucleophilic Aliphatic Substitution Reactions—S_N2 *110*

Box 6.2—S_N2 reactions in biological chemistry   *113*

Nucleophilic Aliphatic Substitution Reactions—S_N1 *114*

Neighboring Group Assistance in S_N1 Reactions   *116*

Nucleophilic Aromatic Substitution—S_NAr *118*

Addition Reactions   *119*

Elimination Reactions—E1 and E2   *121*

Summary   *123*

Case Study—Drugs That Form a Covalent Bond to Their Target   *124*

Exercises   *126*

7. Reactions of Carbonyl Species   *131*
Adam Renslo

Introduction   *131*

Nature of the Carbonyl Group   *131*

Relative Reactivity of Carbonyl-Containing Functional Groups   *133*

Hydration of Aldehydes and Ketones   *134*

Reactions of Aldehydes and Ketones with Alcohols   *136*

Box 7.1—Glucuronidation in the metabolism of drugs   *138*

Imines and Enamines   *139*

Box 7.2—Imines in drug-protein conjugates   *142*

Oximes and Hydrazones   *142*

Chemical Hydrolysis of Ester and Amide Bonds   *144*

Enzymatic Hydrolysis of Peptide Bonds by Proteases   *148*

Box 7.3—Drugs designed to inhibit proteases   *151*

Summary   *152*

Case Study—Odanacatib   *153*

Exercises   *155*

8. Radical Chemistry   *159*
John Flygare & Adam Renslo

Introduction   *159*

Formation, Stability, and Molecular Orbital View of Radicals   *159*

Radical Reactions   *161*

Reactions of Molecular Oxygen   *163*

Iron-Mediated Radical Reactions in Drug Metabolism   *165*

Box 8.1—Fenton chemistry in the action of antimalarial drugs   *167*

Summary   *169*

Case Study—Calicheamicin γ_1 *169*

Exercises   *171*

Solutions to Exercises   *175*

Index   *203*

Contributors

 John Flygare has taught or co-taught courses in organic chemistry, biochemistry, and medicinal chemistry at Stanford University since 1997, with a combined total enrollment of over 5,000 students. He is also a project leader at Genentech in South San Francisco where he leads drug discovery teams in disease areas including oncology, infectious diseases, and neurodegeneration. Several compounds from these programs are currently in human clinical trials. He received his PhD in organic chemistry from Northwestern University and was an NIH Postdoctoral Fellow at Stanford University.

 Dmitry Koltun received his undergraduate education at Higher Chemical College of the Russian Academy of Sciences and his PhD degree from University of Minnesota with Prof. Thomas Hoye in 1999. He began his career at MediChem Life Sciences in Chicago, then moved to CV Therapeutics in Palo Alto, California. He is currently a senior research scientist in the Medicinal Chemistry Department at Gilead Sciences in Foster City, California. He lives in Foster City, California with his wife Elena and daughters Vera and Sonya.

 Jie Jack Li earned his PhD in organic chemistry in 1995 at Indiana University. After a postdoctoral fellowship at MIT, he worked as a medicinal chemist at Pfizer and Bristol-Myers Squibb from 1997 to 2012. Since then he has been an associate professor of chemistry at the University of San Francisco, teaching organic and medicinal chemistry. He has published 23 books for specialist and lay audiences, covering topics ranging from organic and medicinal chemistry to the history of drug discovery.

 Susan M. Miller received her PhD in organic chemistry and mechanistic enzymology from the University of California Berkeley. After postdoctoral work in biological chemistry at the University of Michigan in Ann Arbor, she joined the School of Pharmacy at the University of California, San Francisco, in 1993 where she is now professor of pharmaceutical chemistry. Her research interests lie broadly in mechanistic and structure/function studies of redox enzymes and enzymes involved in biosynthetic pathways for antimicrobials. She teaches aspects of mechanistic organic chemistry and enzymology in both professional pharmacy and graduate chemistry and biophysics programs.

 Adam Renslo earned a BA in chemistry from St. Olaf College in 1993 and a PhD in organic chemistry from Massachusetts Institute of Technology in 1998. After postdoctoral studies at the Scripps Research Institute, he worked as a medicinal chemist in the pharmaceutical industry for 6 years. In 2006 he joined the faculty in the Department of Pharmaceutical Chemistry at the University of California, San Francisco. His research interests include the development of new approaches for targeted drug delivery in infectious disease and cancer. He teaches synthetic organic and medicinal chemistry in both the professional pharmacy and graduate chemistry and chemical biology programs.

Preface

The chemistry of carbon-based molecules—their structures, intermolecular interactions, and reactivity—underlies life as we know it and thus also the beneficial (and sometimes undesired) effects of the medicines we use. The fact that rather simple organic molecules can be profoundly effective in treating human disease in all its complexity must rank among the most significant findings of medicine and basic science. For many students, this realization foments a desire to pursue a career in one of the various fields related to the discovery, study, or appropriate administration of medicines. In my own case, this meant embarking on the study of organic chemistry and learning how to synthesize organic molecules in the laboratory. Later, as a medicinal chemist working in the pharmaceutical industry, I experienced the thrill of seeing a few milligrams (mere specks!) of a newly synthesized compound cure an otherwise lethal infection in a mouse. A few such compounds would later be destined for studies in human patients, beginning the long and often perilous path toward the approval of a new drug.

This textbook is informed by my experiences as a practicing medicinal chemist and as an educator of pharmacy students at the University of California, San Francisco. In its organization and content, the text is largely based on a semester-long course in organic chemistry taught to first-year PharmD students at UCSF. It is intended as a teaching textbook, a companion for students of pharmacy or medicinal chemistry, that can be covered in its entirety in a single semester. Given this, the text is necessarily limited in its scope and is not intended to replace any of the excellent and comprehensive handbooks of medicinal and pharmaceutical chemistry that are available. What *is* covered here are those topics we have found most relevant and instructive in providing students of pharmacy with a solid grounding in organic chemistry as it relates to drug structure and action.

The first four chapters of the text cover the fundamentals of drug *structure* and *binding*—the nature of the chemical bonds in drug structure, the types of non-covalent intermolecular interactions drugs form with their targets, and their three-dimensional shape and conformations. The final four chapters are concerned with chemical *reactivity* relevant to drug action—the reactivity of (some) drugs toward their targets, the metabolism of nearly all drugs, and the reactions carried out by the enzymes that modify drugs or can be targeted by them. Throughout the text, the discussion is intertwined with illustrative examples of drug synthesis, action, or metabolism. Also, each chapter concludes with a drug "case study" selected to emphasize and reinforce the concepts introduced in that chapter.

I am indebted to a number of individuals without whom this project could never have happened. It has been a distinct privilege to interact with the bright and inquisitive PharmD students that UCSF is fortunate enough to attract. Their willing feedback as to what is and is not working in the classroom has shaped how we teach organic chemistry at UCSF, and this in turn is reflected in the final form of the book. I must likewise acknowledge current and former UCSF colleagues (Susan M. Miller, Thomas Scanlan, and Paul Ortiz de Montellano) who contributed to developing the organic chemistry curriculum in the PharmD program. The editors and production designers at McGraw-Hill Education have been a pleasure to work with. I would especially like to thank Michael Weitz, Peter Boyle, and Ruchika Abrol for their assistance and encouragement. I am grateful to Professor Peter Beak (University of Illinois at Urbana-Champaign) for reading the final manuscript. Last but not least, I must thank my coauthors and contributors (John Flygare, Dmitry Koltun, Jie Jack Li, and Susan M. Miller), top-notch researchers and educators who put their own stamp on the chapters to which they contributed. We hope that this first edition of *The Organic Chemistry of Medicinal Agents* will prove useful for students and instructors alike and we welcome suggestions for improvements and additions to future editions.

Adam Renslo

Chapter **1**

The Nature of Bonding in Organic Molecules

Adam Renslo & Dmitry Koltun

CHAPTER OUTLINE

1.1 Introduction
1.2 The Nature of Covalent and Ionic Bonds
   Box 1.1—Drawing organic molecules
1.3 Polarization of Covalent Bonds
1.4 Atomic Orbitals and Valence Bond Theory
1.5 Hybridization of Orbitals and Tetrahedral Carbon

1.6 Hybrid Orbitals of Oxygen and Nitrogen and Common Functional Groups
   Box 1.2—Functional groups containing Phosphorus or Sulfur
1.7 Aromaticity
1.8 Heteroaromatic Ring Systems in Drug Structures
1.9 Summary
1.10 Exercises

1.1 Introduction

In this chapter, we will review fundamental concepts of chemical structure and bonding in the organic molecules that make up drugs and their biological targets. By "organic," we mean molecules that are constructed primarily from the element carbon (C). Carbon exhibits striking versatility in its ability to form various different bonding arrangements with other carbon atoms as well as with other biologically relevant elements such as nitrogen (N), oxygen (O), sulfur (S), and phosphorus (P). It is this versatility that allowed carbon-based life to emerge on our planet. Thus, to understand the molecules of life—proteins, lipids, nucleic acids, hormones, etc.—and the drugs that interact with them, we must start with a solid understanding of structure and bonding in organic molecules. In this chapter, we will begin by contrasting the nature of ionic and

covalent bonding and will describe the polarization of covalent bonds. We will then dive deeper into the nature of the covalent bond, discussing atomic and molecular orbitals, the "hybridization" of orbitals, and aromaticity. Finally, we will review some important functional groups and organic ring systems that figure prominently in the structures of biological molecules and drugs.

In the chapters that follow we will learn more about the intermolecular interactions, mostly non-covalent, that govern the binding of a drug molecule to its intended (and sometimes unintended) biological targets. For now, it is important to recognize that a drug molecule's particular structure—its shape and the nature and connectivity of its atoms—determines what biological activities it will have. If a molecule's structure leads to interactions in the body that correct an abnormality, restore normal function of a cell, or kill a pathogenic

1

or cancerous cell, a new medicine is born. The seemingly endless ways in which organic molecules can be assembled has allowed scientists to create our current pharmacopeia and affords confidence that still more new medicines will be developed to address currently unmet medical needs.

1.2 The Nature of Covalent and Ionic Bonds

Atoms are comprised of a nucleus containing positively charged protons and uncharged neutrons surrounded by negatively charged electrons. On account of their very low mass, electrons behave as both particles and waves. The peculiar wave-like nature of the electron is what prevents this negatively charged particle from simply "falling" into the positively charged nucleus, to which it is clearly attracted. Wave-like electrons are spatially confined to specific atomic "orbitals" surrounding the nucleus. While atomic and molecular orbitals (Sections 1.4 and 1.5) underlie our current understanding of chemical bonding, their existence was hinted at much earlier by a certain periodicity in the chemical reactivity of the elements. It was this observation that allowed Mendeleev to construct his periodic table of the elements. A partial periodic table including just the first three "periods" (rows) of elements most relevant to organic chemistry is provided here (Figure 1.1).

The periodic table arranges the elements in order of increasing number of protons (atomic number, Z) and by "groups" (columns) of elements with similar chemical reactivity. This periodicity led to an understanding of chemical reactivity and bonding as being related to the filling of electron "shells" surrounding the nucleus. To understand why chemical bonds form at all, it is useful to consider those few elements that generally *do not form bonds*—the noble gases. Found at the far right-hand side of the periodic table, noble gases such as helium (He), neon (Ne), and argon (Ar) are "nobly unreactive" because their outermost electron shell is perfectly filled. If helium requires only two electrons to complete its outermost shell, then neon and argon require an additional 8 and 16 electrons, respectively, to do so. The driving force for chemical bonding can thus be understood as a desire of atoms to achieve perfectly filled electron shells (a noble gas "configuration") by forming bonds to other atoms. This can be achieved in one of two ways—by the *exchange of electrons* in an **ionic bond** or by the *sharing of electrons* in a **covalent bond**.

The chemistry of carbon involves covalent bonding and so we will discuss ionic bonding only briefly here. Common table salt (sodium chloride, Na^+Cl^-) provides the most familiar example of an ionic bond between two atoms. Looking at the periodic table we see that both sodium and chlorine are just one column away (and thus one electron away) from a noble gas configuration. Transfer of an electron from sodium to

		1A (1)							8A (18)
	1	1 **H** $1s^1$	2A (2)	3A (13)	4A (14)	5A (15)	6A (16)	7A (17)	2 **He** $1s^2$
	2	3 **Li** [He] $2s^1$	4 **Be** [He] $2s^2$	5 **B** [He] $2s^2 2p^1$	6 **C** [He] $2s^2 2p^2$	7 **N** [He] $2s^2 2p^3$	8 **O** [He] $2s^2 2p^4$	9 **F** [He] $2s^2 2p^5$	10 **Ne** [He] $2s^2 2p^6$
	3	11 **Na** [Ne] $3s^1$	12 **Mg** [Ne] $3s^2$	13 **Al** [Ne] $3s^2 3p^1$	14 **Si** [Ne] $3s^2 3p^2$	15 **P** [Ne] $3s^2 3p^3$	16 **S** [Ne] $3s^2 3p^4$	17 **Cl** [Ne] $3s^2 3p^5$	18 **Ar** [Ne] $3s^2 3p^6$

(left axis label: Period)

Figure 1.1 Periodic table of the first 18 elements (atomic number $Z = 1$ through 18). Groups (columns) 1–8 represent the "main group" elements and are the elements most relevant to organic chemistry and drug structures. Electronic configurations are provided in condensed format, with configuration of valence electrons shown explicitly and inner sphere electrons indicated by the corresponding noble gas configuration, either [He] or [Ne].

chlorine produces a sodium **cation** (Na^+) and chloride **anion** (Cl^-), each with the electronic configuration of neon (i.e., a filled outer electron shell). The "bond" in Na^+Cl^- can be thought of as the electrostatic attraction between the sodium and chloride ions. The benign, unreactive nature of Na^+Cl^- can be contrasted with elemental sodium metal (Na), which reacts violently with water, and elemental chlorine gas (diatomic Cl_2), which was used as a warfare agent in World War I.

Carbon does not form ionic bonds because achieving a noble gas configuration would require that it acquire and stabilize four additional electrons, resulting in a tetra-anion with an overall charge of ⁻4. Small atoms such as C, N, and O are not capable of existing in such highly charged states. Instead, carbon achieves a noble gas configuration by forming four covalent bonds. Each bond comprises two electrons, one provided by the carbon atom and one provided by its bonding partner. With four bonds of two electrons each, a carbon atom has obtained the eight electrons (an octet) required to exactly fill its outermost electron shell. While we commonly shown bonds as simple lines, the chemist Gilbert N. Lewis developed a notation in which a bond is shown as a pair of dots, meant to represent the pair of shared electrons that make up the bond. Lewis structures can be used to show not only single bonds but also double and triple bonds, as illustrated (Figure 1.2). While this notation has clear limitations for drawing larger molecules, we still use Lewis notation to show and keep track of nonbonded lone pair electrons.

Since carbon must form four bonds to achieve a noble gas configuration, we say that carbon has a **valence** of four. By inspecting the periodic table (Figure 1.1), we can furthermore predict that nitrogen should have a valence of three and oxygen a valence of two, since

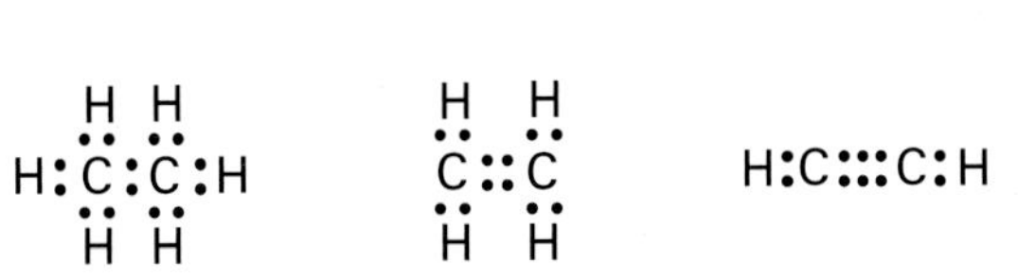

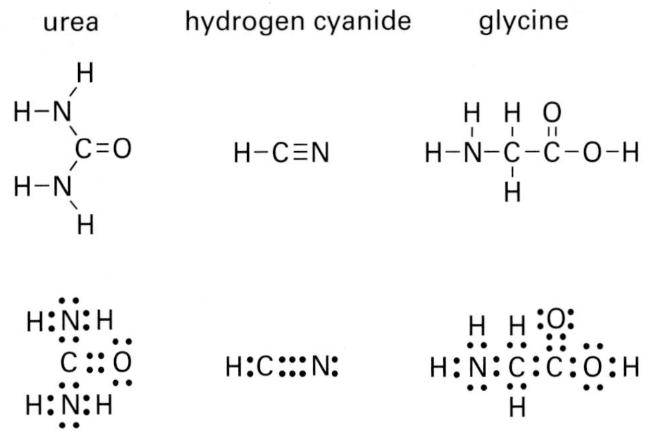

Figure 1.3 Structures of simple organic molecules shown as line drawings and complete Lewis structures.

nitrogen and oxygen will require three or two additional shared electrons, respectively, to achieve a noble gas configuration. Hydrogen is only one column removed from helium in the first row of the periodic table and so it has a valence of one. Similarly, the halogens (Cl, Br, I) have a valence of one since this group (column) is immediately adjacent to the noble gasses and thus is just one shared electron away from a filled shell.

Even with this rather crude notion of filling electron "shells," we can already make sense of a great variety of organic compounds formed from combinations of C, N, O, and H. Some biologically relevant molecules are shown (Figure 1.3) using Lewis structures to illustrate bonding and the filling of electron shells for H (two electrons required) and C, N, and O atoms (eight electrons required). Note that all the bonding and nonbonding electrons associated with a given atom count toward the total shared electron count. Thus the triple bond in hydrogen cyanide (HCN) contributes six shared electrons to both the C and N atoms. These six electrons, when combined with a pair of electrons in the H–C bond and the nonbonded electron pair on the nitrogen atom, produce a total electron count of eight for both C and N (Figure 1.3).

It's a good idea to become proficient in drawing Lewis structures as this approach helps us understand the locations of bonded and nonbonded electrons and reinforces the idea that bonds are comprised of pairs of shared electrons. Of course, using Lewis structures for drug-sized molecules is not practical and so chemists have developed short-hand notations for drawing chemical structures. These are reviewed in Box 1.1 and this standard notation will be used throughout most of this text.

Figure 1.2 Ethane, ethylene, and acetylene shown as Lewis drawings and as line drawings.

Box 1.1 Drawing organic molecules.

Chemists have adopted a drawing convention that avoids the need to explicitly show hydrogen atoms or even write a "C" for each carbon atom. A carbon atom is implicit at each "joint" in a structure, or at an unlabeled terminus. Hydrogen atoms are similarly implicit—each carbon is assumed to contain as many bound hydrogens as necessary to achieve tetravalency. Atoms other than carbon and hydrogen are shown explicitly, as are hydrogen atoms on non-carbon atoms (e.g., the hydroxyl group –OH in 1-butanol). It is also helpful to show hydrogen atoms explicitly on certain functional groups such as aldehydes. Common aromatic rings like phenyl and pyridine are best depicted with alternating double and single bonds.

1-butanol

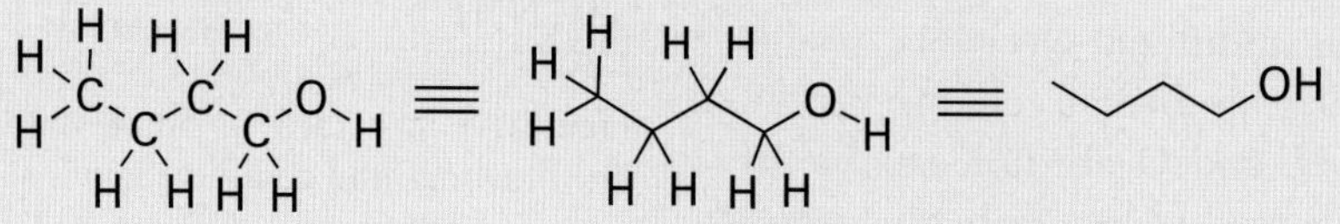

pyridine

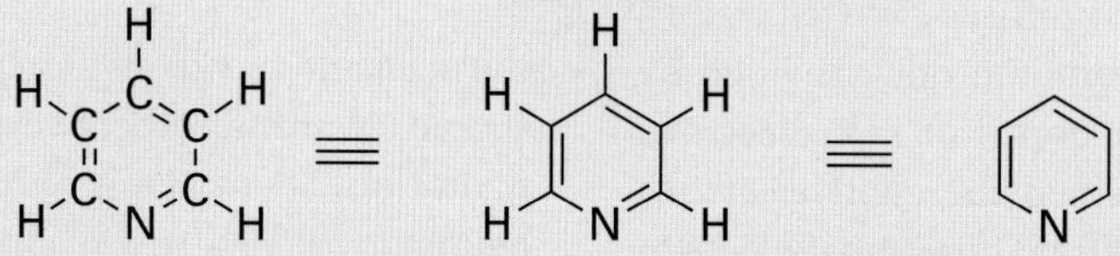

methyl group (Me)

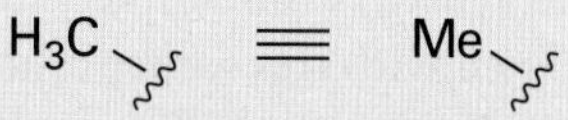

ethyl group (Et)

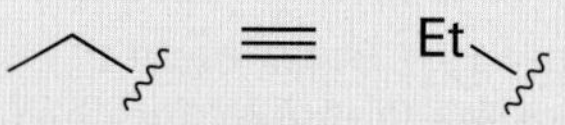

isopropyl group (*i*-Pr)

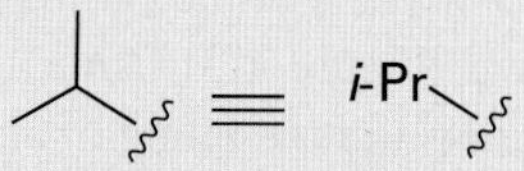

tert-butyl group (*t*-Bu)

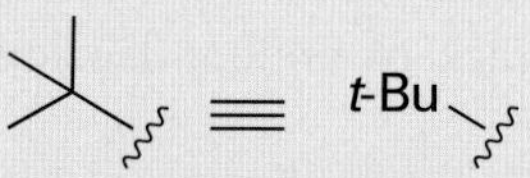

methoxy group (OMe)

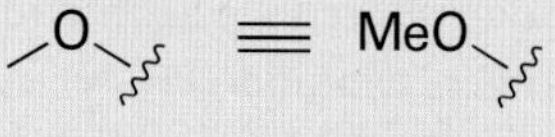

carboxyl group (CO$_2$H)

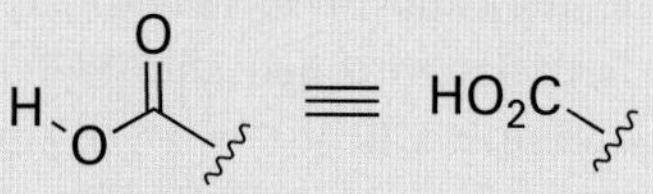

phenyl group (Ph)

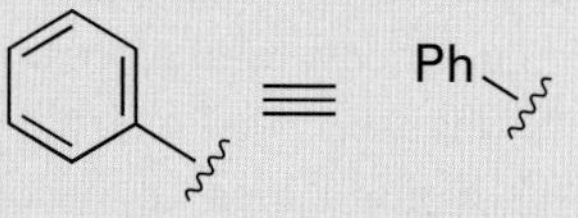

methyl ester group (CO$_2$Me)

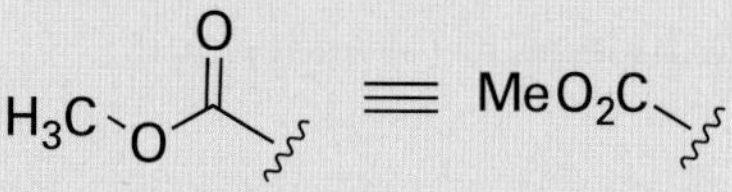

1.3 Polarization of Covalent Bonds

In our discussion of covalent bonding in the previous section, we described the electrons involved in a covalent bond as being shared between the two atoms involved in the bond. If the bonded atoms are identical then the electrons in that bond will indeed be shared equally. However, when two different atoms form a covalent bond, the electrons in the bond will usually not be shared equally between the bonded atoms and the bond is said to be **polarized**. Polarization of covalent bonds occurs because certain atoms have more power to pull electrons toward their nucleus than others. Generally, atoms located further to the right in a period (row) of the periodic table exert a stronger pull on electrons and are said to be more **electronegative**. Fluorine for example is more electronegative than carbon, and oxygen is more electronegative than nitrogen. We can illustrate the polarization of a C–F bond in one of two ways, as shown below. The $\delta+$ nomenclature indicates a partial positive charge and the $\delta-$ a region of partial negative charge. This polarization of the C–F bond (with greater electron density on fluorine) can also be illustrated using the special arrow shown below at right. Both of these notations will be used in subsequent sections and chapters of this text.

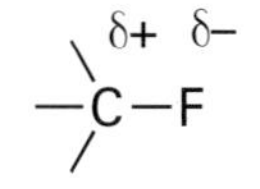

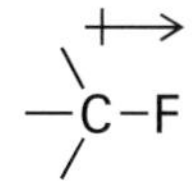

To a first approximation, we can estimate electronegativity using the concept of effective charge, which is equal to the total positive charge of the nucleus minus the negative charge of the non-valence ("inner shell") electrons. For example, lithium (Li) has an atomic number of three ($Z = 3$), and thus three protons in the nucleus and a nuclear charge of +3. Lithium has a single valence electron and two inner shell electrons so the effective charge of lithium is +1 ($3 - 2 = 1$). Being in the same row of the periodic table as lithium, fluorine also has only two inner shell electrons. With an atomic number 9 however, fluorine has an effective charge of +7 ($9 - 2 = 7$). Thus, if one negatively charged electron of Li is experiencing the pull of a single positive charge from the nucleus, an electron from F is experiencing a pull that is seven times greater.

Effective charge is useful for estimating relative electronegativity for elements in the same period (row) of the periodic table, but it is less predictive when comparing atoms from different periods and different groups, like sulfur and nitrogen. In these cases, the Pauling electronegativity scale becomes indispensable. Devised by Linus Pauling, the table assigns each atom an electronegativity coefficient, and the covalent bond is always polarized in the direction of an atom with a larger coefficient (Table 1.1). From the Pauling electronegativity scale we see that nitrogen (Pauling coefficient of 3.0) is more electronegative than sulfur (2.5). We will frequently refer to the electronegativity scale in subsequent chapters as this concept is very powerful in helping to understand chemical reactivity and intermolecular interactions of functional groups.

Table 1.1 Pauling Electronegativity Scale for Selected Elements Most Relevant to Organic Chemistry and Drug Action.

| Period | Group number | | | | | | |
	1A	2A	3A	4A	5A	6A	7A
1	H						
	2.1						
2	Li	Be	B	C	N	O	F
	1.0	1.5	2.0	2.5	3.0	3.5	4.0
3	Na	Mg	Al	Si	P	S	Cl
	0.9	1.2	1.5	1.8	2.1	2.5	3.0
4	K	Ca					Br
	0.8	1.0					2.8
5							I
							2.5

1.4 Atomic Orbitals and Valence Bond Theory

The concept of valence and the Lewis view of covalent bonding is useful to help us understand why elements like H, C, N, and O combine in various ways in organic molecules. Unfortunately, this view fails to explain many other important features of organic molecules, such as the three-dimensional arrangement of bonds and the fact that rotation about C–C single bonds is generally facile while rotation about C–C double or triple bonds is not. In this section we will introduce the concept of the **atomic orbital** as well as **valence bond theory**, in which covalent bonds are understood as arising from the "overlap" of atomic orbitals to form **molecular orbitals**. At least notionally, the overlap of atomic orbitals to form bonds can be equated with the sharing of electrons as posited in the Lewis description of the covalent bond.

Quantum mechanics is the field of physics that deals with matter and energy at very small scales, where the dual wave-particle nature of matter becomes important. According to quantum mechanics, electrons do not circle the nucleus in a fixed orbit like a planet around its sun, but rather are "spread out" in three-dimensional space around the nucleus as defined by specific solutions to the Schrödinger equation.

$$H\psi = E\psi$$

Each solution to this equation is associated with a particular wave function (ψ), also called an atomic

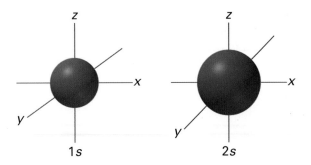

Figure 1.4 Boundary surface of 1s and 2s atomic orbitals. The spherical surfaces shown represent the boundary within which the probability of finding an electron is high (>90%). (Reproduced, with permission, from Carey FA, Giuliano RM. *Organic Chemistry.* 9th ed. New York: McGraw-Hill Education; 2014.)

orbital. The easiest way to visualize an atomic orbital is to consider its probability density, the square of the wave function (ψ^2), which corresponds to the probability that an electron will be found in a particular region of space surrounding the nucleus. The lowest energy atomic orbital for the hydrogen atom (and by extension all other atoms) is the 1s orbital, which has a spherical probability density (Figure 1.4) and can accommodate at most two electrons, provided they have opposite "spin" as dictated by the Pauli exclusion principle. The filling of a 1s orbital with two electrons is the more accurate picture of what is going on with He and its filled electron "shell." Next highest in energy is the 2s orbital, which is also spherical but with its electrons, on average, spending more time further from the nucleus. Next higher in energy are three energetically equivalent 2p orbitals, often denoted $2p_x$, $2p_y$, and $2p_z$. The p orbital has a bilobed or "dumbbell" shaped probability density, with a node of zero probability at the nucleus,

where the wave function changes sign. The three p orbitals are oriented along different axes when shown on a typical coordinate system (Figure 1.5). Each 2p orbital can accommodate up to two spin-paired electrons, for a total of six 2p electrons.

At this point, the power of quantum mechanics to describe the physical world of atoms should be apparent. Specific solutions to the Schrödinger equation provide discrete energy states (e.g., 1s, 2s, 2p orbitals) that are consistent with and help explain the particular arrangement of elements in the empirically derived periodic table. As atomic number increases, electrons are added to atomic orbitals in the order 1s, 2s, 2p, 3s, 3p, and so on according to the relative energies of the atomic orbitals, as determined by solutions to the Schrödinger equation. Let us then revisit the electronic configuration of the noble gas neon (Ne, Z = 10), using an atomic orbital diagram, with relative energies of the atomic orbitals displayed on either a vertical or horizontal axis (Figure 1.6). To complete the electronic configuration of Ne, we add 10 electrons sequentially to the 1s, then 2s, and finally the three 2p orbitals, using an up or down arrow to indicate electron spin (and being sure to show paired electrons with opposite spin). As expected for a noble gas, each orbital is filled with exactly two electrons, producing perfectly filled 1s, 2s, and 2p orbitals. We say that the electronic configuration of Ne is $1s^2 2s^2 2p^6$. The electronic configuration for all elements in the first three periods of the periodic table is shown in Figure 1.1 and in tabular format for the first 12 elements in Table 1.2.

Now consider the ionic bond in Na^+F^-. We can examine the electronic configurations of Na ($1s^2 2s^2 2p^6 3s^1$) and F ($1s^2 2s^2 2p^5$) as illustrated in energy diagrams (Figure 1.7). Sodium has a single unpaired electron in a higher energy 3s orbital, meaning that

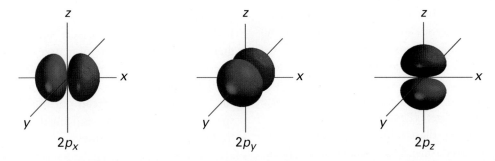

Figure 1.5 Boundary surface of 2p atomic orbitals. The 2p orbital has a node at the nucleus. Three 2p orbitals are oriented along the three axes of a typical three coordinate system. (Reproduced, with permission, from Carey FA, Giuliano RM. *Organic Chemistry.* 9th ed. New York: McGraw-Hill Education; 2014.)

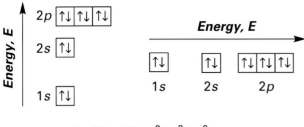

Ne (Z = 10) $1s^2\ 2s^2\ 2p^6$

Figure 1.6 Electronic configuration of the noble gas neon (Ne) shown in two versions of an energy diagram. While the horizontal orientation at right is useful in the way it recalls the periodic table, it incorrectly suggests that the three $2p$ orbitals are of different energies. In fact the energies of the three $2p$ orbitals are equal, as is accurately captured in the vertically displayed diagram at left.

on average this electron spends more time further away from the nucleus as compared to electrons in a $2p$ orbital. In transferring this $3s$ electron to a fluorine atom a cationic sodium ion (Na$^+$) and a fluoride anion (F$^-$) are produced, each with a new electronic

configuration of $1s^2\ 2s^2\ 2p^6$—the same electronic configuration as Ne.

The valence bond description of the covalent bond involves the mathematical combination of two wave functions (i.e., the "overlap" of atomic orbitals) to produce two new **molecular orbitals** (Figure 1.8). This is most simply illustrated for the formation of two new molecular orbitals (MOs) by the combination of two hydrogen $1s$ atomic orbitals (AOs). One of the new molecular orbitals is lower in energy than the $1s$ atomic orbitals while the other is higher in energy. Since one electron is contributed by each of the two $1s$ AOs, we will have two electrons in total to occupy the new MOs of the H–H molecule. These electrons will naturally occupy the MO with lower energy, which is called a **bonding orbital** since its filling represents the formation of a stable bond (being lower in energy than either of the $1s$ AO). The higher energy MO is called an **antibonding orbital** since it is higher in energy than the AOs and filling it would not be expected to result in the formation of a stable bond. Note that electrons

Table 1.2 Electron Configuration of the First 12 Elements.

Element	Atomic number Z	Number of electrons in indicated orbital					
		1s	2s	2p$_x$	2p$_y$	2p$_z$	3s
Hydrogen	1	1					
Helium	2	2					
Lithium	3	2	1				
Beryllium	4	2	2				
Boron	5	2	2	1			
Carbon	6	2	2	1	1		
Nitrogen	7	2	2	1	1	1	
Oxygen	8	2	2	2	1	1	
Fluorine	9	2	2	2	2	1	
Neon	10	2	2	2	2	2	
Sodium	11	2	2	2	2	2	1
Magnesium	12	2	2	2	2	2	2

Source: Reproduced, with permission, from Carey FA, Giuliano RM. *Organic Chemistry.* 9th ed. New York: McGraw-Hill Education; 2014.

Figure 1.7 Electronic configurations of sodium and fluorine in the ground state. Transfer of an electron from sodium to fluorine produces a pair of ions, Na$^+$ and F$^-$, each with the same electron configuration as the noble gas neon ($1s^2\ 2s^2\ 2p^6$).

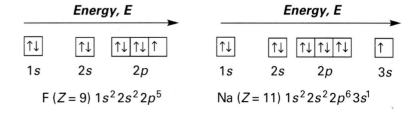

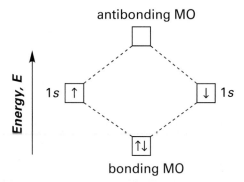

Figure 1.8 The combination of two partially filled hydrogen 1s orbitals leads to two new molecular orbitals, one a bonding MO and the other an antibonding MO. The two electrons fill the bonding orbital, leading to a stable covalent bond in H–H (H_2, molecular hydrogen).

fill MOs in pairs with opposite spin, since the exclusion principle applies to MOs as well as to AOs. Just as valence bond theory can explain the formation of the molecule H–H, it can also explain why the molecule He–He is not observed. With two electrons contributed from each 1s orbital of He, a total of four electrons would need to be placed into the MOs of He–He. This would involve filling both the bonding and antibonding orbitals and any energetic benefit accomplished by filling the former would be more than offset by filling the latter.

A second important tenant of valence bond theory is that stronger bonds are those in which orbital overlap is maximized. Orbital overlap is best visualized using the probability density or boundary surface representations of the AOs involved. From this perspective the combination of two 1s orbitals is equivalent to bringing

two spheres together until their surfaces intersect with a circular cross-section. We might expect orbital overlap to be maximal when this circular cross-section is greatest. For the H–H bond in H_2, this occurs when the nuclei of the two hydrogen atoms are separated by a distance of about 74 picometers or 0.74 Ångstroms (Å). The two 1s orbitals have been replaced by a bonding MO that is egg-shaped, with a circular cross-section and the highest probability of finding electron density between the two hydrogen nuclei. This type of MO is known as a sigma (σ) orbital and the resulting bond a σ bond. Note that rotation of a σ bond does not change the extent of orbital overlap (the cross-section remains circular), and thus σ bonds generally undergo free rotation.

The formation of a σ orbital as described above results from the "in-phase" combination of two 1s atomic orbitals. The corresponding higher-energy antibonding orbital is called a σ* ("sigma star") orbital and arises from "out-of-phase" combination of the 1s atomic orbitals. Note that the antibonding σ* orbital has a node of zero electron density between the two H atoms, whereas electron density is maximal at this same location in a bonding σ orbital (Figure 1.9).

1.5 Hybridization of Orbitals and Tetrahedral Carbon

With an understanding of atomic orbitals and valence bond theory we might hope we could explain bonding in simple organic molecules. However, if we examine the electronic configuration of carbon (Figure 1.10) we quickly discover an apparent problem. Carbon has a

(a) Add the 1s wave functions of two hydrogen atoms to generate a bonding molecular orbital (σ) of H_2. There is a high probability of finding both electrons in the region between the two nuclei.

(b) Subtract the 1s wave function of one hydrogen atom from the other to generate an antibonding molecular orbital (σ*) of H_2. There is a nodal surface where there is a zero probability of finding the electrons in the region between the two nuclei.

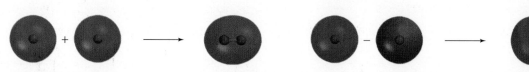

Figure 1.9 Graphical illustration of the formation of a bonding σ orbital and an antibonding σ* orbital by the combination of two 1s atomic orbitals of hydrogen. While the dumbbell shape of the σ* orbital resembles a *p* orbital, these must not be confused. The σ* orbital is a *molecular* orbital with a node between two different atoms whereas the *p* orbital represents electron density surrounding a single atom. (Reproduced, with permission, from Carey FA, Giuliano RM. *Organic Chemistry*. 9th ed. New York: McGraw-Hill Education; 2014.)

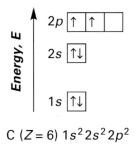

C (Z = 6) $1s^2 2s^2 2p^2$

Figure 1.10 Energy diagram showing the relative energies of atomic orbitals for carbon. Valence electrons available for bonding include two electrons in a 2s orbital and two unpaired electrons in 2p orbitals.

total of four valence electrons in its 2s and 2p orbitals, but the only unpaired electrons are the two found in 2p orbitals. We can imagine how each 2p orbital might combine with a 1s orbital of an H atom to form two filled MOs (two C–H σ bonds). However, it's not obvious how the other two electrons in the 2s orbital could be engaged in new bonds since they are already paired in a relatively low energy AO. Moreover, the geometrical arrangement of p orbitals about the carbon nucleus (Figure 1.5) would predict that two C–H σ bonds should be separated by an angle of 90°. However, we know from experimental data that carbon forms four bonds, not just two, and that typical bond angles in carbon-based molecules are ~180°, ~120°, or ~109.5°.

Linus Pauling proposed a solution to this problem by suggesting that the valence 2s and 2p orbitals on carbon might "mix" to form new **hybrid orbitals** with different energies and geometries depending on how the s and p orbitals are combined. While this proposal

was made in an effort to rationalize experimental observations, quantum mechanical calculations do in fact support the notion of hybrid atomic orbitals formed by mixing s and p orbitals. Here, we will use energy diagrams and boundary surface illustrations to describe this "hybridization" of carbon. There are three ways in which carbon can be hybridized—by mixing the single 2s orbital with either one, two, or all three of the 2p orbitals (Figure 1.11). The result of mixing one 2s and one 2p orbital is a pair of sp hybrid orbitals, each with equal s and p "character." This leaves the remaining two p orbitals unchanged (unhybridized) and so we can say that sp hybridized carbon consists of two sp hybrid orbitals and two 2p orbitals. If instead we mix the single 2s orbital with two 2p orbitals, the result is three sp^2 hybrid orbitals and a single 2p orbital. Finally, if we mix the 2s orbital with all three 2p orbitals, we obtain four sp^3 hybrid orbitals and no unhybridized p orbitals.

Several points are worth noting at this point. Most importantly, you may have noted in Figure 1.11 that each of the three hybridization schemes results in four orbitals, each with a single unpaired electron. This nicely fits with the known valence of carbon and makes it quite easy to see how these four orbitals might be combined with other atoms to form molecular orbitals (and four bonds). Another important point is that the number of new hybrid orbitals formed in each case exactly matches the number of s and p orbitals used for hybridization. Thus for sp hybridization we combined one s and one p orbital to produce two sp orbitals. Finally, we should note that hybridization occurs because it ultimately leads to molecular orbitals (and bonds) with favorable energies. In other words, hybridization of atomic orbitals is

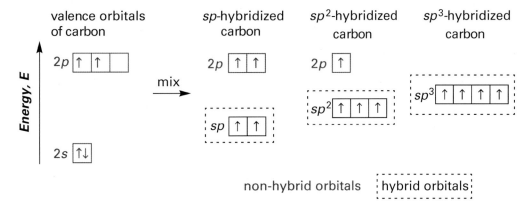

Figure 1.11 Energy diagram illustrating three different ways of hybridizing carbon by mixing the valence 2s orbital with either one, two, or all three of the valence 2p orbitals. The resulting forms of hybridized carbon each have four unpaired electrons and are thus capable of forming four bonds with other atoms.

Figure 1.12 Bonding in methane (CH_4) involves the orbital overlap of half-filled sp^3 hybrid orbitals on carbon with half-filled $1s$ orbitals on hydrogen. (Reproduced, with permission, from Carey FA, Giuliano RM. *Organic Chemistry*. 9th ed. New York: McGraw-Hill Education; 2014.)

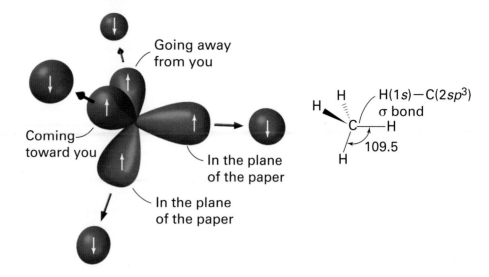

a phenomena of atoms *in molecules*, where orbital overlap leads to the formation of bonds.

The most useful aspect of hybridization is that it allows us to rationalize the experimentally observed geometries of tetravalent carbon. Thus, sp^3-hybridized carbon as in methane (CH_4) comprises four sp^3 hybrid orbitals, each pointing toward the corners of a tetrahedron (bond angle ~109.5°). Having 25% s character and 75% p character, the sp^3 orbital takes on the dumbbell shape of a p orbital, but with one lobe much larger in size than the other (Figure 1.12). Recalling the tenants of valence bond theory, we would say that methane is formed by combining four sp^3 orbitals on carbon with the $1s$ orbitals of four hydrogen atoms. Each hydrogen $1s$ orbital overlaps with one of the four sp^3 orbitals, forming four C–H σ bonds. Overlap occurs on the larger lobe of the sp^3 orbital since this maximizes orbital overlap, resulting in a stronger bond. The C–C bonds in related hydrocarbons such as ethane and propane are simply σ bonds formed by overlap of carbon sp^3 hybrid orbitals.

Next, consider sp^2-hybridized carbon and the structure of ethylene (C_2H_4). Each of the two carbon atoms in ethylene comprises three sp^2 orbitals lying in the same plane and pointing toward the vertices of an equilateral triangle, a so-called "trigonal-planar" arrangement with bond angles of ~120°. The lone p orbital on each carbon atom is exactly orthogonal to the plane of sp^2 hybrid orbitals. The C–H bonds in ethylene are σ bonds formed by end-on overlap of carbon sp^2 hybrid orbitals with hydrogen $1s$ orbitals (Figure 1.13). The double bond in ethylene has two components. The first is a normal σ bond formed by end-on overlap of sp^2 orbitals on the

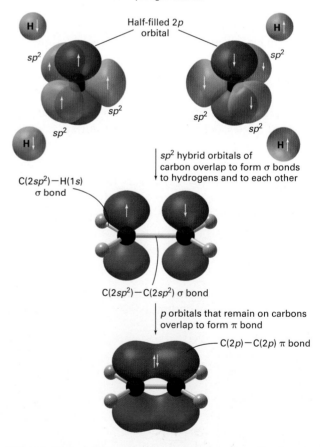

Figure 1.13 Bonding in ethylene illustrating the orbital interactions involved. The double bound comprises a σ bond (MO) and a π bond (MO), with two electrons in each molecular orbital. (Reproduced, with permission, from Carey FA, Giuliano RM. *Organic Chemistry*. 9th ed. New York: McGraw-Hill Education; 2014.)

two carbon atoms. The second component involves *side-on overlap* of the unhybridized *p* orbitals on the two carbon atoms, resulting in what is called a π bond. The π electrons in the π bond of ethylene reside above and below the plane formed by the σ bonds, as illustrated (Figure 1.13). This same plane is a node of the *p* orbital, where the probability of finding a π electron is zero. Unlike in a σ bond, rotations about the axis of a π bond would result in reduction and ultimately loss of orbital overlap. Thus, the need to maintain side-on overlap of *p* orbitals in forming a π bond explains why rotation about double bonds is generally forbidden.

Finally, we consider *sp* hybridized carbon in the molecule acetylene (C_2H_2). In *sp* hybridized carbon, two *sp* orbitals project outward in a linear arrangement, 180° opposed from one another. If an *sp* hybrid orbital were arbitrarily aligned on the x-axis of a three-coordinate system, then the remaining two unhybridized *p* orbitals would reside, one each, on the y-axis and z-axis. The C–H bonds of acetylene are σ bonds formed from

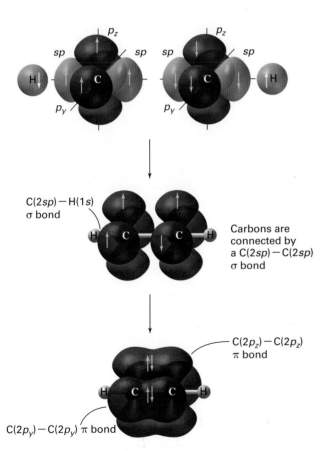

Figure 1.14 Bonding in acetylene based on *sp* hybridized carbon. The triple bond comprises one σ bond and two π bonds. (Reproduced, with permission, from Carey FA, Giuliano RM. *Organic Chemistry.* 9th ed. New York: McGraw-Hill Education; 2014.)

overlap of the carbon *sp* orbital and 1*s* hydrogen orbital. The triple bond of acetylene has three components, one σ bond formed by end-on overlap of *sp* orbitals, and two orthogonal π bonds formed by side-on overlap of the two sets of *p* orbitals (Figure 1.14).

As a final note, remember that the combination (overlap) of two atomic orbitals, whether they are hybrid orbitals or not, must produce exactly two new MOs—a bonding MO (σ or π orbital) as well as an antibonding MO (σ* or π* orbital). In all of the examples provided above, two half-filled AOs were combined, contributing a total of two electrons to the new bond and thus exactly filling a σ or π orbital and forming a stable covalent bond.

1.6 Hybrid Orbitals of Oxygen and Nitrogen and Common Functional Groups

Hybridization of orbitals is important in other main group elements as well, and we will discuss in this section nitrogen and oxygen, which aside from carbon and hydrogen are the most commonly encountered atoms in organic chemistry and drug structure (common functional groups of sulfur and phosphorus are described in Box 1.2). Nitrogen lies next to carbon in the periodic table, with an atomic number of 7 ($Z = 7$) and an electronic configuration of $1s^2\ 2s^2\ 2p^3$. We can mix the valence 2*s* and 2*p* orbitals of nitrogen just as we did with carbon, resulting in *sp*, *sp²* and *sp³* hybridization (Figure 1.15). Note that in each of these arrangements nitrogen has three unpaired electrons while a fourth orbital harbors a pair of electrons, called a **lone pair**. Thus we predict that nitrogen should form a total of three bonds comprising σ bonds or some combination of σ and π bonds, depending on the form of hybridization. The presence of lone pair electrons on nitrogen atoms has profound implications for the reactivity, intermolecular interactions, and acid-base chemistry of nitrogen containing molecules, as we will see throughout this text.

The nitrile functional group (CN) is the major example of *sp* hybridized nitrogen in organic chemistry. By analogy with the linear triple bond in acetylene, the nitrogen atom in a nitrile forms one σ bond and two π bonds with an *sp* hybridized carbon atom. The nonbonding *sp* orbital on nitrogen points opposite the C–N bond, and contains a lone pair of electrons (represented using Lewis nomenclature as a pair of dots, Figure 1.15). Like *sp²* carbon in ethylene (Figure 1.13),

Box 1.2 Functional groups containing phosphorus or sulfur.

Among the other main group elements of high significance in biology and drug structures are phosphorus (P, $Z = 15$) and sulfur (S, $Z = 16$). These elements are found in the third row of the periodic table, phosphorus in the same group as nitrogen and sulfur in the same group as oxygen. In biological and drug-like molecules P and S most commonly adopt tetrahedral geometries. You can imagine sp^3 hybrid orbitals of P and S being derived from the valence $3s$ and $3p$ atomic orbitals, much as $2s$ and $2p$ orbitals are combined in sp^3 N and O. However, because third row elements have vacant $3d$ orbitals that can also participate in hybridization and bonding, P and S form functional groups that would appear to violate the octet rule when shown as typical line drawings or Lewis structures. Let's look at some examples.

The most common sulfur-containing functional groups you are likely to encounter in drug structure

are the thiol, sulfide, sulfoxide, sulfone, sulfonamide, sulfonic acid (sulfonate when deprotonated), and sulfate groups. Thiol and sulfide groups present no particular problem as they are directly analogous to their oxygen counterparts—alcohols and ethers (in fact, sulfides are often referred to as thioethers). Other sulfur functional groups however possess additional bonds to oxygen and/or nitrogen atoms. As noted above, these additional bonding interactions are made possible by the presence of vacant $3d$ orbitals in sulfur that can participate in bonding. As illustrated below, the lone pair on sulfur in the sulfoxide group is sometimes shown with a line connecting it to the sulfur atom. This nonstandard representation is reserved for sulfur and is meant to suggest the tetrahedral geometry of sp^3 hybridized sulfur. This type of drawing becomes especially important when representing different stereoisomers (as we will see in Chapter 3).

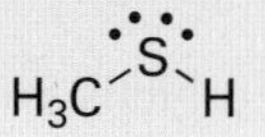

thiol 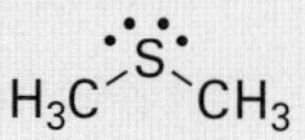   sulfide 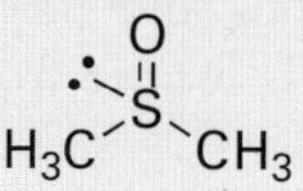   sulfoxide 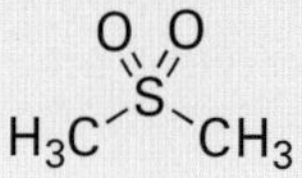   sulfone

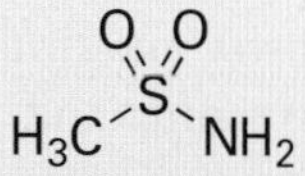

sulfonamide 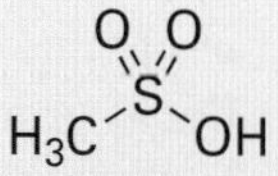   sulfonic acid 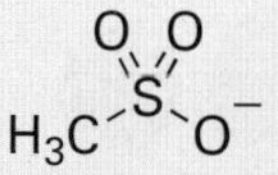   sulfonate 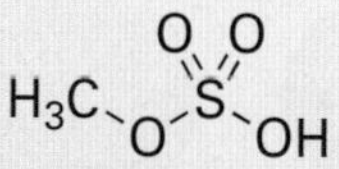   alkyl bisulfate

By constructing resonance hybrids of the sulfone and sulfoxide groups we can produce specific resonance forms that do not violate the octet rule. These forms do exhibit significant charge separation within the molecule however, which is generally unfavorable. It is the involvement of $3d$ orbitals that allows the

valence shell of sulfur to accommodate additional bonding interactions such as the double bonds between sulfur and oxygen in these functional groups. As with any resonance hybrid, the true nature of the S—O bond in these structures is best represented by the combination of the individual resonance forms.

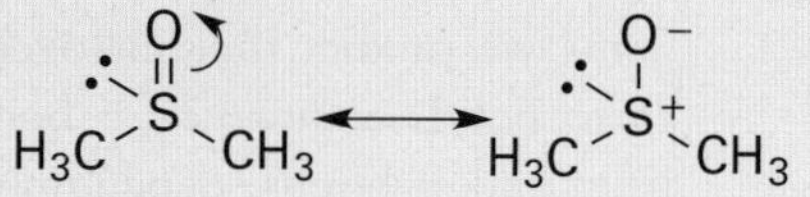

sulfoxide 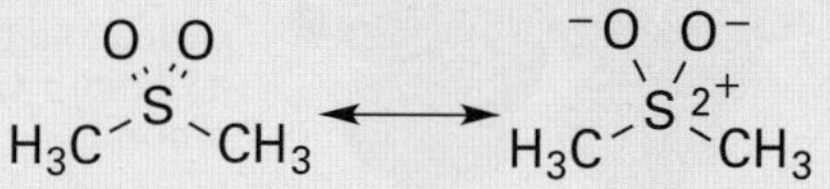   sulfone

Phosphorus is most commonly encountered in biology in the form of phosphate, as in phospholipids, adenosine triphosphate (ATP) and in the phosphate groups that form the backbone of DNA. Phosphate is also employed in the structures of some drugs, often to improve aqueous solubility. The phosphonate group, which possesses a P—C bond, is found in

some widely used drugs, such as "bisphosphonates" used to treat osteoporosis (e.g., alendronate sodium, Fosamax®). As with the sulfur functional groups, it is possible to draw resonance forms of the phosphate and phosphonate functional groups that conform to the octet rule, though these groups are almost universally shown with a P=O double bond.

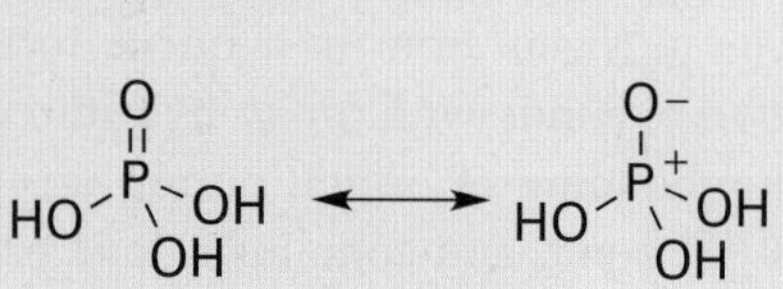

phosphate 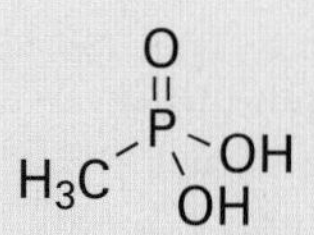   phosphonate 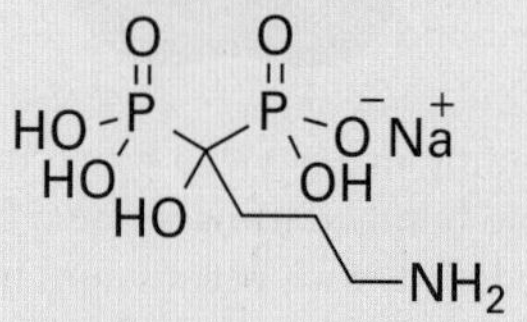   alendronate sodium

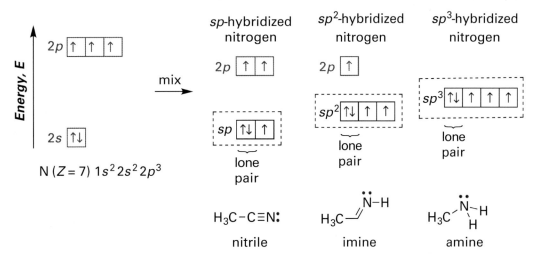

Figure 1.15 Energy diagram illustrating the mixing of nitrogen valence orbitals into sp, sp^2, and sp^3 hybridized forms. With one additional valence electron as compared to carbon, hybridized forms of nitrogen all possess one orbital containing a lone pair of electrons, shown in red. Common functional groups containing sp, sp^2, and sp^3 hybridized nitrogen, respectively, are shown at the bottom of the figure.

nitrogen sp^2 orbitals are disposed in a trigonal-planar arrangement, with an orthogonally located p orbital containing one unpaired electron. Again, the key difference with nitrogen is that one of the sp^2 orbitals bears a lone pair of electrons. This form of nitrogen is found in functional groups containing C=N double bonds, such as in imines, oximes, and hydrazones (discussed in Chapter 7) and in a wide variety of aromatic heterocycles (Section 1.8). Finally, sp^3 hybridized nitrogen is found in common "saturated" amines, which are commonly encountered in drug structures because they can contribute both to target binding, and in their protonated (charged) form can improve aqueous solubility. Nitrogen with sp^3 hybridization has tetrahedral geometry, with the lone pair occupying one of the four corners of a tetrahedron.

Oxygen ($Z = 8$; $1s^2\ 2s^2\ 2p^4$) is most commonly encountered in sp^2 and sp^3 hybridized forms in organic molecules and in drug structures. With two additional valence electrons as compared to carbon, hybridized forms of oxygen possess two orbitals with unpaired electrons and two orbitals bearing lone pairs (Figure 1.16). Thus oxygen typically forms two σ bonds (two single bonds) or one σ and one π bond (a double bond) in its bonding interactions. The C=O double bond is called a **carbonyl** and is found in a wide variety of important functional groups, including aldehydes, ketones, and amides to name a few. The importance of this group is such that an entire chapter (Chapter 7) is devoted to carbonyl chemistry. We can understand bonding in carbonyl compounds (Figure 1.16) by analogy with the

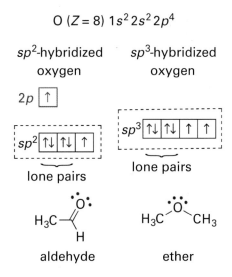

Figure 1.16 Energy levels of valence electrons in sp^2 and sp^3 hybridized oxygen. In each case two orbitals are available for bonding while two contain lone pairs, shown in red. Common functional groups containing sp^2 and sp^3 hybridized oxygen, respectively, are shown at the bottom of the figure.

bonding in ethylene. In an aldehyde, for example, overlap of sp^2 hybridized orbitals on C and O form the σ component of the double bond, while side-on overlap of the p orbitals contributes the π component. The carbon atom has two additional half-filled sp^2 orbitals and these form two additional σ bonds (one to C and one to H in the case of an aldehyde). The two remaining oxygen sp^2 orbitals each contain a lone pair of electrons, which lie in the plane formed by the σ bonds. The oxygen atom in alcohols and ethers is sp^3 hybridized, with roughly tetrahedral geometry and with the two lone pairs occupying two of the four corners of a tetrahedron.

At this point it is worth noting some peculiar aspects of bonding in the amide functional group. Amides are especially important in the context of drugs and drug action since amide bonds make up the peptide backbone in proteins, and are also commonly encountered in drug structure. If we consider the amide bond in a simple molecule like formamide (Figure 1.17), we would predict that the nitrogen atom should be sp^3 hybridized, since it forms three σ bonds and has a lone pair of electrons. However, experimental data tells us that the geometry of the nitrogen atom in formamide and many other amides is closer to trigonal-planar than tetrahedral. As well, the energetic barrier to rotation about the C–N bond in amides is three to fourfold higher than for typical single bonds. Both of these experimental observations suggest that the C–N bond in amides has "double bond character" and the nitrogen atom exhibits hybridization closer to sp^2 than sp^3. The explanation for this behavior in molecular orbital terms is that the nitrogen lone pair electrons reside in a $2p$ orbital and that extra stability is afforded by overlap of this filled orbital with the π bond of the neighboring carbonyl function (Figure 1.17).

Another way to illustrate the double bond character of the C–N bond in amides is to show a **resonance hybrid**, by which we mean a collection of alternative structures

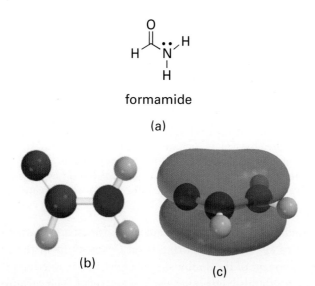

formamide

(a)

(b)

(c)

Figure 1.17 Chemical structure (a) and ball and stick representation (b) of formamide. The nitrogen atom in formamide is sp^2 hybridized with the lone pair residing in a p orbital, such that overlap with the carbonyl π system is possible (c). (Parts b and c reproduced, with permission, from Carey FA, Giuliano RM. *Organic Chemistry*. 9th ed. New York: McGraw-Hill Education; 2014.)

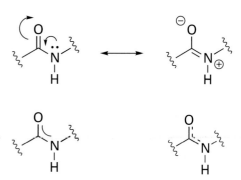

Figure 1.18 A resonance hybrid structure for an amide bond is shown at top and is made up of two resonance forms. Resonance forms need not contribute equally to a resonance hybrid and often do not. Other representations of an amide (at bottom) are sometimes encountered and are intended to indicate resonance stabilization in a single structure.

(or **resonance forms**) in which only the distribution of electrons is changed (H or other atoms do not move). Double-ended arrows are typically used to indicate that the collection of resonance forms together form a resonance hybrid structure (Figure 1.18, top). When drawing resonance forms it is helpful to use curly arrows to keep track of the movement of *pairs of electrons*. If, for example, we show the lone pair electrons on nitrogen in an amide contributing to a double bond with carbon, we must also break one of the C–O bonds so that the octet rule is not violated. This produces a new representation of the amide bond in which there is a C–O single bond and a C–N double bond (Figure 1.18). Neither of these resonance forms is strictly correct in describing an amide bond. Rather, it is some combination (hybrid) of the various resonance forms that together provide a more accurate picture of an amide bond. Sometimes resonance stabilization is indicated in a single structure by using a quarter circle or dotted lines, as illustrated for an amide bond here (Figure 1.18, bottom). While such structures are sometimes useful they can be confusing and are best avoided if possible. The concepts of resonance stabilization and the formation of more extended π systems encompassing more than two atoms will be further developed in the next section as we discuss the special stability enjoyed by aromatic ring systems.

1.7 Aromaticity

In the previous section, we saw how **delocalization** of electrons in p orbitals explains the partial double-bond character of the amide bond. The electrons in aromatic ring systems are another important example of the delocalization of electrons in p orbitals. Hydrocarbons such as benzene, toluene, and naphthalene (below) were originally described as being "aromatic" because of their generally distinctive and (to some) pleasing smell. What truly distinguish such compounds however are not their aromas but rather the special stabilization that is afforded by a specific arrangement of p orbitals and a particular number of electrons shared by them. Benzene is the prototypical aromatic compound, and was first isolated by Michael Faraday in the early 19th century. Subsequently, various structures were proposed to account for the molecular formula, which was known to be C_6H_6. In 1865, Kekulé proposed the cyclic structure of alternating double and single bonds that remains, to this day, the most common and useful representation of benzene.

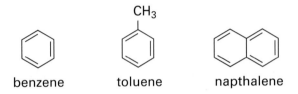

benzene   toluene   napthalene

The Kekulé structure of benzene does not however tell the full story of this remarkable molecule. First, it is known experimentally that all the C–C bonds in benzene are of equal length (140 pm, 1.40 Å) and intermediate between that of a typical single (1.46 Å) and double bond (1.34 Å). Furthermore, benzene is more stable and less reactive than a comparable polyene that is not cyclic, such as hexa-1,3,5-triene. Thus, it is not strictly correct to show benzene as a cyclohexatriene with alternating double and single bonds. A resonance hybrid structure of benzene with two equally contributing resonance forms nicely solves this problem as it predicts that all the bonds in benzene are equivalent (below). Another drawing convention was introduced by Thiele and shows the benzene ring with a circle drawn within a hexagon (Figure 1.19, top right). This representation of benzene emphasizes the equal nature of all bond lengths and is still used in the literature occasionally. The problem with Thiele-type drawings is that polyaromatic compounds such as naphthalene cannot be represented accurately— while the Kekulé drawing of naphthalene above clearly shows all 5 double bonds (and 10 π electrons), the Thiele-type representation of naphthalene could be misinterpreted as representing two independent 6-electron π systems, for a total of 12 π electrons. Correctly identifying the number of electrons in a π system is crucial because, as we will see, this determines whether or not a conjugated ring system is aromatic.

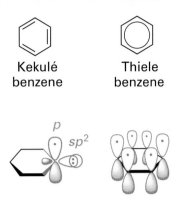

Kekulé   Thiele
benzene   benzene

Figure 1.19 Top: Kekulé (left) and Thiele (right) drawings of benzene. The Kekulé form is preferred as it unambiguously represents the number of π electrons and is also much more useful for drawing reaction mechanisms. Bottom: Bonding in benzene illustrating in blue the two C–C σ bonds and single C–H σ bond formed via sp^2 hybrid orbitals on each ring carbon. In addition, six singly occupied p orbitals combine (overlap) to form molecular orbitals with special stabilization.

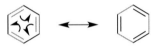

Now let's shift from the resonance hybrid description of benzene to the view of valence bond theory. We would expect based on the Kekulé structure of benzene that each carbon atom should be sp^2 hybridized, since this fits with the planar structure and 120° bond angles observed in benzene. Each carbon atom forms two σ bonds with adjacent carbon atoms (by end-on overlap of sp^2 hybrid orbitals) and one C–H σ bond by overlap with a $1s$ orbital of H (Figure 1.19, bottom left). This leaves six p orbitals, one on each carbon and each with a single electron to contribute to the π system. Rather than forming three distinct π bonds, the six p orbitals combine to form π molecular orbitals that contain all six electrons. The overlap of p orbitals and sharing of the six π electrons thus explains the equal bond lengths in benzene. To explain the special stability enjoyed by aromatic systems however, we must dig a little deeper and examine how atomic p orbitals combine to form π molecular orbitals.

A number of criteria must be met to produce a molecule that benefits from the special stability associated with aromaticity. These include the presence of a cyclic, coplanar array of contiguous p orbitals that together contain a total of $4n + 2$ π electrons, where n is an integer. The peculiar fact that aromaticity is associated with certain numbers of π electrons was first noted by Erich Hückel in 1931 and is now known as **Hückel's rule**. The

Figure 1.20 Energy diagram showing the favorable filling of π MOs in benzene. The energy of the bonding π MOs is lower than that of the *p* AOs from the six carbon atoms of the ring.

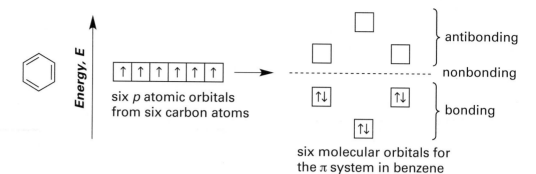

insight was made through Hückel's examination of the molecular orbitals of various cyclic polyenes. Hückel's rule correctly predicts that benzene will be aromatic (6 π electrons, $4n + 2$ where $n = 1$) and that cyclobutadiene (4 π electrons) and cyclooctatetraene (8 π electrons) will not benefit from aromatic stabilization. In fact, interaction of the *p* orbitals in cyclobutadiene is destabilizing rather than stabilizing and such molecules are said to be anti-aromatic. Cyclooctatetraene is neither aromatic nor anti-aromatic because it does not have a coplanar array of *p* orbitals (it adopts a boat-like conformation); its π bonds do not interact and instead behave like isolated double bonds. Such molecules are termed non-aromatic.

To understand the basis for Hückel's rule and the dramatically different stabilities of benzene and cyclobutadiene we must examine the π molecular orbitals (MOs) that are formed from the *p* atomic orbitals (AOs) of these molecules. If we combine the six *p* orbitals of benzene, we can produce an equal number of MOs, as illustrated in the figure (Figure 1.20). In this case three of the MOs are bonding (π orbitals) and three are anti bonding (π* orbitals). The six electrons from the *p* AOs exactly fill the three bonding π MOs, leading to a highly stable π system and explaining the special stability of this aromatic ring system.

Next, let us consider the MOs that might form from the four *p* AOs of butadiene (Figure 1.21). In this case, the four new MOs include one bonding and one antibonding MO as well as two "nonbonding" MOs. Filling the MOs of cyclobutadiene with the available four π electrons leads to one filled bonding orbital and two half-filled (unpaired) nonbonding orbitals. These two unpaired electrons located in nonbonding orbitals make cyclobutadiene highly reactive and the molecule can only be observed transiently before it reacts with itself to form dimeric species.

You may have noted that the placement of MOs in Figures 1.20 and 1.21 is the same as the vertices of hexagonal benzene and square cyclobutadiene rings, as drawn in the figures. It turns out that for any planar, fully conjugated, monocyclic polyene, a relevant MO energy diagram can be constructed by inscribing the relevant polygon in a circle, with one of the vertices pointing exactly down. These are known as **Frost circles** and are useful for analyzing the MOs and possible aromaticity of planar polyene rings (generally 3–7 membered rings, and rings larger than ~10 atoms). As an example, consider the cyclopentadienyl *anion* and the cycloheptatrienyl *cation*, shown as Frost circles (Figure 1.22).

Figure 1.21 Energy diagram showing the energy levels for π MOs of cyclobutadiene.

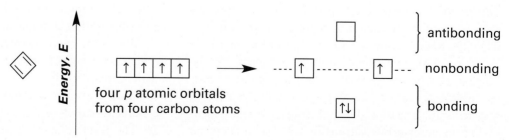

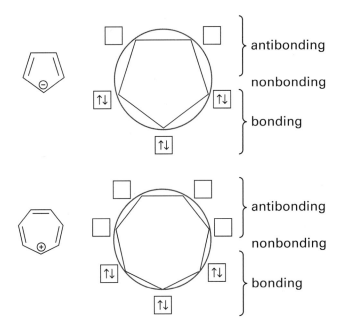

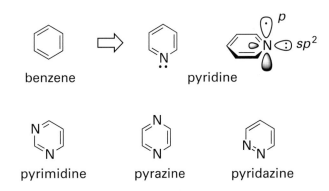

pyrimidine   pyrazine   pyridazine

Figure 1.23 Electronic structure of the nitrogen atom in pyridine is shown at top. Nitrogen contributes a single electron in a p orbital to the π system, completing a sextet (for clarity, the p orbitals on the carbon atoms are not shown). A lone pair of electrons resides in one of the three sp^2 hybrid orbitals on nitrogen. Aromatic heterocycles containing two nitrogen atoms are shown at bottom.

Figure 1.22 Frost circles illustrating the aromaticity of cyclopentadienyl anion (top) and cycloheptatrienyl cation (bottom). While the negative and positive charges are shown on single carbon atoms in the Kekulé-like structures at left, the six π electrons in each ion are fully delocalized, leading to equal C–C bond lengths, as in benzene.

Since both of these ions have a contiguous array of p orbitals and six π electrons, they are aromatic. Recall that Hückel's rule relates to the total number of π electrons, not the number of ring atoms. As charged ions of carbon, these aromatic ions are still more reactive than the neutral parent molecules cyclopentadiene and cycloheptatriene, neither of which is aromatic. The main consequence of the ions being aromatic is that they can be formed much more easily from the neutral hydrocarbon than one might otherwise predict.

1.8 Heteroaromatic Ring Systems in Drug Structures

Aromaticity is important not only in the structures of benzene and related carbocyclic ring systems but also in a huge variety of heteroaromatic ring systems—aromatic rings containing nitrogen, oxygen, or sulfur atoms in various combinations. Such ring systems are found in the structures of many drugs, where they serve roles as structural scaffolding and can also form various intermolecular interactions (as we will see in Chapter 2). To begin, let us consider replacing a single carbon atom in benzene with nitrogen to form pyridine (Figure 1.23). We might predict based on the ~120° bond angles that

the nitrogen atom in pyridine must be sp^2-hybridized, just like the carbon atoms in the ring. Recalling the energy diagram of sp^2-hybridized nitrogen (Figure 1.15), we can see that the nitrogen atom can contribute one electron in a lone p orbital to the delocalized aromatic π system of pyridine, for a total of six π electrons (thus satisfying Hückel's rule). Two of the three nitrogen sp^2-hybrid orbitals will form bonds to neighboring carbon atoms, while the third will contain a lone pair of electrons projecting out in the plane of the ring. By adding a second nitrogen atom to the ring at various positions we can produce additional six-membered aromatic heterocycles, such as the pyrimidine, pyrazine, and pyridazine ring systems (Figure 1.23). The bonding in these systems is exactly analogous to that in pyridine, with each nitrogen atom contributing a single electron in a p orbital to the aromatic π system and with a lone pair of electrons in an sp^2-hybrid orbital lying in the plane of the ring.

Next let us consider five-membered aromatic heterocycles containing nitrogen, oxygen, or sulfur atoms (Figure 1.24). Recall that Hückel's rule applies to the total number of electrons in a π system, not the number of atoms in the ring. Thus, five-membered rings can be aromatic, provided that a total of six electrons are contributed to the π system by the five ring atoms. Thus, sp^2-hybridized oxygen in furan contributes two electrons to the π system via its lone p orbital, thereby completing a sextet of π electrons and making furan aromatic. The remaining four valence electrons of oxygen in furan are distributed just as in the nitrogen atom of pyridine—one each in two sp^2-hybrid orbitals bonded to neighboring carbon atoms and a lone pair of electrons in the third

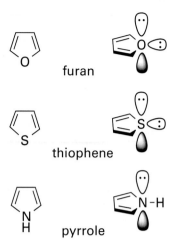

Figure 1.24 Electronic structure is shown for the oxygen, sulfur, and nitrogen atoms in the five-membered aromatic heterocycles furan, thiophene, and pyrrole. In these ring systems the heteroatom contributes a pair of electrons to the π system, which together with four electrons contributed by the four carbon atoms (carbon *p* orbitals not shown) complete a sextet of π electrons and make the ring systems aromatic.

sp²-hybrid orbital. The bonding situation is very similar for sulfur in thiophene, except that the electron pair contributed to the aromatic system lies in a larger *3p* orbital (as compared to the *2p* orbitals of N, C, and O). The bonding of the nitrogen atom in pyrrole is noteworthy in that it is distinct from that found in six-membered nitrogen heterocycles like pyridine. Hence to achieve a sextet of π electrons, the nitrogen atom must contribute *two* electrons in its *p* orbital, rather than the one electron required to achieve aromaticity in pyridine or pyrimidine. The three nitrogen *sp²* orbitals form bonds

with two ring carbon atoms, while the third forms a bond with a hydrogen atom (or with a carbon atom in the case of *N*-substituted pyrroles).

A number of additional aromatic heterocyclic ring systems are known bearing one or more heteroatom. Some examples common in drug structures are provided below (Figure 1.25). Two particularly important heterocycles are the imidazole and pyrazole ring systems, both five-membered ring systems with two nitrogen atoms. In these ring systems one nitrogen atom has pyridine-like bonding while the other has pyrrole-like bonding. To satisfy Hückel's rule in these ring systems requires that one nitrogen atom donate a pair of electrons while the other donates a single electron. This can be contrasted with the case of the oxadiazole ring system, in which the oxygen donates a pair of electrons and so both nitrogen atoms are pyridine-like (donating one electron each). Finally, note that fusion of five- and six-membered rings leads to a variety of aromatic systems with 10 π electrons (4*n*+2, where *n* = 2). Here too you will see examples of both pyridine-like and pyrrole-like nitrogen atoms contributing one or two electrons as required to satisfy Hückel's rule.

In this chapter we have seen how the early view of covalent bonding as the sharing of an electron pair was further developed through quantum mechanics and valence bond theory into our modern understanding of bonding in organic molecules. In this text, we will generally employ simple line drawings with Lewis lone pairs to represent organic molecules. When viewing and drawing such simplified structures however, one must remain cognizant of the true nature of the bonds and lone pairs being represented.

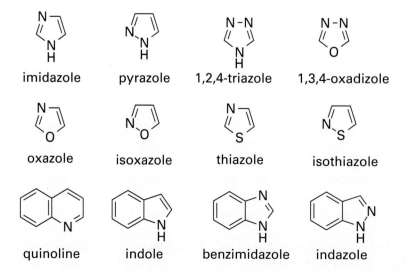

Figure 1.25 Examples of other aromatic heterocycles found commonly in the structures of drugs.

1.9 Summary

Section 1.1 The biological activity of a drug is a direct consequence of its chemical structure—the connectivity of its atoms and its shape.

Section 1.2 The formation of ionic or covalent bonds can be understood as the need for the atoms involved in the bond to achieve filled electron shells and a stable noble gas configuration. This can be achieved by *exchange of electrons* in an **ionic bond**, or by *sharing of electrons* in a **covalent bond**. Covalent bonds can be illustrated using **Lewis structures** in which two dots represent the pair of electrons involved in a covalent bond.

Section 1.3 Covalent bonds involving different atoms are usually polarized, with greater electron density found on the more electronegative of the bonded atoms. The **Pauling electronegativity scale** provides a convenient means to compare electronegativities of bonded atoms and thus predict how the bond is polarized.

Section 1.4 **Valence bond theory** provides a description of bonding as the overlap of atomic orbitals to form molecular orbitals. Specific solutions of the Schrödinger equation are associated with specific atomic orbitals, including spherical s orbitals and bilobed p orbitals. The electronic configuration of a particular atom is obtained by adding the total available electrons to atomic orbitals in the order of their relative energies (i.e., in the order $1s$, $2s$, $2p$, $3s$, etc.).

Section 1.5 The **hybridization** of s and p orbitals into sp, sp^2, and sp^3 hybrid orbitals helps to explain the nature and geometry of bonding in organic molecules. End-on overlap of atomic orbitals leads to σ molecular orbitals (σ **bonds**). Side-on overlap of p orbitals leads to a π molecular orbital (π **bond**). The combination of two atomic orbitals always leads to the formation of two molecular orbitals—one bonding orbital and one anti bonding orbital.

Section 1.6 Other main group elements such as N, O, S, and P also form hybrid orbitals when joined into organic molecules. Important structures containing sp^2 hybridized nitrogen include imines and aromatic heterocycles. An important bond containing sp^2 hybridized oxygen is the carbonyl (C=O), which is found in a variety of important functional groups. The lone pair on nitrogen in an amide bond is located in a p orbital that can interact with the π bond of the carbonyl. This **delocalization** of the nitrogen lone pair electrons lends partial double bond character to the amide C–N bond.

Section 1.7 Compounds such as benzene and naphthalene enjoy special stabilization as a result of resonance delocalization of π electrons. **Hückel's rule** states that planar ring systems with a conjugated array of p orbitals containing $4n +2$ π electrons will enjoy special stability and will be aromatic. **Frost circles** are useful for predicting the molecular orbitals of conjugated polyenes.

Section 1.8 A wide variety of aromatic rings containing N, O, or S atoms are important in the structures of drugs. These are called **heteroaromatic** rings because they contain one or more heteroatoms (non-carbon atoms). The bonding of sp^2 hybridized nitrogen in pyridine and pyrrole is different because nitrogen contributes either one electron (pyridine) or two electrons (pyrrole) to the π system of the ring.

1.10 Exercises

Problem 1.1 Predict the direction of polarization for each of the bonds shown in blue below, using the Pauling electronegativity scale (Table 1.1). Use either the partial charges or arrow nomenclature introduced in Section 1.3 to show the predicted direction of polarization.

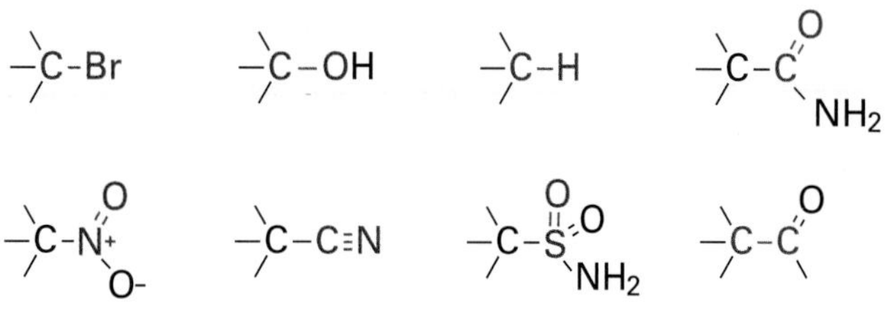

Problem 1.2 Predict the hybridization state for the C, N, and O atoms indicated with an asterisk (*) in the drug structures show below.

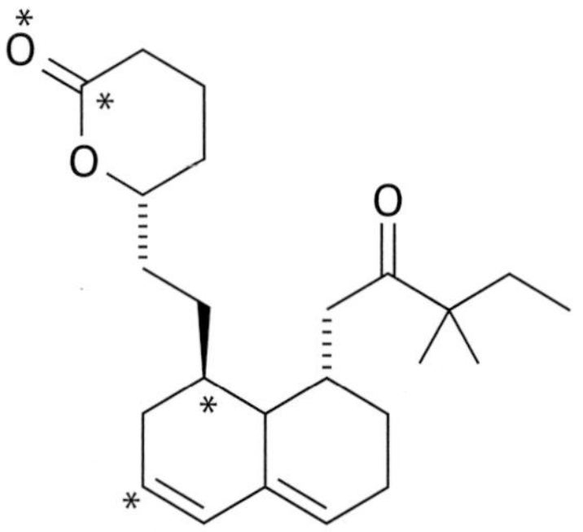

simvastatin

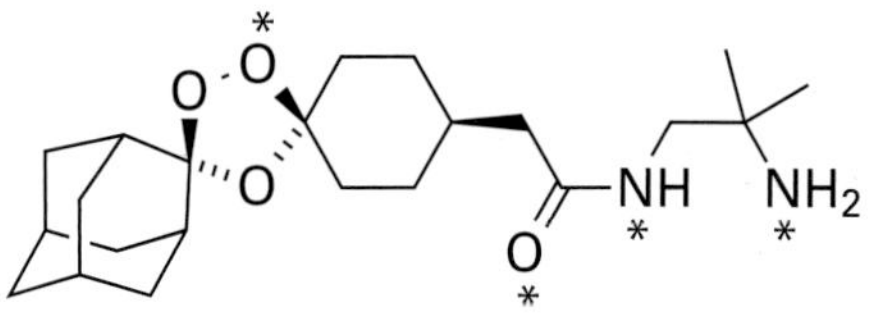

arterolane

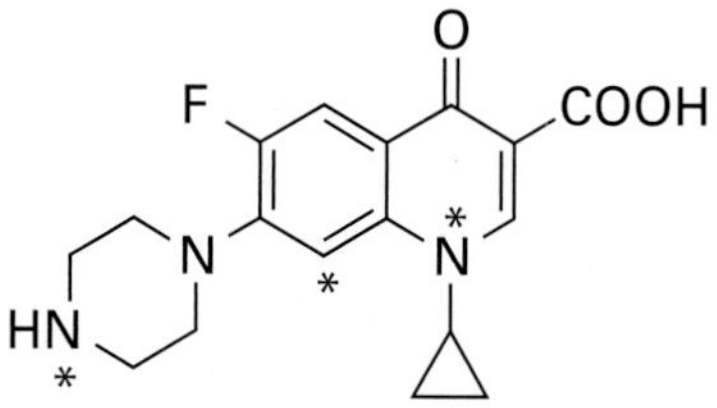

ciprofloxacin

Problem 1.3 State whether each of the following molecules is aromatic, anti-aromatic, or non-aromatic.

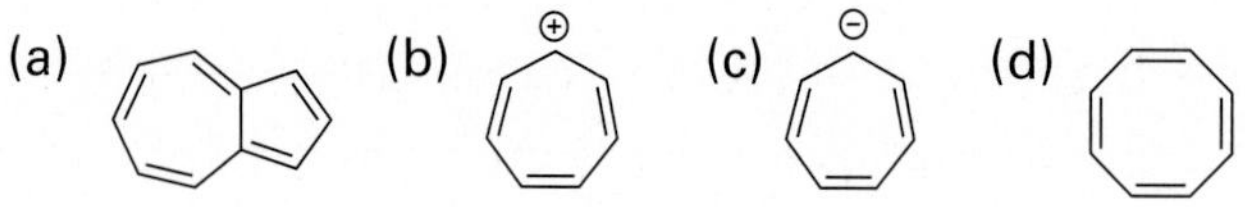

(a) (b) (c) (d)

Problem 1.4   Which of the molecular orbital diagrams below correctly represents the cyclobutadienyl cation shown. Is this species aromatic, anti-aromatic, or neither? Explain your reasoning.

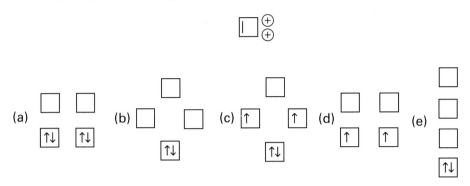

Problem 1.5   Each of the following anions has a negative charge on carbon. Which of the anions do you expect should be more stable? Explain your reasoning in terms of the molecular orbital theory or using a resonance hybrid structure.

Problem 1.6   Is the cyclopropenyl cation shown below aromatic? Explain your answer using a Frost circle to construct a molecular orbital diagram for the cation.

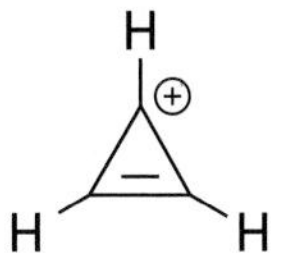

Problem 1.7   Indicate whether each of the nitrogen atoms shown in blue in the drug structures below exhibits pyridine-like or pyrrole-like bonding.

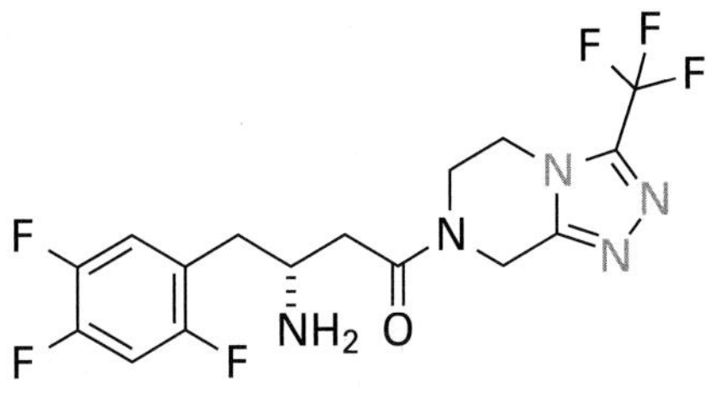

sitagliptin 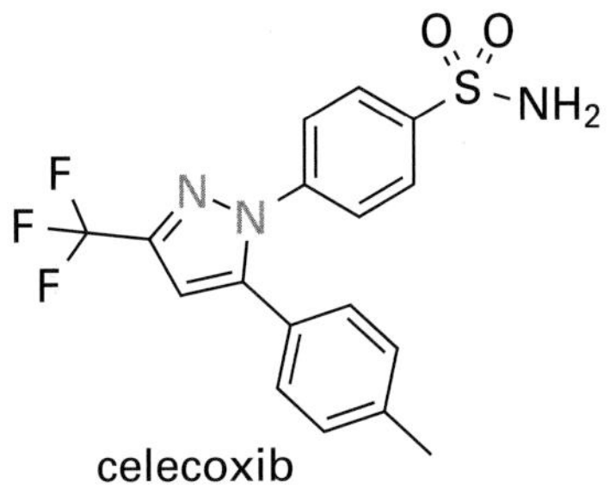   celecoxib

Chapter 2
Non-Covalent Interactions

Adam Renslo

CHAPTER OUTLINE

2.1 Introduction

2.2 Enthalpic and Entropic Contributions to Ligand/Drug Binding

2.3 The Strength of Non-Covalent Interactions

2.4 Desolvation and the Hydrophobic Effect

2.5 Ionic Interactions

Box 2.1—Ionic interactions in a proton channel from influenza virus

2.6 Hydrogen Bonds

2.7 C–H Bonds as Hydrogen Bond Donors

2.8 Aryl Rings as Hydrogen Bond Acceptors

Box 2.2—A π-hydrogen bond in glutathione *S*-transferase

2.9 Aryl-Aryl Interactions

2.10 Cation-π Interactions

Box 2.3—Hydrophobic and cation-π interactions in the binding of neurotransmitters and drugs

2.11 Halogen Bonds

Box 2.4—C–F bonds as hydrogen bond acceptors and in orthogonal interactions with carbonyl groups

2.12 Summary

2.13 *Case Study*—Inhibitors of Factor Xa as Anticoagulants

2.14 Exercises

2.1 Introduction

In the first chapter we described the nature of the covalent chemical bonds in biological molecules and drug substances. In this chapter we will discuss the various *non-covalent* interactions that are important in biological molecules and in their interaction with drug molecules. Although non-covalent interactions are typically orders of magnitude weaker than covalent bonds, this does not imply that they are of less importance. As we will see, these "weak" interactions are what give proteins their particular three-dimensional shape and function, enable the copying of genetic information in DNA, and govern the interactions of drug molecules with their biological targets.

We can glean the importance of non-covalent interactions by looking at the structures of the amino acids that form proteins and the nucleotide bases present in DNA and RNA. Nature creates a huge diversity of structural and functional proteins using the same 20 amino acid building blocks (Table 2.1). Individual amino acids are distinguished by the chemical nature of their side chains. They can be roughly grouped into categories as being hydrophobic (leucine, valine, etc.), aromatic (phenylalanine, tryptophan), hydrophilic/uncharged (serine, glutamine), and hydrophilic/charged (lysine, arginine, aspartate, glutamate). This diversity is no accident—nature has selected for amino acids that are capable of forming a wide range of non-covalent interactions.

While proteins evolved primarily to serve structural and functional roles, the role of the DNA molecule is to store information. Here too nature has employed non-covalent interactions (hydrogen bonds and aryl-aryl stacking) that are well suited to the task at hand. The highly complementary yet reversible nature of A:T and

Table 2.1 Structures of the Amino Acids Present in Protein Structure.

Name	Symbol	Structural formula	pK_1	pK_2	pK_3
With aliphatic side chains			α-**COOH**	α-**NH$_3^+$**	**R Group**
Glycine	Gly [G]	H—CH—COO$^-$ | NH$_3^+$	2.4	9.8	
Alanine	Ala [A]	CH$_3$—CH—COO$^-$ | NH$_3^+$	2.4	9.9	
Valine	Val [V]	H$_3$C \\ CH—CH—COO$^-$ / | H$_3$C NH$_3^+$	2.2	9.7	
Leucine	Leu [L]	H$_3$C \\ CH—CH$_2$—CH—COO$^-$ / | H$_3$C NH$_3^+$	2.3	9.7	
Isoleucine	Ile [I]	CH$_3$ \\ CH$_2$ \\ CH—CH—COO$^-$ / | CH$_3$ NH$_3^+$	2.3	9.8	
With side chains containing hydroxyl (OH) groups					
Serine	Ser [S]	CH$_2$—CH—COO$^-$ | | OH NH$_3^+$	2.2	9.2	about 13
Threonine	Thr [T]	CH$_3$—CH—CH—COO$^-$ | | OH NH$_3^+$	2.1	9.1	about 13
Tyrosine	Tyr [Y]	See below.			
With side chains containing sulfur atoms					
Cysteine	Cys [C]	CH$_2$—CH—COO$^-$ | | SH NH$_3^+$	1.9	10.8	8.3
Methionine	Met [M]	CH$_2$—CH$_2$—CH—COO$^-$ | | S—CH$_3$ NH$_3^+$	2.1	9.3	
With side chains containing carboxylic acids or their amides					
Aspartic acid	Asp [D]	$^-$OOC—CH$_2$—CH—COO$^-$ | NH$_3^+$	2.1	9.9	3.9
Asparagine	Asn [N]	H$_2$N—C—CH$_2$—CH—COO$^-$ || | O NH$_3^+$	2.1	8.8	
Glutamic acid	Glu [E]	$^-$OOC—CH$_2$—CH$_2$—CH—COO$^-$ | NH$_3^+$	2.1	9.5	4.1
Glutamine	Gln [G]	H$_2$N—C—CH$_2$—CH$_2$—CH—COO$^-$ || | O NH$_3^+$	2.2	9.1	

Table 2.1 Structures of the Amino Acids Present in Protein Structure. (*continued*)

Name	Symbol	Structural formula	pK_1	pK_2	pK_3
With side chains containing basic groups					
Arginine	Arg [R]	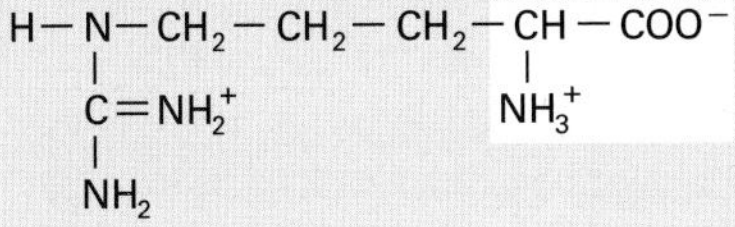 H—N—CH₂—CH₂—CH₂—CH—COO⁻ (C=NH₂⁺, NH₂; CH bears NH₃⁺)	1.8	9.0	12.5
Lysine	Lys [K]	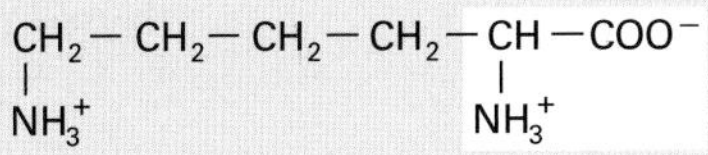 CH₂—CH₂—CH₂—CH₂—CH—COO⁻ (NH₃⁺; NH₃⁺)	2.2	9.2	10.8
Histidine	His [H]	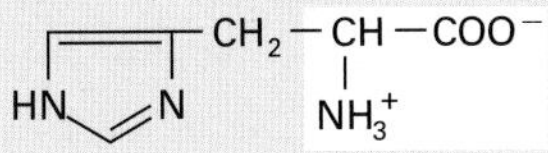 (imidazole, HN N)—CH₂—CH—COO⁻ (NH₃⁺)	1.8	9.2	6.0
Containing aromatic rings					
Histidine	His [H]	See above.			
Phenylalanine	Phe [F]	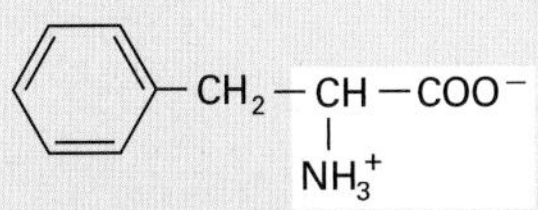 (phenyl)—CH₂—CH—COO⁻ (NH₃⁺)	2.2	9.2	
Tyrosine	Tyr [Y]	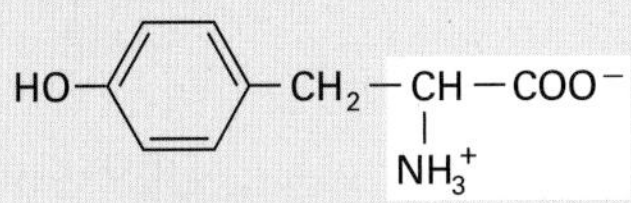 HO—(phenyl)—CH₂—CH—COO⁻ (NH₃⁺)	2.2	9.1	10.1
Tryptophan	Trp [W]	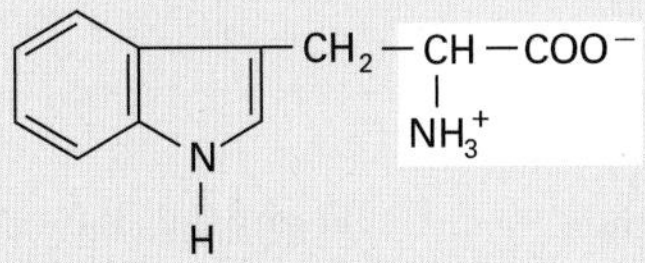 (indole)—CH₂—CH—COO⁻ (NH₃⁺)	2.4	9.4	
With a secondary amino group					
Proline	Pro [P]	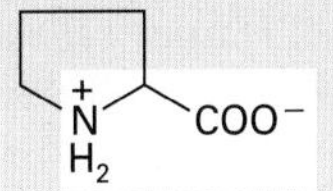 (pyrrolidine N H₂⁺)—COO⁻	2.0	10.6	

Source: Reproduced, with permission, from Murray RK, Bender D, Botham KM, Kennelly PJ, Rodwell VW, Weil PA. *Harper's Illustrated Biochemistry.* 29th ed. New York: McGraw-Hill Education; 2012.

G:C base pairing ensures high fidelity in the storage and copying of genetic information (Figures 2.1 and 2.2).

For a drug molecule to be safe and effective it must bind to its biological target with high affinity and fidelity. Most drugs bind via non-covalent interactions and even those that bind covalently must first "recognize" their intended target via non-covalent interactions. The structures of drugs are therefore imbued with many of the same chemical features found in their biological targets, including hydrophobic regions, hydrophilic regions, hydrogen bond donors/acceptors, aromatic rings, and charged atoms. Moreover, since most drugs are synthetic substances, they can be designed to exploit other non-covalent interactions that are less common,

or even absent, in biological macromolecules. In this chapter we will discuss a wide range of non-covalent interactions, with an emphasis on their importance in the binding of drugs to their biological targets.

2.2 Enthalpic and Entropic Contributions to Ligand/Drug Binding

Any favorable non-covalent binding interaction is associated with a negative free energy of binding (ΔG). This is true of two interacting proteins, two interacting small molecules, or the interaction of a small molecule

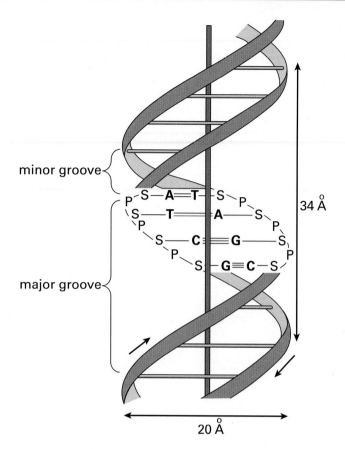

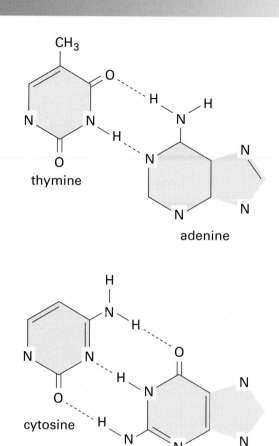

Figure 2.1 The familiar double helix structure of DNA is formed by two complementary strands of DNA held together by non-covalent interactions that include hydrogen bonds and aryl-aryl stacking interactions. The dimensions and location of minor and major groove are shown. A, adenine; C, cytosine; G, guanine, P, phosphate; S, sugar [deoxyribose]; T, thymine. (Reproduced, with permission, from Murray RK, Bender D, Botham KM, Kennelly PJ, Rodwell VW, Weil PA. *Harper's Illustrated Biochemistry.* 29th ed. New York: McGraw-Hill Education; 2012.)

Figure 2.2 Base pairing between complementary adenine-thymine and cytosine-guanine involves hydrogen bonding (dashed lines). (Reproduced, with permission, from Murray RK, Bender D, Botham KM, Kennelly PJ, Rodwell VW, Weil PA. *Harper's Illustrated Biochemistry.* 29th ed. New York: McGraw-Hill Education; 2012.)

(drug) with its biological target. The free energy of binding is in turn dependent on changes in enthalpy (ΔH) and entropy (ΔS) according to the familiar equation $\Delta G = \Delta H - T\Delta S$. What this equation reveals is that binding events can be enthalpically and/or entropically driven. Enthalpy-driven interactions tend to be those that require precise positioning of the interacting partners, as is the case, for example, with hydrogen bonds (Section 2.6) and halogen bonds (Section 2.11). Entropically driven interactions often involve the displacement of water molecules from a protein surface into bulk solution, thus increasing the overall disorder (entropy) of the system.

Another interesting consequence of the relation $\Delta G = \Delta H - T\Delta S$ is that weak binding interactions (small ΔG) can result from large but counteracting ΔH and ΔS values. In fact, drug binding often results from a balancing of entropic and enthalpic factors that are in opposition. This counterbalancing is sometimes referred to as entropy-enthalpy compensation and while it is not a rule of intermolecular interactions it is quite common. To see why this might be so, consider that an exothermically favorable interaction such as a well-positioned hydrogen bond will necessarily require precise spatial orientation of the interacting molecules. While these constraints on motion and orientation make for an exothermic hydrogen bond (favorable ΔH), they also reduce entropy. Conversely, consider the interaction of an aliphatic side chain in a drug with a hydrophobic surface on a protein. The enthalpy of binding in this case may be small or even endothermic, but in the event several water molecules are expelled from the hydrophobic surface into bulk solution and a significant gain in entropy is the result.

As we review various types of non-covalent interactions in the sections below, it is important to remember that these interactions do not happen in a vacuum (at least not in living organisms). We will see in Section 2.4 that the enthalpy and entropy of water molecules are often crucial factors in the overall free energy of drug binding.

2.3 The Strength of Non-Covalent Interactions

The strength of a non-covalent interaction will depend on various factors, among which is the distance between the interacting groups. Generally, the strength of interaction will increase as the two groups approach one another in space, reaching a maximum attraction at some specific distance r, and becoming less attractive and eventually repulsive as the groups are forced still closer together (Figure 2.3). The specific relationship between distance and attraction is not the same for all types of non-covalent interactions. The strength of ionic interactions, for example, is inversely proportional to the distance between charges ($1/r^2$) whereas the strength of van der Waals interactions and hydrogen bonds are proportional to $1/r^6$. Ionic interactions therefore can be attractive over a significant distance whereas hydrogen bonds are attractive only over a very narrow range of distances. The strength of non-covalent interactions is also inversely

related to the "dielectric" of the medium (i.e., solvent) in which the interaction occurs. A high-dielectric medium such as water will favorably surround (or "solvate") ionic species, whether positively or negatively charged. This will tend to weaken the electrostatic attraction of the charges and indeed, such ionic interactions (Section 2.5) tend to be weak when they occur on the surface of a protein, near water. The same interaction will be much stronger should it occur in the interior of a protein, an environment more akin to a low-dielectric organic solvent.

The positioning of interacting groups in space is also important, and as with distance, the requirements vary for different types of non-covalent interactions. Ionic interactions, for example, can be approximated as an interaction of two point charges in space. The relative orientation of such point charges is not important, only the distance between them matters. We might say that such interactions are nondirectional in nature. If the interacting groups are not point charges but polarized bonds (dipoles), then we might expect the relative positioning to be very important (and at least as important as distance). This is the case for hydrogen bonds, where a polarized carbonyl bond interacts with a polarized N–H or O–H bond. We can therefore say that hydrogen bonds are directional interactions. Between the examples of two interacting point charges and two interacting dipoles lie many other interactions with geometric requirements that fall between these two extremes.

2.4 Desolvation and the Hydrophobic Effect

The tendency of hydrophobic solutes to associate in an aqueous solution is a consequence of both favorable **van der Waals** interactions between the hydrophobic surfaces and more importantly, the exclusion of water molecules from those hydrophobic surfaces. This latter effect is known as the **hydrophobic effect** and is a consequence of some special properties of the water molecule. Water is the smallest molecule capable of both donating and accepting a hydrogen bond. This allows for a complex yet dynamic network of hydrogen bonding interactions between water molecules in solution (Figure 2.4). This arrangement is optimal from both an enthalpic and entropic perspective because every water molecule is free to move through bulk solution while continually breaking and reforming enthalpically favorable hydrogen bonds along its travels. This ideal is disrupted when a more hydrophobic solute (e.g., a drug or protein) is introduced to the solution. In response, water

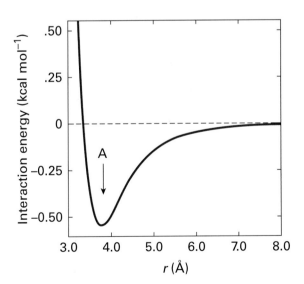

Figure 2.3 Potential energy diagram illustrating how the strength of van der Waals interactions vary as a function of the distance r in Ångstroms. (Reproduced, with permission, from Murray RK, Bender D, Botham KM, Kennelly PJ, Rodwell VW, Weil PA. *Harper's Illustrated Biochemistry.* 29th ed. New York: McGraw-Hill Education; 2012.)

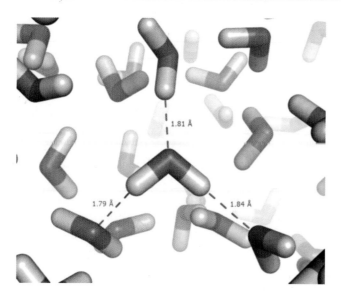

Figure 2.4 Image illustrating hydrogen bonding interactions in water molecules in solution. The central water molecule is shown donating two hydrogen bonds and accepting one hydrogen bond. Reproduced under terms of the Creative Commons Attribution-Share Alike 3.0 Unported license, commons.wikimedia.org. Copyright Thomas Splettstoesser, www.scistyle.com.

molecules will tend to form a highly organized "shell" around the solute so as to minimize its interaction with bulk solution. When more than one hydrophobic solute is present, it becomes energetically favorable for them to associate since fewer water molecules are required to surround the aggregate than the individual solutes. The net result of association is then the release of water molecules from the organized solvation shell and back into bulk solution, where their entropy is much greater. This is the classical description of the hydrophobic effect—an entropy-driven process that tends to minimize the amount of solvated hydrophobic surface area.

The classical, entropy-driven hydrophobic effect holds for "idealized" solutes—what we might imagine as tiny, molecule-sized drops of oil in water. Of course proteins and drugs are not spherical drops of oil and, in fact, the shape and chemical nature of a protein surface affects the entropy and enthalpy of the water molecules surrounding it. In the case of narrow crevices in proteins or flat aromatic surfaces in drugs, the hydrophobic effect can even be enthalpy-driven. This so-called "nonclassical hydrophobic effect" occurs when water molecules surrounding a surface are unable to form good hydrogen bonding contact with other water molecules. Upon release from such surfaces, the water molecules are able to form exothermically favorable hydrogen bonding geometries and distances in bulk solvent. If the distinction between the classical and nonclassical hydrophobic effects is still not clear, do not fret. The most important

thing to remember is that the entropy and enthalpy of water molecules surrounding a solute (drug or protein) will have a significant effect on the association of those solutes. When it comes to the chemistry of life, water is never an unconcerned spectator.

The hydrophobic effect is hugely important in both protein folding and the binding of drugs to their biological targets. In a folded protein, peptide sequences composed of hydrophobic amino acids (Val, Leu, etc.) will naturally tend to form hydrophobic contacts so that water is released to bulk solution. An example from protein structure is the formation of α-helices that further assemble into bundles of α-helices (Figure 2.5). The formation of such structures involves both polar and hydrophobic interactions. Hence the backbone amide bonds in the α-helix form specific, directional hydrogen bonds that stabilize the helical structure. Assembly of multiple helices is often driven by the desolvation of hydrophobic side chains on the interacting helices and is thus an example of the hydrophobic effect at work.

The binding of a drug to the active site of an enzyme or receptor usually involves the desolvation of hydrophobic patches on both drug and enzyme/receptor. The magnitude of the effect can be estimated by calculating the total hydrophobic surface area that is "buried" (made inaccessible to water) upon drug binding. In fact, buried hydrophobic surface area has been found to be the best single predictor of drug binding affinity across diverse drug-target interactions. Of course drug binding sites

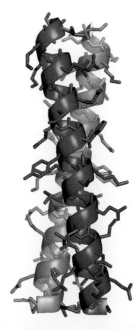

Figure 2.5 Association of two α-helices in a "leucine zipper." The association of the two helices is driven by the burial of hydrophobic surfaces on one side of each α-helix.

are not uniformly hydrophobic and different binding sites vary widely in their hydrophobic and hydrophilic character. The hydrophobic effect will tend to be most important when hydrophobic and/or narrow and poorly solvated surfaces are desolvated upon drug binding.

2.5 Ionic Interactions

Ionic interactions are probably the easiest type of non-covalent interaction to understand. We know that opposite charges attract one another while like charges are repulsive. Some other notable characteristics of these interactions are that their strength decreases gradually with distance and that they are nondirectional interactions. This means that ionic interactions can have attractive or repulsive effects over considerable distances and that the interacting groups do not need to be precisely positioned to exert their effects. The strength of an ionic interaction will also depend on the dielectric constant of the environment surrounding the interacting groups. For example, imagine a protein with lysine and aspartate residues in proximity on the surface of a protein. Both groups will be highly "solvated," meaning they will be surrounded by water molecules. The positively charged amine on lysine will interact favorably with the lone pair electrons on water molecules while the negatively charged carboxylate on aspartate will interact with the more electropositive hydrogen atoms of the surrounding water molecules. These interactions with solvent will weaken the strength of the ionic interaction. If on the other hand the Lys and Asp residues are found in the hydrophobic interior of a protein, the ionic interaction will be very strong indeed. Such interactions are called

salt bridges in the language of protein structure and usually contribute significantly to the stability of a particular protein conformation (or "fold").

The hydrophobic nature of protein interiors can also affect the ionization state of amino side chains. We usually think of aspartate and glutamate side chains as anionic groups and this is indeed the predominant ionization state for these residues in water at neutral pH. The basic side chains of lysine and arginine in contrast are positively charged in aqueous solution at neutral pH. Ionization of these groups is much less favorable however in low-dielectric organic solvents or in the hydrophobic interior of proteins. The result is that acidic and basic side chains are more likely to be found in their neutral (non-ionized) state in the protein interior than when exposed to water on the surface of a protein. Another factor that can influence ionization state is the relative proximity of two or more ionizable groups. For example, when two anionic carboxylate side chains are in close proximity they will tend to repel one another. A consequence of this repulsion can be that the acidity one of the residues is reduced such that only one of the two side chains is in its ionized form. Another example of proximity effects on the acidity of amino acid side chains is described in Box 2.1.

2.6 Hydrogen Bonds

A **hydrogen bond** is a non-covalent interaction most typically formed between a lone pair of electrons on oxygen or nitrogen and the hydrogen atom of a polarized H–X bond (Figure 2.6). When describing a hydrogen bond the

---

Box 2.1 Ionic interactions in a proton channel from influenza virus.

Both attractive and repulsive ionic interactions can play a role in the function of biological macromolecules. A good example of the latter is found in the M2 protein of the influenza A virus. This viral protein is an ion channel that permits a flow of protons into the virus, but only when the virus is in an acidic environment. Protons move through a central pore in the channel that is formed by a bundle of four α-helices (see below, panel (a)). To detect acidity (pH), the M2 channel uses a pH "sensor" comprised of four histidine residues (shown in orange) that circumscribe the inside of the channel. Because of their proximity to one another, the four histidine residues have quite different pKa values—estimated to be 7.6, 6.8, 4.9, and 4.2. At neutral pH, only one or two histidines will be protonated and the channel remains closed.

At lower pH, as is found in the endosome of the host cell (pH~5), a third histidine becomes protonated. The repulsive ionic interaction between the protonated histidines causes a conformational change that opens the channel, acidifying the inside of the viral particle and leading to release of viral RNA into the infected cell. Since the M2 proton channel is essential at various stages of the viral life cycle, it makes for a good drug target. In fact, the drug amantadine works by inhibiting the M2 channel. The spherical shape of amantadine allows it to insert into a hydrophobic region of the M2 channel, with its amino group directly interacting with the histidine residues of the pH sensor (panel (b)). Binding of amantadine disrupts the protonation equilibrium of the histidine residues, effectively locking the channel in its closed state.

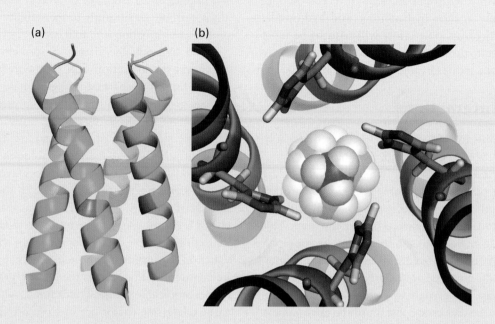

Panel (a) shows the α-helical structure of the influenza M2 protein in cartoon form. The locations of the four histidine residues that constitute the pH sensor are shown in orange. Panel (b) shows a view looking down the pore, with four histidine residues in the foreground and the antiviral drug amantadine in the background, blocking the pore.

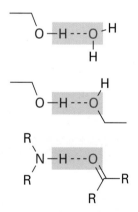

Figure 2.6 Examples of hydrogen bonds between molecules of water and ethanol (top), two molecules of ethanol (middle), and between a carbonyl group and polarized N–H bond (bottom).

H–X bond is said to be the **hydrogen bond donor** while the atom contributing the lone pair electrons is the **hydrogen bond acceptor**. We have already noted the complex network of hydrogen bonds formed by water molecules in solution, a situation made possibly by the fact that an individual water molecule contains both an hydrogen bond acceptor (O atom) and two hydrogen bond donors (H–O bonds). Hydrogen bonds are also of great importance to the structure and molecular recognition properties of biological macromolecules. In particular, biology employs hydrogen bonds where specificity is required. Recall, for example, the structure of DNA with its distinct hydrogen bonding patterns for complementary nucleotide base pairs (Figure 2.2). In protein structure, hydrogen bonding is crucial for the proper formation of secondary structure like the α-helix and the β-sheet (Figure 2.7). Given the importance of hydrogen bonds in biology, it is no surprise that most drugs form hydrogen bonding interactions with their biological targets and that these contribute to the specificity of the interaction.

Perhaps the most salient feature of hydrogen bonds is their directional nature—that is, the requirement that donor and acceptor atoms possess a particular geometrical arrangement in space. In most cases, the preferred orientation of a hydrogen bond will be along the direction of the lone pair orbital on the acceptor atom. A hydrogen bond to a carbonyl oxygen, for example, is usually found at a ~120° angle relative to the C=O bond. Note also that hydrogen bonds to sp^2-hybridized acceptor atoms tend to lie in the same plane

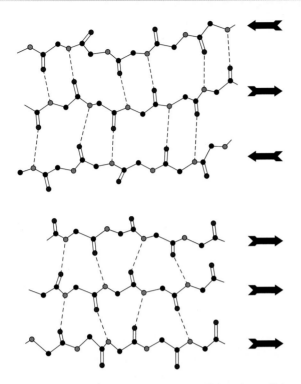

Figure 2.7 Hydrogen bonding in antiparallel and parallel β sheets that comprise an important structural motif in many proteins. (Reproduced, with permission, from Murray RK, Bender D, Botham KM, Kennelly PJ, Rodwell VW, Weil PA. *Harper's Illustrated Biochemistry.* 29th ed. New York: McGraw-Hill Education; 2012.)

as the double bond or aromatic ring containing the acceptor atom. Hydrogen bonds to the S=O function in contrast tend to form along the axis of the sulfur oxygen bond itself. The geometric requirements for sp^3 hybridized acceptor atoms such as the oxygen atom in ethers have somewhat less strict geometric requirements than do sp^2 hybridized donors, though a trajectory along the direction of the lone pair orbital can to a first approximation be assumed to be favorable.

The intrinsic strength of a hydrogen bond can be understood in terms of an electrostatic interaction. The more electron-withdrawing the X group in an H–X donor, the stronger the hydrogen bond. In general, H–O donors form stronger H–bonds with shorter distances to the acceptor atom than H–N donors, because of the greater electronegativity of oxygen as compared to nitrogen. With respect to the hydrogen bond acceptor, *greater* electron density on the acceptor atom will generally result in a stronger hydrogen bond. For example, in the case of a pyridine ring nitrogen atom as acceptor we should expect a stronger hydrogen bond in cases where the pyridine ring is substituted with electron-donating substituents and a weaker hydrogen bond in

the case of an electron-withdrawing substituent on the ring (Figure 2.8). The steric environment surrounding an acceptor atom will also affect the strength of a hydrogen bond. Thus, cyclic systems will be better hydrogen bond acceptors or donors than the comparable acyclic forms because the acceptor/donor atom is more exposed in the cyclic form (Figure 2.8).

The discussion of hydrogen bonding strength above holds for hydrogen bonds in isolation but ignores the fact that in biological systems, hydrogen bonds to water molecules must be broken in order to form a hydrogen bond to a particular protein residue or drug molecule. The enthalpy associated with the hydrogen bond is therefore counter-balanced by a "desolvation penalty" resulting from the enthalpy lost in stripping water molecules from the interacting groups. As a result, hydrogen bonding interactions between a drug and its target often contribute relatively little to the overall binding free energy of the interaction. Hydrogen bonds do however contribute significantly to the specificity and fidelity of binding of a drug to its intended target.

Notwithstanding the discussion above, there are cases where hydrogen bonds can contribute significantly

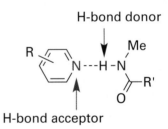

Figure 2.8 Electronic and steric effects on the strength of hydrogen bond acceptors and donors. In all cases donors are colored red and acceptors blue.

to the free energy of binding. Not surprisingly, this is most likely to occur in cases where the hydrogen bond is located in the interior of a protein, away from bulk water. Imagine, for example, a peptide (amide) bond buried in a hydrophobic cavity within a protein and unable to form hydrogen bonds to other residues in the protein. We could say that the hydrogen bond acceptor (carbonyl O atom) and hydrogen bond donor (H–N) of the amide are "unsatisfied" since they do not have hydrogen bonding partners. Solvation by water in this case is will not be favorable since a water molecule in the protein interior would be isolated from bulk solution and forced to interact with hydrophobic residues. Thus, a drug molecule that binds to this site and forms hydrogen bonds to the amide function would be associated with significant favorable enthalpy for the hydrogen bonds formed. There will be little if any desolvation penalty and the hydrogen bond acceptor and/or donor functions in the binding site are now "satisfied," having found suitable hydrogen bonding partners.

2.7 C–H Bonds as Hydrogen Bond Donors

The most prevalent and widely recognized types of hydrogen bonds are those formed between H–N or H–O donors and O= or −N= acceptor atoms, as described in Section 2.6. However, certain H–C bonds can serve as hydrogen bond donors as well, interacting favorably with O=, −N=, and other hydrogen bond acceptor atoms. The importance of such C–H hydrogen bonds in protein structure and drug binding has become better appreciated in recent years. Since carbon is less electronegative than oxygen or nitrogen, we would expect that H–C donors will form weaker hydrogen bonds than H–O or H–N donors. While this is true, it is also the case that H–C donors pay a smaller desolvation penalty than H–O or H–N donors and thus the overall free energy of the interaction can be comparable. Hydrogen bonds involving H–C donors are still directional in nature and thus can be important in determining the specificity of drug binding and in protein folding.

Important examples of H–C type donors in biological molecules include the α-H atoms of the peptide backbone (i.e., **H–C–NH–C=O–**) and hydrogens on carbon atoms adjacent to oxygen or nitrogen atoms in amino acid side chains and sugars (**H–C–O–** or **H–C–N–**). The electron-withdrawing effects of the neighboring oxygen or nitrogen atoms serve to make these particular H–C bonds more polarized (greater positive character on H)

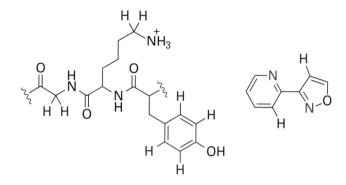

Figure 2.9 Examples of H–C type donors in proteins include H atoms in the peptide backbone and polarized C–H bonds in certain amino acid side chains (shown in red). Polarized H–C bonds in drug structures (in red, at right) can also participate in hydrogen bonds with nearby hydrogen bond acceptors (shown in blue), forming intramolecular hydrogen bonds.

and thus better donors of a hydrogen bond (Figure 2.9). Even unactivated H–C bonds such as in the side chains of Leu and Ile have been observed to form hydrogen bonds in cases where stronger donors are unavailable for hydrogen bonding. Of the 20 amino acids, Gly and Ala residues are among the most common donors of H–C hydrogen bonds, since their alpha positions are the least hindered (and because Gly uniquely possesses two H–C bonds at the alpha position). A more unique aspect of H–C donors is that they form favorable hydrogen bonds over a wider range of angular orientations as compared to H–O and H–N donors. Thus hydrogen bonds to H–C donors can be observed to form with O···H–C angles of between ~110° and 170° whereas H–O and H–N hydrogen bonds are more typical in the range of ~160°–180°.

The sp^2 hybridized H–C bonds in aromatic amino acids and in drug structures can also serve as H–C hydrogen bond donors (Figure 2.9). The best donors are those that are more polarized, for example, the H–C= bonds in the aromatic side chains of phenylalanine and tyrosine. In drug structures, H–C donors will most typically be found in aromatic or heteroaromatic rings (**H–C=C** or **H–C=N–**). The more electron-deficient such ring systems are, the stronger the potential H–C hydrogen bonds. The importance of H–C donors in drug molecules is illustrated by the importance of O···H–C hydrogen bonds in the binding of many kinase inhibitors. Finally, polarized H–C bonds within drug-like molecules can play a role in stabilizing particular conformations of a drug substance through the formation of hydrogen bonds to acceptor atoms in the same molecule, forming **intramolecular** hydrogen bonds.

2.8 Aryl Rings as Hydrogen Bond Acceptors

Aromatic rings can also serve as acceptors of hydrogen bonds from various types of donors (H–O, H–N, and H–C). These interactions are sometimes called π-**hydrogen bonds** since they involve the π electrons of the aromatic ring as the acceptor. The preferred geometry of this interaction is that in which the H–X bond of the donor lies above the plane of the aromatic ring, in a T-shaped orientation. In proteins, less than 10% of aromatic amino acids are found to participate in π-hydrogen bonds, and so these interactions are much less common than traditional hydrogen bonds. While computations predict that O–H---aryl and N–H---aryl interactions are somewhat stronger than C–H---aryl interactions, in reality C–H---aryl interactions are much more common than π-hydrogen bonds involving H–O or H–N donors. The reasons for this are twofold. First, as stronger donors, H–O and H–N groups will in general prefer to interact with stronger hydrogen bond acceptors such as O= and –N=, or water. Second, the lower desolvation cost for a typical H–C donor means that even a relatively weak C–H---aryl interaction may be preferred over the solvated state. The topic of C–H---aryl interactions will be more extensively explored in the next section. An example of an O–H---aryl interaction is provided in Box 2.2.

Box 2.2 A π-hydrogen bond in glutathione *S*-transferase.

The enzyme glutathione *S*-transferase plays an important role in cellular detoxification by facilitating the conjugation of the tri-peptide glutathione to foreign substances. The interaction of GSH (shown in green) with GST (orange) provides an example of a π-hydrogen bond involving an O–H donor from a Thr residue with an aryl acceptor on a Tyr residue. In accepting this π-hydrogen bond, electron density in the aryl ring is polarized, which in turn makes the phenolic H–O group more acidic and thus a better hydrogen bond donor to the neighboring thiolate of bound GSH (green, sulfur atom in yellow). This network of hydrogen bonds thus contributes binding energy and specificity to the GSH/GST interaction and also modulates the acidity and reactivity of GSH. In later chapters we will discuss the role of GSH in the elimination of some drugs and drug metabolites.

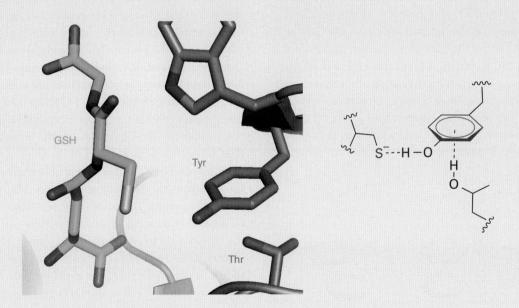

Example of an O–H π-hydrogen bond between Thr and Tyr side chains in the X-ray structure of glutathione *S*-transferase (orange) bound to glutathione (green). The π-hydrogen bond from Thr makes the O–H function in Tyr a better hydrogen bond donor to the thiolate anion of bound GSH. At right hydrogen bond donors are colored red and acceptors blue.

2.9 Aryl-Aryl Interactions

In this section we will discuss the interactions of multiple aryl rings, which can occur with **edge-to-face, face-to-face**, or **parallel-displaced** geometries. (Figure 2.10) In the previous section we saw that sp^2 hybridized **H–C=C–** bonds can serve as hydrogen bond donors while the π-face of an aromatic ring can serve as acceptor of a π-hydrogen bond. The edge-to-face arrangement can thus be understood as an example of a π-hydrogen bond. Like other hydrogen bonds, this interaction will be strengthened when the donor X–H bond is more polarized, for example, when a C–H donor is part of an electron-deficient heteroaromatic ring system. Computational and experimental studies suggest that in aqueous solution the edge-to-face interaction is energetically preferred over stacked geometries by a small margin. Surveys of protein structures have indicated that ~60% of aromatic amino acid side chains are involved in aryl-aryl interactions of one type or another (by comparison, recall that only ~10% of such side chains participate in π-hydrogen bonding, Section 2.7).

Aryl-aryl stacking interactions can be subdivided into two subtypes: face-to-face and parallel-displaced (Figure 2.10). Stacking interactions are less directional in nature than hydrogen bonds, since the aryl rings involved can rotate coaxially without disrupting the interaction. The favorable binding free energy of a stacking interaction derives from a combination of van der Waals forces, the hydrophobic effect, and the polar moments (dipoles or quadrupoles) of the interacting rings. Dipoles and quadrupoles can be thought of as uneven distributions of charge in the π system. A favorable aryl-aryl interaction will be one in which these regions of uneven charge are attractive. Aside from protein structure, aryl-aryl interactions are of obvious importance in the base-pair stacking interactions of DNA and RNA, and in the association of various aromatic enzyme cofactors in proteins.

Most drugs contain at least one aromatic or heteroaromatic ring and many are known to interact with aromatic surfaces in their target proteins or, in the case of DNA-intercalating drugs, with stacked nucleoside bases. Aryl-aryl interactions within proteins are necessarily limited to interactions of just a handful of aromatic amino acids, primarily Phe, Tyr, and Trp. In contrast, aryl-aryl interactions between drugs and their targets are much more diverse, for the simple reason that an almost unlimited variety of aromatic and heteroaromatic rings can be incorporated into the structures of drug molecules. Thus, altering the nature of the interacting aromatic ring in a drug structure can enhance edge-to-face or stacking interaction between a drug and its target. In the case of an edge-to-face interaction this might be accomplished by adding an electron-withdrawing group to further polarize the aromatic C–H donor. Similarly, strengthening a stacking interaction with a Tyr residue (electron-rich) might be accomplished by employing electron-poor heteroaromatic rings in the drug structure. Potent anticancer cytotoxins such as doxorubicin and the duocarmycins possess large flat aromatic surfaces that are ideally suited to stack with the nucleoside bases of DNA. This DNA "intercalation" is essential to the function of these agents and the potent cellular toxicities that they exhibit.

2.10 Cation-π interactions

Cation-π interactions involve the association of positively charged groups with aromatic ring systems. The fundamental nature of this interaction is an electrostatic one between the positively charged cation and the electrons in the π-system of the aromatic ring. Thus, for inorganic ions in the gas phase, the rank-order of binding free energy to benzene is $Li^+ > Na^+ > K^+$. This is what one would expect for a simple electrostatic interaction—the smaller Li^+ ion lies closest to the aromatic ring and thus forms the tightest interaction. Similarly, the ammonium cation H_4N^+ binds benzene more strongly than the larger tetramethylammonium cation Me_4N^+. The distance dependence of cation-π interactions is analogous to ionic interactions, or approximately $1/r^2$ (where r is the distance between interacting groups). Thus, cation-π interactions can be attractive over much greater distances than van der Waals forces or hydrogen bonds.

The cation-π effect operates in biological systems too, although discerning its effects is more challenging due to solvation. In aqueous solution, cation-π interactions involving Me_4N^+ are stronger than those involving H_4N^+ (the reverse of the situation in the gas phase). In water, the hydrophobic effect and a high

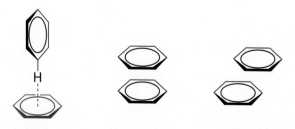

edge-to-face   face-to-face   parallel-displaced

Figure 2.10 Examples of the three main varieties of aryl-aryl interactions.

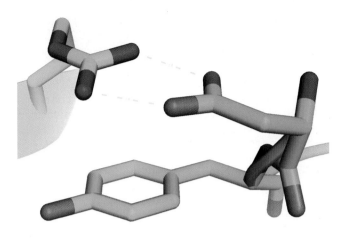

Figure 2.11 Hydrogen bonding interaction between Asp and Arg side chains. The π faces of the acid and guanidine functions provide a relatively lipophilic surface that stacks on the aryl ring of a nearby Tyr residue.

penalty for desolvating the ammonium ion overwhelm the mostly electrostatic effect of the cation-π interaction. Inorganic cations such as Na^+ and K^+ are so favorably hydrated in aqueous solutions that they do not interact with aromatic rings at all. However, the cation-π interaction is important in the association of cationic amino acid side chains (Lys, His, and Arg) with aromatic amino acids (Phe, Tyr, and Trp). For example, the guanidine function (in Arg) and the imidazole ring (in His) will often stack on aromatic side chains, such that their hydrophobic π surfaces are in contact. This stacking is

driven by a combination of the hydrophobic effect and electrostatic cation-π interaction. In a remarkable yet common motif in protein structure, the side chain of an Arg residue forms ionic/hydrogen bonding interactions with the carboxylate side chain of Asp residues, while simultaneously stacking on an aromatic side chain of a third residue (Figure 2.11). Other examples of cation-π interactions in drug molecules are described in Box 2.3.

2.11 Halogen Bonds

The halogen atoms chlorine (Cl), bromine (Br), and iodine (I) are capable of forming non-covalent interactions called **halogen bonds**. Fluorine participates in intermolecular interactions quite distinct from the other halogens, as detailed in Box 2.4. In a halogen bond, the C–X bond (X = Cl, Br, I) serves as the "donor" of a halogen bond while a lone pair of electrons on a carbonyl, alcohol, or carboxylate oxygen serves as the acceptor of the halogen bond. The electron density around the halogen atom in a C–X bond is polarized, with more electronegative character around the periphery and more electropositive character at the pole, opposite the carbon atom. It is this electropositive region that interacts favorably with lone pair electrons of the halogen bond acceptor. The preferred geometry of the interaction is thus similar to a hydrogen bond, with a roughly linear C–X---O=C geometry being favored (Figure 2.12). The angle between the donor halogen atom X and the acceptor carbonyl (X---O=C angle) is typically around 120°, which reflects the sp^2 hybridized

---

Box 2.3 Hydrophobic and cation-π interactions in the binding of neurotransmitters and drugs.

Certain receptors, enzymes, and ion channels utilize cation-π interactions to fulfill their biochemical or signaling function. Notable examples include the enzymes and receptors that bind acetylcholine. Acetylcholine is a neurotransmitter that acts as an **agonist** (activating ligand) of nicotinic and muscarinic acetylcholine receptors. The tetraalkylammonium group in acetylcholine forms cation-π interactions with a number of aromatic Tyr and Trp residues in the nicotinic acetylcholine receptor. Nicotine also acts as an agonist of this receptor, as do drugs like

varenicline (Chantix®) that are used to treat nicotine addiction. At physiological pH, the aliphatic amines in these compounds will exist in their protonated form (as illustrated) and can thus mimic the tetramethylammonium group of acetylcholine. The enzyme acetylcholine esterase hydrolyzes the ester bond in acetylcholine, thus terminating signal transmission across the synapse. This enzyme possesses a complement of four aromatic side chains that interact with the cationic tetraalkylammonium group of its acetylcholine substrate.

acetylcholine   nicotine   varenicline

Box 2.4 C–F bonds as hydrogen bond acceptors and in orthogonal interactions with carbonyl groups.

The highly polarized C–F bond forms intermolecular interactions that are different in many ways from those formed by C–X bonds of the other halogens. The C–F bond can accept hydrogen bonds from various donors, and can do so with a range of different geometries between donor and acceptor. An example is found in the successful diabetes drug sitagliptin (Januvia®), which targets the protease enzyme dipeptidyl peptidase-4 (DPP-4). Specifically, it is the ortho fluorine atom on the phenyl ring of sitagliptin (shown in blue below) that accepts N–H hydrogen bonds from the side chains of Asn and Arg residues of DPP-4. An altogether different type of interaction is that between a C–F bond and a carbonyl function. The preferred T-shaped geometry of this interaction clearly implies a different type of interaction than for other C–X to carbonyl halogen bonds. The C–F/carbonyl interaction may involve molecular orbital overlap between lone pair electrons on F and the π-antibonding orbital of the carbonyl bond (a so-called $n \rightarrow \pi^*$ interaction).

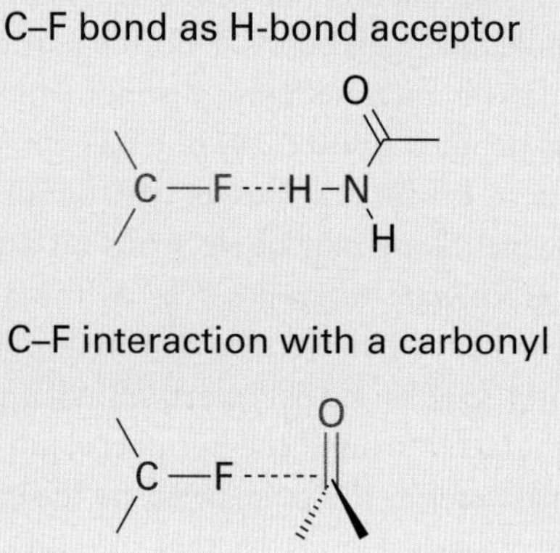

C–F bond as H-bond acceptor

C–F interaction with a carbonyl

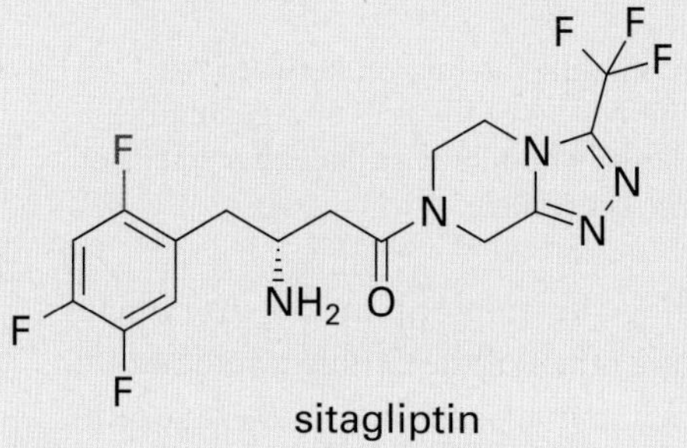

sitagliptin

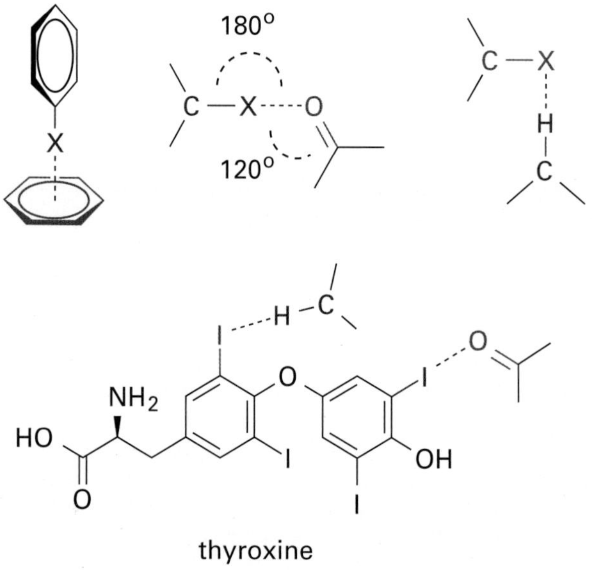

oxygen atom bearing the lone pair electrons (Figure 2.12). Aryl rings can also serve as acceptors of a halogen bond just as they can accept a π-hydrogen bond. In this case the preferred geometry will be T-shaped, with the electropositive region on the halogen interacting with the π electrons of the aryl ring (Figure 2.12).

While the end of a C–X bond can mimic a hydrogen bond donor, the periphery of the halogen atom in a C–X bond has a very different character. This diffuse and polarizable electron density will instead prefer to interact in van der Waals and hydrophobic interactions with aliphatic C–H bonds of proteins. The diverse character of halogen interactions is illustrated in the binding of the thyroid hormone thyroxine to its transport protein transthyretin. Remarkably, transthyretin employs distinct intermolecular interactions to recognize the two iodine-containing rings of thyroxine (Figure 2.12). Thus, the central ring binds in a site lined with aliphatic side chains and forms predominantly van der Waals and hydrophobic interactions. In contrast, the C–I bonds on the terminal ring interact with backbone carbonyl residues, forming halogen bonds. Thus nature employs two different types of intermolecular interactions to recognize the different C–I bonds in thyroxine, and in this way the specificity of hormone binding is enhanced.

thyroxine

Figure 2.12 Top: preferred geometries for halogen bonds between C–X bonds (X = Cl, Br, I) and aryl rings or carbonyl groups. Halogen atoms can also interact around their periphery with C–H bonds in a van der Waals type interaction (top, right). Bottom: the thyroid hormone thyroxine interacts with its transport protein transthyretin via both halogen bonds and van der Waals interactions.

2.12 Summary

Section 2.1 A variety of non-covalent interactions can be involved in the recognition of a drug substance by its biological target.

Section 2.2 A binding event between drug and target molecule can be described by the relation $\Delta G = \Delta H - T\Delta S$. Thus, a favorable binding free energy (ΔG) can result from a favorable binding enthalpy (ΔH), increased entropy (ΔS), or both. The nature of the non-covalent interactions involved in drug binding will determine if the process is entropy or enthalpy-driven.

Section 2.3 The strengths of non-covalent interactions are related to the distance between the interacting groups. Some interactions are favorable only over short distances (**hydrogen bonds, van der Waals** forces) whereas others (ionic interactions) are effective over longer distances.

Section 2.4 The **hydrophobic effect** is the largest single energetic driving force in most drug binding events. The classical description of the hydrophobic effect is an entropy-driven process that desolvates a hydrophobic surface, releasing water molecules into bulk solution.

Section 2.5 **Ionic interactions** result from the electrostatic attraction of positively and negatively charged groups. Such interactions are strongest when the interacting groups are not highly solvated, such as in the hydrophobic interior of a protein.

Section 2.6 A **hydrogen bond** describes the non-covalent interaction between a polarized H–X bond as the "donor" and a Lewis base (most often a lone pair on O or N) as the acceptor. The interaction is ubiquitous in biological macromolecules and in drug binding, where the directional nature of the interaction affords binding specificity and fidelity.

Section 2.7 Sufficiently polarized C–H bonds can also serve as donors of hydrogen bonds. Examples include C–H bonds at the α-carbon of amino acids and those with a neighboring heteroatom (X–C–H, where X = N or O). While generally weaker than N–H or O–H donors, hydrogen bonds based on C–H donors usually pay a smaller desolvation penalty.

Section 2.8 The π face of aryl rings can serve as the Lewis base acceptor of a hydrogen bond from N–H, O–H, and especially C–H donors. These interactions are sometimes called **π-hydrogen bonds** to distinguish them from more typical hydrogen bonds involving lone pair acceptors.

Section 2.9 Interactions of two aryl rings tend to involve edge-to-face or stacking geometries. Edge-to-face interactions are an example of a π-hydrogen bond and have specific geometric requirements. Aryl-aryl stacking interactions can occur via different geometries and arise from a combination of hydrophobic, van der Waals, and quadrupole interactions.

Section 2.10 Positively charged organic or inorganic cations can form a favorable electrostatic interaction with the π face of aromatic rings. Like other ionic interactions, π-**cation interactions** can be felt over relatively large distances. These interactions play an important role in the binding of cationic neurotransmitters such as acetylcholine.

Section 2.11 **Halogen bonds** are non-covalent interactions between a C–X bond donor (X = Cl, Br, I) and a lone pair of electrons on a carbonyl function as acceptor. The geometric requirements of the interaction are similar to those of traditional hydrogen bonds. The interaction of C–F bonds with carbonyl functions, however, is of a different nature, with an orthogonal T-shaped geometry being preferred.

2.13 Case Study—Inhibitors of Factor Xa as Anticoagulants

In this chapter we have discussed a wide variety of intermolecular interactions that can play a role in the binding of a drug to its target. In this case study we will discuss a new class of oral anticoagulants approved in the past decade for the treatment and prevention of blood clots and stroke. Examples of this new class include rivaroxaban (Xarelto®), apixaban (Eliquis®), and betrixaban which as of 2014 was still in clinical trials (Figure 2.13). These compounds inhibit the coagulation factor Xa (fXa), which lies at the intersection of signaling pathways common to both the intrinsic and extrinsic branches of the coagulation cascade.

Factor Xa is a serine protease that converts prothrombin to thrombin, ultimately leading to the formation of a blood clot. Both prothrombin and thrombin are proteases, enzymes designed to break one or more peptide (amide) bonds in their protein substrates (Chapter 6 will include a more extensive discussion of proteases and their enzymatic mechanisms). To carry out the bond breaking hydrolysis reaction at the appropriate site, a protease must first "recognize" a specific amino acid sequence in the substrate. Typically, a substrate protein will bind to the protease with specific amino acid side chains bound in complementary binding pockets in the protease active site. These various side chain binding sites are named by convention S3···S2···S1···*cleavage site*···S1'···S2'···S3' etc., where the peptide bond to be broken is situated between the S1 and S1' sites. Protease inhibitors are usually designed to mimic the interactions formed between the protease and its normal substrate.

The active site of fXa features a box-shaped S4 pocket formed by three aromatic side chains (Figure 2.14, in cyan). This pocket is an excellent

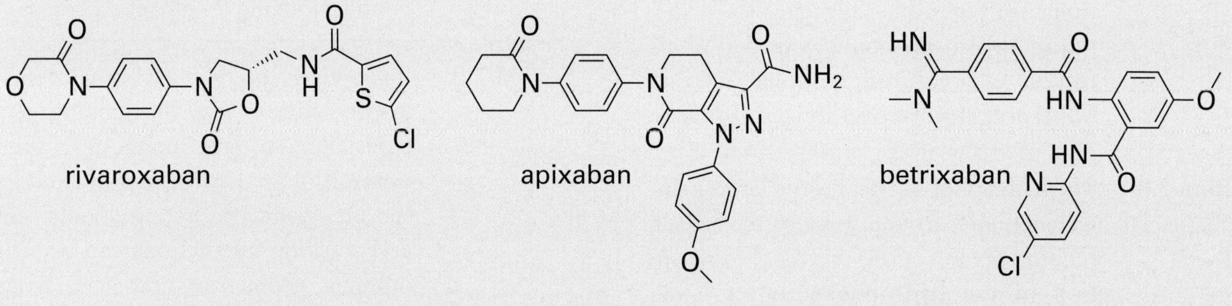

Figure 2.13 Structures of factor Xa inhibitors rivaroxaban, apixaban, and betrixaban.

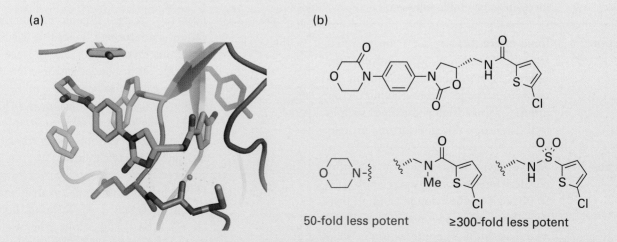

50-fold less potent   ≥300-fold less potent

Figure 2.14 (a) Binding mode of rivaroxaban (shown in green) to factor Xa as determined by X-ray crystallography. Key aromatic side chains of the S4 pocket of fXa are shown in cyan (Tyr99, Trp215, Phe174) while a key aromatic side chain in the S1 pocket (Tyr228) is colored magenta. (b) Relatively small changes to the structure of rivaroxaban lead to significant loss of activity, for the reasons discussed in the text.

example of a poorly solvated protein surface. In most fXa inhibitors then, filling of the S4 pocket contributes significantly to the overall free energy of binding. The S4 pocket is filled by a morpholinone ring in rivaroxaban that expels water molecules while also forming favorable C–H-π interactions with the surrounding aromatic side chains of Tyr99, Trp215, and Phe174. The electron-withdrawing carbonyl group in the morpholinone ring polarizes the neighboring C–H bonds, making them more effective C–H donors. Indeed, a close analog of rivaroxaban lacking the carbonyl group was found to bind fXa about 50 times more weakly (Figure 2.14)!

The S1 pocket of factor Xa is another important binding subsite for most fXa inhibitors. Important features of the S1 pocket include the aromatic side chain of Tyr 228 and an anionic side chain (Asp189) that binds an Arg side chain in the prothrombin protein substrate. Several early fXa inhibitors were designed to form an ionic interaction with Asp189 and thus had cationic functionality in their structures. While such charged compounds were indeed potent inhibitors of fXa, they often had poor oral bioavailability. This problem was avoided in rivaroxaban by eliminating the ionic interaction with Asp189 and instead exploiting a halogen bond between a chlorine atom on the thiophene ring and Tyr228 in fXa (Figure 2.14).

The morpholinone and chlorothiophene rings of rivaroxaban are connected by an aryloxazolidinone ring system that forms hydrogen bonding contacts within the fXa active site (Figure 2.14, yellow hashed lines). The carbonyl of the oxazolidinone ring accepts a hydrogen bond from the backbone NH bond of Gly219 while the thiophene amide donates a hydrogen bond to the backbone carbonyl of Gly219. These intermolecular interactions of rivaroxaban with fXa are highly cooperative—the hydrogen bonding interactions anchor the core of the inhibitor in a way that allows the thiophene and morpholinone rings to project into the S1 and S4 pockets, respectively. When the amide connection to the thiophene ring was replaced with a sulfonamide or N–Me amide, a ~300-fold loss of potency resulted (Figure 2.14). Changes this dramatic are unlikely to result from the loss of a single hydrogen bond. More likely, the change to a sulfonamide or N–Me amide negatively affects binding cooperativity by less optimally positioning the morpholinone and chlorothiophene rings in the S4 and S1 binding pockets.

Having discussed the binding of rivaroxaban in some detail, it will be interesting to inspect the structures of the other factor Xa inhibitors presented in Figure 2.13. Can you predict which ring systems in apixaban and betrixaban might bind in the S1 and S4 pockets of fXa? Would the interactions of these other inhibitors at S1 and S4 be similar to rivaroxaban or different in some way? Also, can you predict which atoms in apixaban and betrixaban might accept or donate a hydrogen bond from the backbone amide of Gly219? Do you predict any differences for these inhibitors compared to rivaroxaban? Getting the "right" answers to these questions is less important than the act of generating hypotheses about how these related but different inhibitors interact with their common target.

2.14 Exercises

Shown below are the structures of drugs along hypothetical target interactions indicated by dashed lines to specific amino acids. For each dashed line, suggest one or more intermolecular interaction(s) that could reasonably form between the specific amino acid and indicated portion of the drug structure. For specific interactions such as hydrogen bonds, draw out the interaction and clearly label the hydrogen bond donor and acceptor atoms.

Problem 2.1

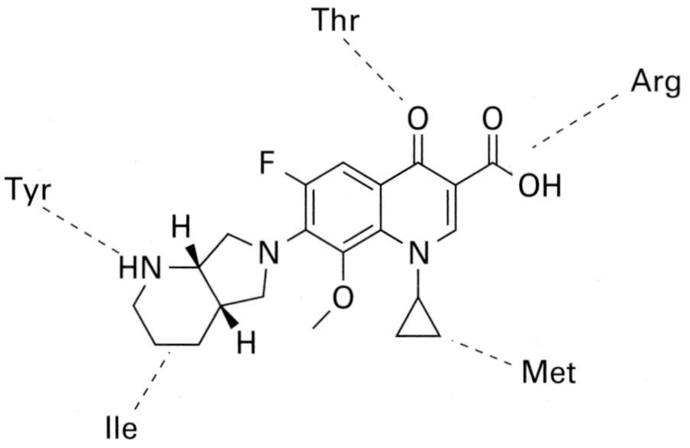

Problem 2.2

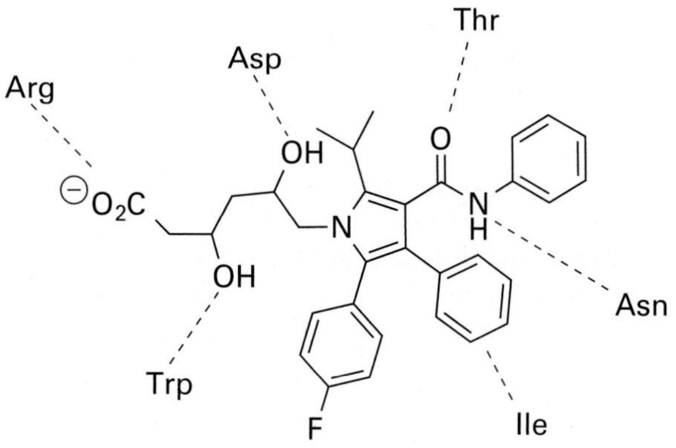

Problem 2.3

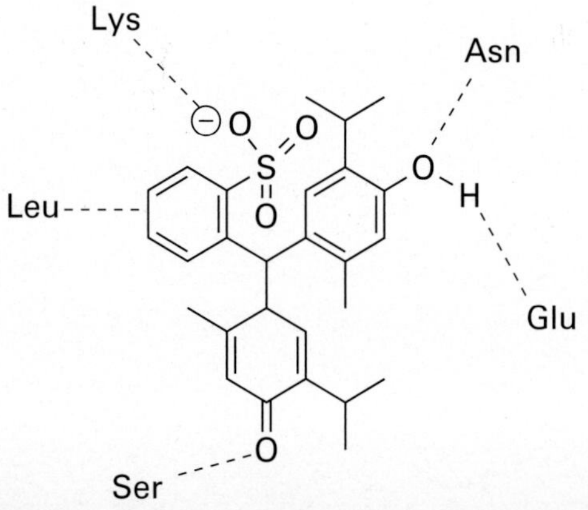

Problem 2.4

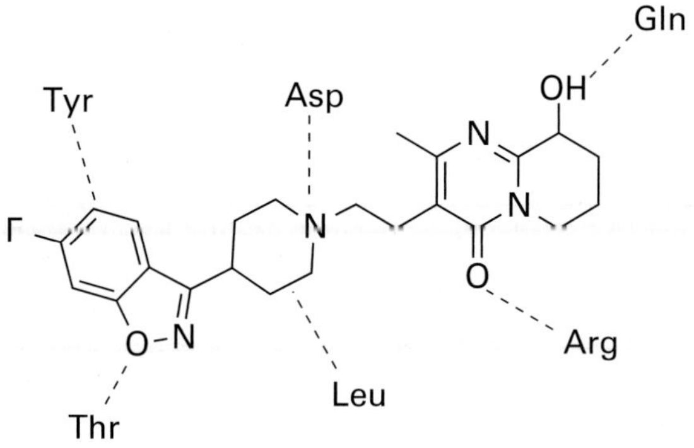

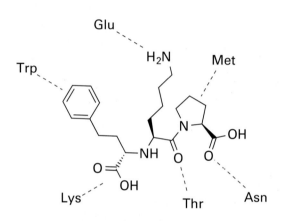

Problem 2.5

Problem 2.6

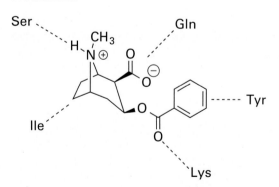

Chapter 3
Stereochemistry

Adam Renslo

CHAPTER OUTLINE

3.1 Introduction

3.2 Chirality and the Shape of Molecules

3.3 Stereoisomers—Some Important Definitions

   Box 3.1—Determining isomeric and stereo-chemical relationships between molecules

3.4 Avoiding Confusion

3.5 Stereoisomers of 1,3-Dimethylcyclohexane

3.6 Chirality Centers

3.7 Assigning the Configuration of Chirality Centers

   Box 3.2—Cahn–Ingold–Prelog rules in brief

3.8 Configurational Assignment and Stereochemical Relationships

3.9 Meso Compounds

3.10 Chirality Centers at Non-Carbon Atoms

3.11 Other Sources of Chirality and Stereoisomerism

   Box 3.3—Atropisomerism

3.12 Summary

3.13 *Case Study*—Racemic and Non-Racemic Drugs

3.14 Exercises

3.1 Introduction

In this chapter we will consider the stereochemistry of organic molecules, a topic that is concerned with how the atoms of a molecule are arranged in three dimensions. This is an important topic in pharmaceutical chemistry because the shape of a drug molecule affects both its desired biological activity and its potential for exhibiting undesired effects. To introduce the topic of stereochemistry, consider the three chemical drawings shown below (Figure 3.1). Each of these representations

describes a six-membered carbon ring with two methyl groups attached at defined positions—all three drawings describe the molecule 1,3-dimethylcyclohexane. However, as one moves from the first to second drawing, additional important information is conveyed. Whereas the first drawing tells us only about the connectivity of carbon atoms, the second tells us about the relative orientation of the two methyl groups—one is projecting out of the plane of the paper whereas the other is receding behind it. This drawing describes a specific **stereoisomer** of 1,3-dimethylcyclohexane. An even more informative representation is provided in the third drawing, which tells us not only about the relative orientation of the methyl groups but also about the relative positioning of all the carbon atoms in the cyclohexane ring. This third drawing attempts to illustrate the actual three dimensional shape of 1,3-cyclohexane, including its **conformation**, a topic we will cover in detail in the following chapter.

In considering the drawings of 1,3-dimethylcyclohexane above it may have occurred to you that other stereoisomers of 1,3-dimethylcyclohexane might also exist. For example, what if both the methyl groups

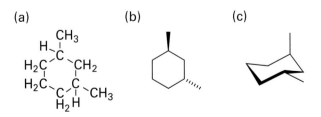

(a)   (b)   (c)

Figure 3.1 Three depictions of the molecule 1,3-dimethylcyclohexane. Drawings (b) and (c) convey additional stereochemical and conformational information not provided by drawing (a).

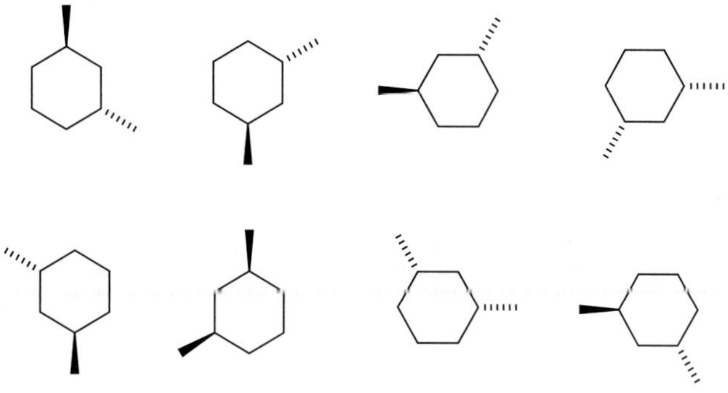

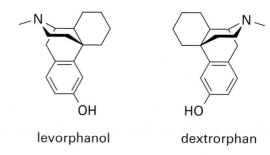

Figure 3.2 Several different stereochemical representations of 1,3-dimethylcyclohexane. Not all of the structures shown represent distinct stereoisomers. Can you spot the duplicates? How many distinct stereoisomers are present in this set?

levorphanol   dextrorphan

Figure 3.3 An example of two mirror-image molecules (enantiomers), both of which happen to be useful drugs. The two molecules have very different biological activities however, as is often the case with enantiomers.

projected from the same side of the ring? What if the methyl groups were found on different carbons of the ring but still in a 1,3-relationship? There would appear to be many possible stereoisomers of 1,3-dimethyl-cyclohexane (Figure 3.2). But, are all of these molecules truly different? Are some of these not equivalent representations of the same molecule? How many unique stereoisomers of 1,3-dimethylcyclohexane exist and how are they related to each other? These are the questions we seek to answer in studying the stereochemistry of molecules.

3.2 Chirality and the Shape of Molecules

Stereochemistry is of critical importance to drug action because the shape of a drug molecule is an important factor in determining how it interacts with the various biological molecules (enzymes, receptors, etc.) that it encounters in the body. Take, for example, the two very similar molecules shown above (Figure 3.3). At first glance they may appear to be identical but in fact they are related to one other in the same way a right hand is to a left hand. That is, each molecule is the mirror image of the other. You can see this by imagining (or actually placing) a mirror between the molecules on the page. Just as the mirror image of your right hand is a left hand, so is the mirror-image form of some molecules distinct. Objects or molecules that possess this property of being different from their mirror image are said to be **chiral**. Objects or molecules that are indistinguishable from their mirror image are **achiral** (not chiral).

To understand why chirality is important in the action of drugs, consider the chiral, mirror-image drug molecules levorphanol and dextrorphan (Figure 3.3). Levorphanol

activates opioid receptors and has powerful analgesic properties. However, its activity at multiple opioid receptors means that it is also a highly addictive substance and therefore is used only in the treatment of severe pain. In contrast, dextrorphan has no significant analgesic properties and is nonaddictive, but does has antitussive activity (it is the active metabolite of dextromethorphan, a widely used cough suppressant). Mirror-image molecules tend to have different pharmacological properties because biological macromolecules are themselves chiral and hence are affected differently by the mirror-image forms of a chiral drug molecule. A helpful analogy is that of hands and gloves—both chiral objects. A right-handed glove best fits a right hand so we might say that a right-handed glove can distinguish a right hand from a left. So too can biological macromolecules distinguish between the mirror-image forms of chiral drug molecules.

3.3 Stereoisomers—Some Important Definitions

It will be helpful at this stage to introduce some terms that are useful in describing relationships between stereoisomers. First, one must be clear about the distinction between **constitutional isomers** and stereoisomers. Constitutional isomers have a different connectivity of atoms. For example, 1,2-dimethylcyclohexane and 1,3-dimethylcyclohexane are constitutional isomers because the methyl groups on the cyclohexane ring are attached at different positions—their atom connectivity is different (Figure 3.4). Stereoisomers have identical atom connectivity but are distinct in shape (they cannot be perfectly superimposed). If two stereoisomers are also mirror-image molecules, then they are said to be **enantiomers**. The molecules levorphanol and dextrorphan discussed above are enantiomers because they are mirror-image stereoisomers. Since a molecule can have

Figure 3.4 Constitutional isomers have different connectivity of atoms, whereas stereoisomers differ only in shape.

only a single mirror image, enantiomers always come in pairs. Any pair of stereoisomers that are *not* mirror-image molecules are termed **diastereomers**. The relationships between these various terms are summarized in the box (Box 3.1).

3.4 Avoiding Confusion

It is very important to avoid confusing the property of chirality with descriptive terms like enantiomer and diastereomer. Intermingling of these terms and concepts is often a source of confusion for students of stereochemistry. First, note that all chiral molecules will have exactly one enantiomer (the mirror-image molecule). Note also that the mirror image of an achiral molecule will be the same molecule and so an achiral molecule can never have an enantiomer. However, some achiral molecules do have stereoisomers. This may seem surprising since chirality seems so closely tied to stereoisomerism. Consider however the "*cis*" and "*trans*"

isomers of 1,4-dimethylcyclohexane shown below (Figure 3.5). Both molecules are achiral and neither has an enantiomer since both are identical to their mirror image. The two molecules have the same connectivity of atoms but are clearly different, thus meeting our definition of stereoisomers. Since they are not mirror-image isomers, *cis*- and *trans*-1,4-dimethylcyclohexane must be diastereomers.

3.5 Stereoisomers of 1,3-Dimethylcyclohexane

Now let us reconsider all the possible stereoisomers of 1,3-dimethylcyclohexane. It is possible to imagine many possibilities (Figure 3.2) but closer inspection reveals that many of these structures are the same molecule drawn in a different orientation (e.g., upside down, or rotated on the plane of the paper). Since each methyl group can be found in one of two **configurations** (pointing up or down) we need only consider the four structures shown below (Figure 3.6). Inspection of the first two structures reveals them to be the same molecule—a rotation of 180° through the plane of this page will convert one into the other. It is also apparent that this stereoisomer is achiral since it is identical to its mirror image. One way to see this is to recognize that a mirror plane can be placed *within* the molecule. Any molecule (or object) that can be bisected by a mirror plane will be identical to its mirror image and thus, is achiral.

Box 3.1 Determining isomeric and stereochemical relationships between molecules.

The tree diagram below may be helpful in illustrating and determining the relationship between different types of isomers. Start at the top by asking the question whether the two molecules in question are actually different (we will assume that the molecular formulae are the same). If the molecules are truly different then we can say that we are dealing with isomers of one sort or another. If the atom connectivity is also the same, then we are dealing with stereoisomers that differ only in shape. The final question then is whether or not the stereoisomers are mirror image isomers. If yes, they are enantioners, if no, they are diastereomers.

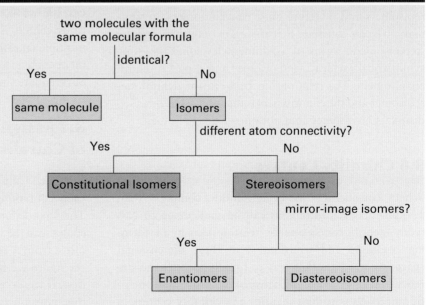

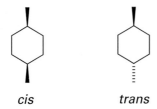

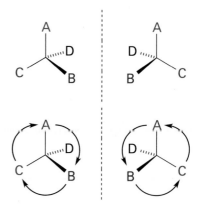

Figure 3.5 An example of stereoisomers that are achiral (not chiral). The *cis* and *trans* isomers of 1,4-dimethylcyclohexane are diastereomers since they are nonsuperimposable stereoisomers but are not mirror-image isomers.

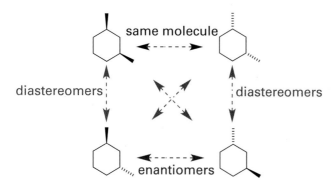

Figure 3.6 Only three distinct stereoisomers of 1,3-dimethylcyclohexane are possible. These include a pair of enantiomers (bottom) and a single achiral stereoisomer (top) that is diastereomeric with each of the chiral stereoisomers.

Figure 3.7 A hypothetical pair of enantiomers based on tetrahedral carbon with four different groups attached. The hashed line indicates a mirror that relates the two enantiomers. The sense of rotation moving from A to B to C is indicated on the drawings at bottom, and is opposite in the two enantiomers.

Now consider the second (lower) pair of isomers in Figure 3.6. In this case, no internal mirror plane is present and no amount of rotation through space will serve to superimpose the two molecules—thus, they are stereoisomers. By reorienting this pair of molecules in space we can show that they are in fact mirror-image stereoisomers and therefore must be enantiomers. In summary, we can conclude that there are only three unique stereoisomeric forms of 1,3-dimethylcyclohexane—one symmetrical (achiral) stereoisomer and a pair of chiral enantiomers. The relationship between the achiral stereoisomer and the enantiomers is that of diastereomers—distinct stereoisomers but not mirror-image isomers.

3.6 Chirality Centers

When considering molecules more complex than 1,3-dimethylcyclohexane, it can be challenging to correctly identify stereoisomeric relationships by performing rotations and translations in three dimensional space. We need another way to rapidly identify the stereochemical relationships between molecules. One helpful approach is to first identify any **chirality centers** in

a molecule and assign their **configuration**. As the name implies, chirality centers are centers within a molecule from which chirality originates. The most typical source of chirality centers in drug molecules are tetrahedral sp^3 hybridized carbon atoms attached to four different substituents. Consider for example the pair of enantiomers shown above in which a carbon atom is attached to four substituents, generically denoted A, B, C, and D (Figure 3.7). The central carbon atom in each enantiomer is a chirality center. It will always be the case that a molecule with a single chirality center will be chiral and will have a single enantiomer. Molecules with more than one chirality center will typically have both an enantiomer and one or more diastereomers. There are special cases however when a molecule with two or more chirality centers is achiral on the whole. This occurs when multiple chirality centers are related by a symmetry element such as a mirror plane. These special cases will be covered later in the chapter.

3.7 Assigning the Configuration of Chirality Centers

Consider again the pair of enantiomers discussed above, each containing a single chirality center (Figure 3.7). The "handedness" of the chirality centers in these molecules can be visualized in an interesting way. If we move from A to B to C in the molecule shown at left in the figure we find we are moving in a clockwise direction. If we do the same exercise with the enantiomer of this molecule (shown at right), we find that the sense of rotation is now counterclockwise. We might say that one molecule is "right handed" while its enantiomer is "left handed" based on the direction of rotation. This difference in rotational direction forms the basis of the Cahn–Ingold–Prelog (CIP) rules for assigning the stereochemical configuration of chirality centers. To successfully employ these rules requires that we properly assign the "priority" of various groups and properly orient the chirality center prior to assessing its configuration. In the example above it was natural to proceed from A to B to C based on the order of these letters in the alphabet. When actual chemical substituents are involved we instead employ the CIP rules to determine a rank-order priority for the substituents.

The CIP rules for assigning priority are quite logical and easy to master. In the simplest case, the substituents attached to a chirality center are assigned priority based on the atomic number (Z) of the atoms directly attached to the chirality center. If the four atoms directly attached are all different, then priority is easily assigned (higher priority for higher atomic number). A more typical case is shown below, where the four atoms directly attached include one hydrogen, two carbons, and one oxygen atom (Figure 3.8). Already we can say on the basis of atomic number that the oxygen substituent ($Z = 8$) is afforded the highest priority and the hydrogen substituent ($Z = 1$) the lowest. However, to distinguish priority between the two carbon substituents we must consider the additional atoms present. Moving out one

additional bond in each of these substituents we arrive at a carbon atom in one case and an oxygen atom in the other. Thus we can say that the substituent with oxygen at the second atom in the chain has higher priority (based on atomic number). Note that it does not matter that the other substituent is linked to *two* carbon atoms—atomic number takes priority over the number of groups attached. Thus, we have now assigned priority for all four groups attached to the chirality center. The next step is to orient the molecule such that the chirality center being analyzed has its lowest priority group (in this case hydrogen) *pointing away* from the perspective of the viewer. In this example the orientation needs no adjustment and we can directly consider the sense of rotation in progressing from high to lower priority (from 1 to 3). In this case the sense of rotation is clockwise and we therefore assign the configuration as *R*, from the Latin for "right"—*rectus*. It may be helpful to imagine the chirality center as a steering wheel with the lowest priority group representing the steering column, receding from view. Using this pictorial device, a "right turn" at the steering wheel (clockwise rotation) indicates the *R* configuration.

Let us now consider another molecule with a single chirality center (Figure 3.9). To assign the configuration of this center we again start by first considering the four atoms *directly* connected to the chirality center. Immediately we can assign the amino substituent ($Z = 7$) highest priority and the hydrogen substituent ($Z = 1$)

clockwise rotation from 1 to 3

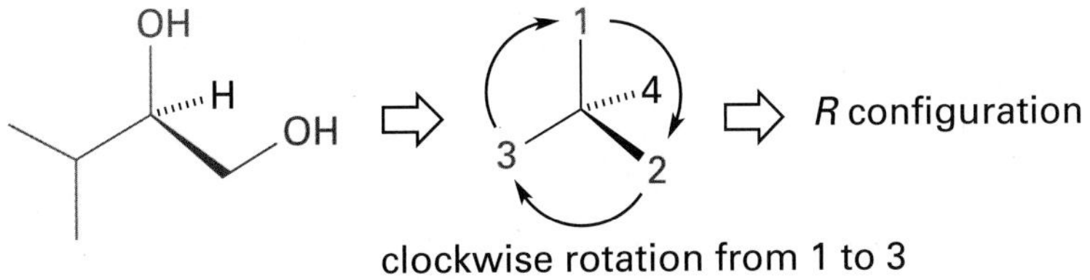

Figure 3.8 Assignment of configuration at a chirality center using the Cahn–Ingold–Prelog rules. Priority of substituents (1-4) is based on atomic number and the molecule is oriented such that the lowest priority group is positioned away from the viewer. A clockwise rotation in moving from 1 to 2 to 3 indicates the *R* configuration.

counterclockwise rotation from 1 to 3

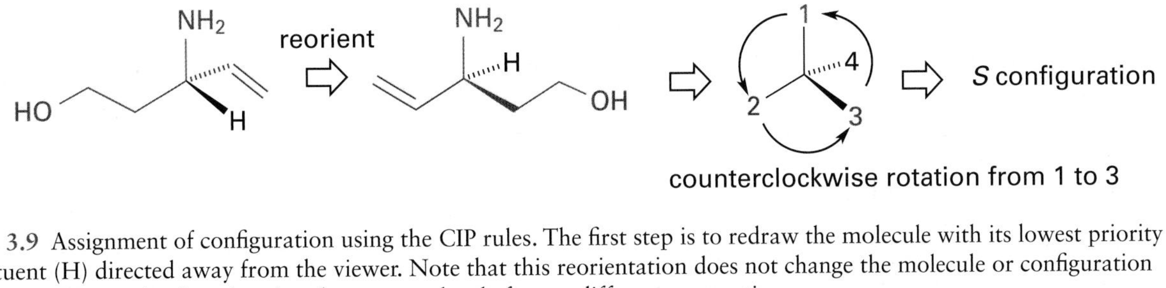

Figure 3.9 Assignment of configuration using the CIP rules. The first step is to redraw the molecule with its lowest priority substituent (H) directed away from the viewer. Note that this reorientation does not change the molecule or configuration in any way. We are simply redrawing the same molecule from a different perspective.

lowest priority on the basis of atomic number. As with the previous example, we cannot immediately assign the priority of the other two substituents since both are attached via carbon atoms. We therefore consider the atoms one bond further out within each substituent and find that carbon is next in both cases. However, according to the CIP rules, a double bond is treated as two single bonds and so the substituent with a double bond to carbon takes priority over that with only a single bond. Note here that the *number* of carbon atoms directly attached becomes relevant only when atomic number alone is not sufficient to determine priority. Note also that the presence of higher atomic number atoms (e.g., oxygen) further out in a substituent is irrelevant if a distinction can be made nearer to the chirality center. Having fully assigned priority, we must now rotate the molecule such that the lowest priority substituent is pointing away from our point of view. After doing this we can see that the sense of rotation according to priority is counterclockwise (a left-hand rotation) and can therefore assign the configuration as *S*, from the Latin for "left"—*sinister*. Everything you need to know about assigning configuration using the CIP rules has been covered in working these two examples. A more formal presentation of the CIP rules for assigning configuration is provided in Box 3.2.

Box 3.2 Cahn–Ingold–Prelog rules in brief.

1. Assign a priority to each substituent based on the atomic number of the atom *directly connected* to the chirality center (e.g., S > O > N > C > H, etc.)

2. For any substituents that cannot be assigned priority based on the first atom, consider the atoms directly connected to the first atom, and so on until priority can be assigned.

3. In assigning priority, atomic number is principle. The *number* of substituents attached should be considered only when atomic number alone cannot distinguish priority.

4. Double and triple bonds are counted as a connection to two and three atoms, respectively.

5. After assigning priority, reorient the chirality center such that the lowest priority group recedes from view.

6. Assign configuration based on the sense of rotation in moving from higher to lower priority substituents (clockwise rotation indicates the configuration is *R*, counterclockwise rotation indicates the configuration is *S*).

3.8 Configurational Assignment and Stereochemical Relationships

Now we will demonstrate how the assignment of absolute configuration (*R* or *S*) at chirality centers can be used to quickly assess stereochemical relationships. Because each chirality center can have one of two configurations, a molecule with n chirality centers will have a maximum of 2^n possible stereoisomers. There may be fewer than 2^n stereoisomers if symmetry elements are present, as we saw above with 1,3-dimethylcyclohexane, which has only three unique stereoisomers out of the maximum possible of $2^2 = 4$.

Consider now the molecule shown below in which two chirality centers produce the maximum of four distinct stereoisomers (Figure 3.10). The stereochemical relationships are indicated along with assignments of absolute configuration at each chirality center. Note first that the four stereoisomers exist as two pairs of enantiomers, and that each of these pairs is diastereomeric with the other. Note also that for enantiomers, the configuration at *both* chirality centers is changed whereas for diastereomers the configuration at only one of the two centers is different. This analysis will be the same no matter how complex a molecule is. For example, the enantiomer of a molecule with 10 chirality centers will have the opposite configuration at all 10 of those centers. A diastereomer of the same molecule will have a different configuration at one or more of the 10 centers, but not at all 10. Thus, when analyzing two suspected stereoisomers one can simply assign the configuration as *R* or *S* at each chirality center and thereby determine if the molecules in question are enantiomers, diastereomers, or in fact are identical and not stereoisomers at all (i.e., have the same configuration at all centers). This is a powerful approach to such problems and therefore it is important to become adept at applying the CIP rules to chirality centers in complex molecules.

3.9 Meso Compounds

As noted above, there are special cases where a molecule can have less than the maximum number (2^n) of possible stereoisomers. When two chirality centers in a molecule are related by a symmetry element such as an internal mirror plane, then the molecule as a whole will be achiral (since it will be identical to its mirror image). Such molecules are termed **meso** compounds, *provided that the complete set of stereoisomers includes chiral members*. This latter requirement means that the

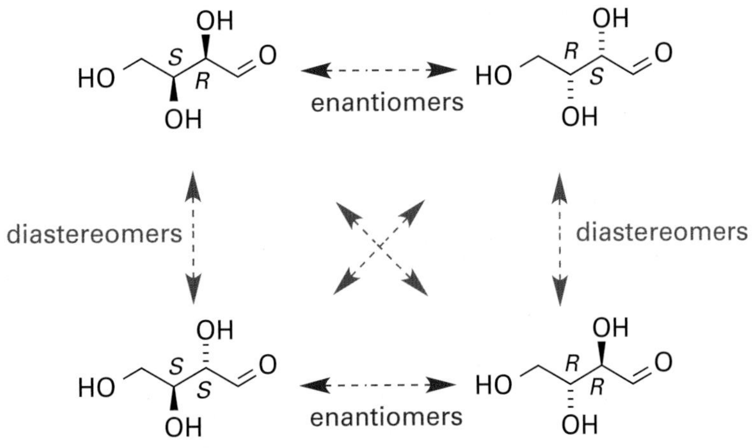

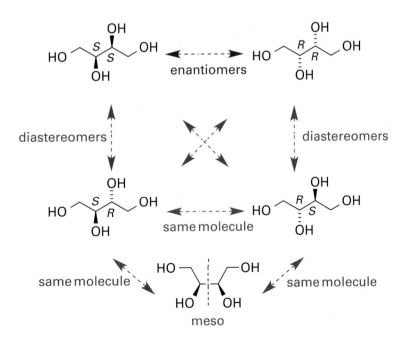

Figure 3.10 Stereochemical relationships in a molecule with two chirality centers. This molecule has the maximum number of stereoisomers ($2^2 = 4$) for a molecule with two chirality centers.

cis and *trans* stereoisomers of 1,4-dimethylcyclohexane (Figure 3.5) are not meso compounds, since no chiral stereoisomers of 1,4-dimethylcyclohexane exist (convince yourself that this is true). To further clarify this point, recall that meso compounds have two or more chirality centers related by a mirror plane. Since neither *cis* nor *trans* 1,4-dimethylcyclohexane have a chirality center, these compounds cannot be meso compounds.

For a specific example of a meso compound, consider the set of stereoisomers shown below (Figure 3.11). These molecules are very similar to the previous set

we considered (Figure 3.10), the difference being that the aldehyde group has been replaced with an alcohol function. This seemingly small change produces some interesting results. First, you might notice that the configuration (*R* or *S*) of some of the chirality centers has changed. This is due to changes in substituent priority stemming from the fact that an aldehyde group (counted as two C−O bonds by CIP rules) has been replaced by an alcohol function (a single C−O bond). Second, replacement of the aldehyde with an alcohol produces an element of symmetry in some of the stereoisomers.

Figure 3.11 Only three of a maximum possible four stereoisomers exists for the molecule shown. These include a pair of enantiomers and a single meso compound. Meso compounds have two or more chirality centers but are achiral overall due to the presence of an internal mirror plane.

As a result, there is now only a single pair of enantiomers in the set (the *S, S* and *R, R* isomers); the other two stereoisomers (*S, R* and *R, S*) are in fact the same molecule! This may not be obvious at first, but inspection will reveal that these molecules can be superimposed via a 180° rotation in the plane of the page. Another way to see this is to imagine rotating the central bond by 180°—an internal mirror plane can then be easily spotted (Figure 3.11).

Based on this analysis, we therefore conclude that only three distinct stereoisomers exist for the molecule in question—a pair of enantiomers and a meso compound that is diastereomeric with the enantiomers. One important thing to note is that configurational assignments cannot be used to spot a meso compound. As drawn, the stereoisomers at the bottom of Figure 3.11 can be assigned as *R, S* and *S, R* and this would normally suggest that the molecules are enantiomers. However, because of internal symmetry, the molecule as a whole is achiral and the *R, S* and *S, R* isomers are in fact identical. Thus, in determining relationships between stereoisomers one must be adept at assigning configurations and also be on the lookout for elements of symmetry within molecules.

3.10 Chirality Centers at Non-Carbon Atoms

Our discussion so far has focused on stereochemistry at carbon because sp^3 hybridized carbon is by far the most common source of chirality in organic molecules. Although tetrahedral sp^3 hybridized *nitrogen* atoms are quite common in organic molecules and drugs, nitrogen atoms with four different groups attached are generally *not* considered to be chirality centers. The reason for this is that sp^3 hybridized nitrogen undergoes rapid inversion at physiological temperatures, making the isolation or separation of stereoisomers impossible. Strictly speaking it is accurate to think of such molecules as rapidly interconverting mixtures of stereoisomers, but for practical purposes chirality at tetrahedral nitrogen centers is ignored and nitrogen is said to be configurationally unstable. Tetrahedral oxygen is also common in organic molecules, but with identical lone pairs of electrons constituting two of the four substituents, an oxygen atom cannot meet the definition of a chirality center. However, sulfur in the sulfoxide oxidation state does exist as a configurationally stable tetrahedral center. Perhaps the most well-known drug molecule with a chirality center at sulfur is the widely used proton pump inhibitor

esomeprazole

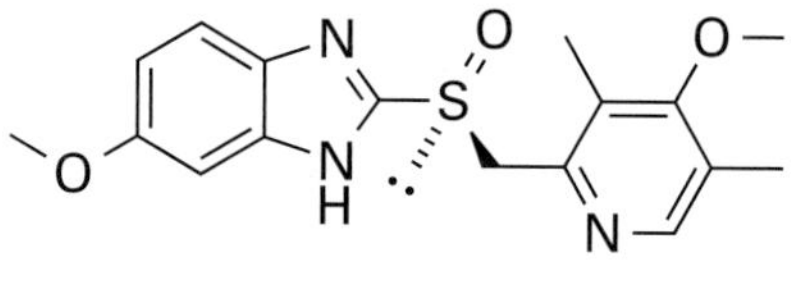

Figure 3.12 Esomeprazole is an example of a drug with a chirality center at a tetrahedral sulfur atom. The sulfoxide oxygen and lone pair electrons comprise two of the four substituents present on the chirality center.

omeprazole, which is better known by the trade name Prilosec®. Like many drugs, omeprazole is used as an equal mixture of *R* and *S* enantiomers (a **racemic** mixture). The cleverly named esomeprazole is the pure *S* enantiomer of omeprazole and is marketed as Nexium® (Figure 3.12).

3.11 Other Sources of Chirality and Stereoisomerism

Although less common, it is possible for chirality in small molecules to arise not from a point or center but from a **chirality axis**. Take, for example, the case of substituted allenes, functional groups formed when two sp^2 hybridized carbon centers are joined by a single sp hybridized carbon atom. The central carbon atom in allenes is often represented by a solid dot, as illustrated in Figure 3.13. The two π bonds in an allene are orthogonal, meaning that the substituents at either end of an allene are not in the same plane, but rather are related by a 90° twist. This arrangement is illustrated in the drawing of a pair of allene-containing enantiomers below (Figure 3.13). These molecules may not look like enantiomers at first glance but more careful inspection will reveal that they are not superimposable. These enantiomeric allenes do not have a chirality center but rather possess a chirality axis that can be imagined as a line running through the three carbon atoms of the allene. A chirality axis is also present in some molecules wherein free rotation about a single bond is not possible or is slow on human time scales. This is illustrated for a pair of enantiomers that contain no sp^3 hybridized carbon atoms at all, but do possess bulky bromine atoms that restrict rotation about a central C−C bond (Figure 3.13). These molecules are rendered chiral by the presence of a chirality axis running through the C−C bond that connects the two aryl rings. An example of an important antibiotic that possesses multiple chirality axes of this type is detailed in Box 3.3.

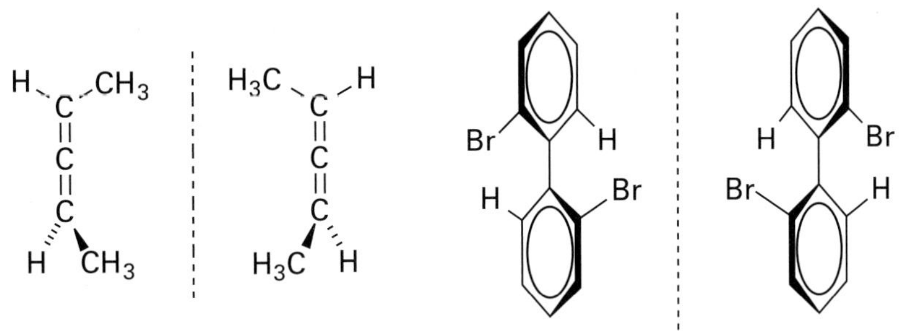

Figure 3.13 Compounds that are chiral by virtue of a chirality axis. The compounds at left are examples of allenes in which a central *sp* hybridized carbon is joined via orthogonal π bonds to two *sp²* hybridized carbon atoms. The compounds at right are enantiomers in which the large bromine atoms prevent free rotation about the C–C bond connecting the aryl rings.

Box 3.3 Atropisomerism.

Isomerism that results from hindered rotation about single bonds is referred to as **atropisomerism**. Usually this occurs when large groups are present in close proximity to a C–C single bond, thus hindering its rotation. Stereoisomers that result from atropisomerism will be either enantiomers or diastereomers, so the term atropisomer does not replace the normal terms we use to describe stereoisomers. Rather atropisomerism describes a mechanism by which isomerism can occur (hindered rotation about a bond). A notable example of atropisomerism is found in the remarkable chemical structure of vancomycin, illustrated

vancomycin aglycone

at right. This "antibiotic of last resort" contains multiple chirality axes stemming from hindered rotations about both C–C and C–O bonds where the various aryl rings are joined.

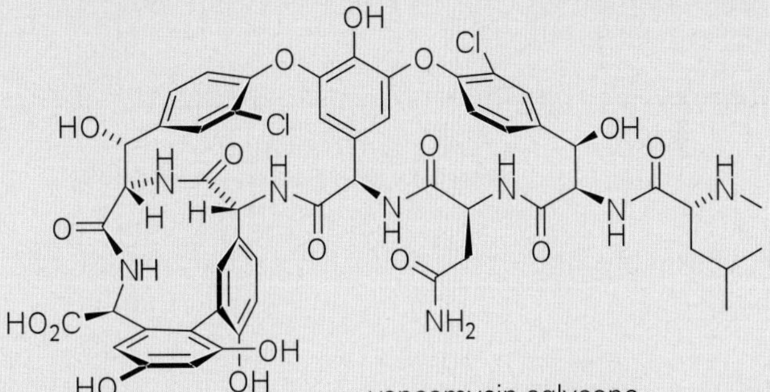

3.12 Summary

Section 3.1   Stereochemistry is concerned with molecular shape and the relationships between molecules with identical atom connectivity but different shapes.

Section 3.2   Chirality is a *property* of objects that are not the same thing as their mirror image. Objects (or molecules) that meet this criteria are said to be **chiral**. Those that are identical to their mirror image are said to be **achiral**.

Section 3.3   Constitutional isomers have different connectivity of atoms whereas stereoisomers have the same atom connectivity but different shapes. Stereoisomers can be further classified as **enantiomers** (mirror-image stereoisomers) or **diastereomers** (non-mirror image stereoisomers) (see also Box 3.1).

Section 3.4 The property of chirality should not be confused with the descriptive terms enantiomer and diastereomer. All chiral molecules have one, and only one, enantiomer. Achiral molecules will never have an enantiomer but may have one or more diastereomers (see Figures 3.5, 3.6, and 3.11).

Section 3.5 The molecule 1,3-dimethylcyclohexane has three distinct stereoisomers—a pair of enantiomers and an achiral diastereomer.

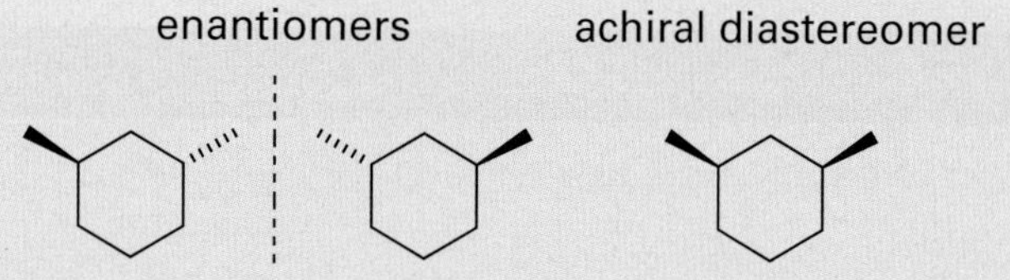

enantiomers   achiral diastereomer

Section 3.6 A **chirality center** is a center (point) from which chirality originates in a molecule. The most common type of chirality center in organic molecules is an sp^3 hybridized carbon atom attached two four distinct substituents.

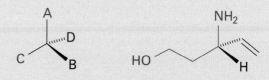

Section 3.7 A chirality center can have one of two configurations, either R or S. The Cahn–Ingold–Prelog (CIP) rules are employed to assign the **configuration** of chirality centers (see Box 3.2).

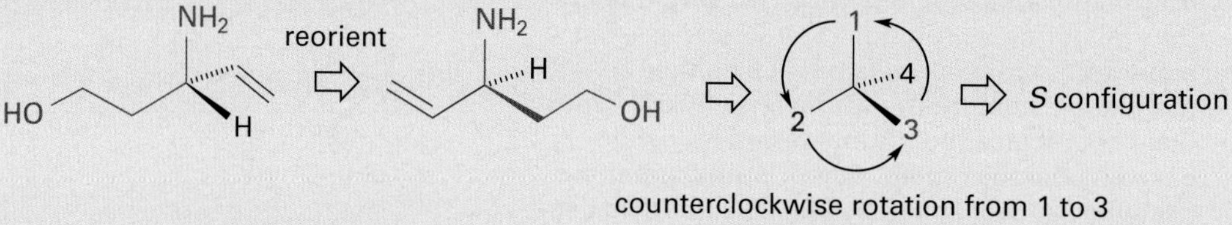

reorient

S configuration

counterclockwise rotation from 1 to 3

Section 3.8 The assignment of configuration at chirality centers is a powerful strategy for determining stereochemical relationships between molecules. Enantiomers have the opposite configuration at all chirality centers. Diastereomers have opposite configuration(s) at one or more chirality centers, but not at all chirality centers (or they would be enantiomers).

Section 3.9 **Meso compounds** are achiral members of a set of stereoisomers that includes at least one chiral member. Meso compounds have two or more chirality centers related by an internal symmetry element such as a mirror plane. Configurational assignment by CIP rules cannot identify meso compounds—visual inspection for symmetry elements is required.

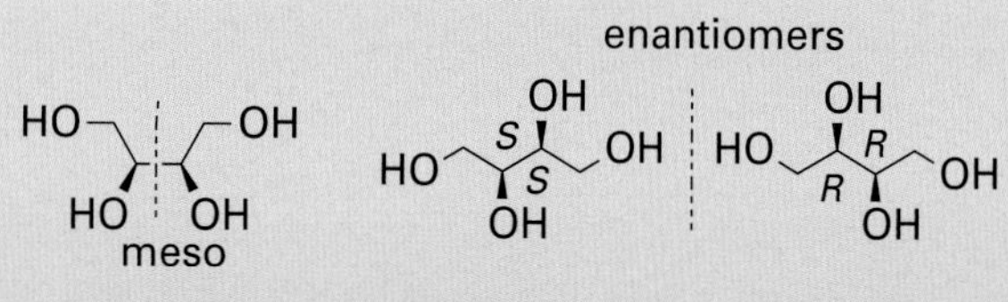

enantiomers

meso

Section 3.10 Any configurationally stable atom with tetrahedral (sp^3) geometry and four different substituents can be considered a chirality center. The most common non-carbon chirality center in drugs is tetrahedral sulfur in the sulfoxide oxidation state.

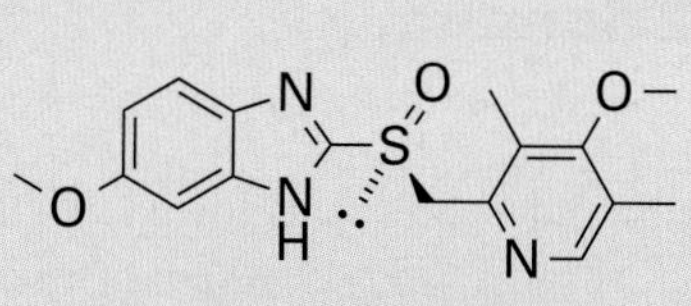

esomeprazole

Section 3.11 Chirality can also originate from a **chirality axis**. Certain allenes and rotationally constrained biaryl systems are chiral by virtue of a chirality axis.

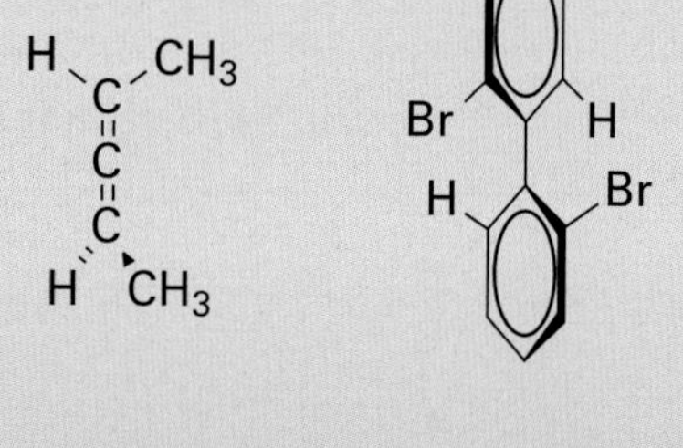

3.13 Case Study—Racemic and Non-Racemic Drugs

Currently, about 80% of the new drug molecules approved for clinical use are chiral, and of these, the vast majority are developed and marketed as single enantiomers. This was not always the case however, and prior to the 1990s most chiral drug substances were manufactured and used as **racemic mixtures** (equal mixtures of *R* and *S* enantiomers). This might seem surprising since we have already noted that the chiral macromolecules of living organisms can usually distinguish between the enantiomeric forms of drug species. It turns out however that the separation of drug enantiomers is not a trivial task, especially when it comes to manufacturing many tons of a drug. Thus, the current availability of single enantiomer drugs is a result of the development in recent decades of synthetic methods and separation technologies that enable the large-scale manufacture of single-enantiomer drugs. In this case study, we will discuss racemic and non-racemic drug substances

by focusing on the specific examples of omeprazole, ibuprofen, ketoprofen, and naproxen.

Omeprazole and Esomeprazole

It can generally be assumed that one enantiomeric form of a drug substance will be more active at a given biological target than the other. In fact, the terms **eutomer** and **distomer** are sometimes used to describe, respectively, the "active" and "inactive" enantiomer of a racemic drug substance. Sometimes however, the situation is more complicated, as is the case with the proton pump inhibitor omeprazole. Omeprazole (marketed as Prilosec®) was the first member of a new class of drugs intended to treat gastroesophageal reflux disease by directly inhibiting the proton pump (a H+/K+ ATPase) responsible for secreting protons (H+) into the stomach. As we noted in Section 3.10, omeprazole contains

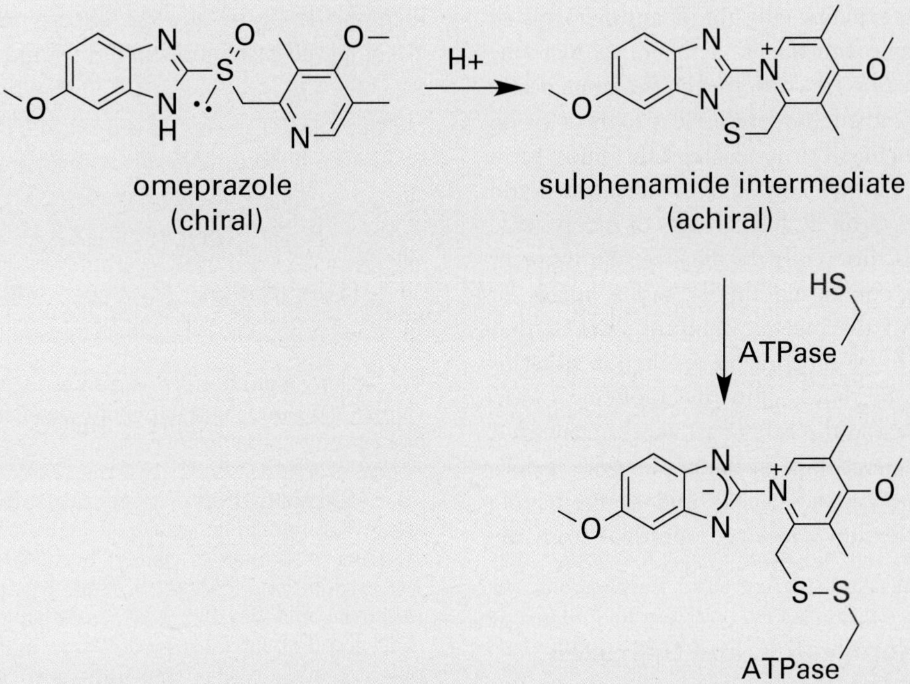

omeprazole
(chiral)

sulphenamide intermediate
(achiral)

Figure 3.14 The chiral proton pump inhibitor omeprazole is converted in the parietal cells of the stomach into an achiral sulphenamide intermediate. The sulphenamide is electrophilic and reacts with a thiol (–SH) function on the proton pump (a H+/K+ ATPase) to form a disulfide bond, thereby inhibiting the pump and slowing the secretion of protons into the stomach.

a chirality center at the tetrahedral sulfur atom and thus can exist in two enantiomeric forms (*R* and *S*). Omeprazole was originally developed and marketed as a racemic mixture and became a hugely successful product, with annual sales exceeding US$6 billion in the year 2000.

Interestingly, the *R* and *S* forms of omeprazole have equivalent inhibitory activity against the H+/K+ ATPase. This is because omeprazole itself is not the chemical species directly responsible for inhibition of the proton pump. As illustrated below (Figure 3.14), omeprazole first undergoes an acid promoted rearrangement to afford a reactive sulphenamide intermediate (some steps are omitted in the reaction scheme below). The sulphenamide intermediate next reacts with a thiol (–SH) group on the ATPase, forming a covalent disulfide bond and thereby inhibiting the enzyme (Figure 3.14).

You may have noted that the sulfur atom in the active sulphenamide intermediate is no longer attached to four different substituents and is therefore no longer a chirality center. Indeed, whereas omeprazole is chiral, the active sulphenamide intermediate is not, and this explains why the *R* and *S* forms of omeprazole have equivalent activity against the ATPase (both forms are converted to the same active intermediate). One might therefore expect little or no therapeutic benefit from a single-enantiomer form of omeprazole. However, in ~3% of Caucasians and 10–15% of Asians the *R* and *S* forms of omeprazole are metabolized differently in the liver. Subsequent clinical studies comparing the *R* and *S* forms of omeprazole with the racemic mixture showed that administration of (*S*)-omeprazole resulted in superior drug exposure in these "slow metabolizing" individuals. Thus, while the benefit is associated with a relatively small percentage of the population, it does constitute a therapeutic benefit and esomeprazole (marketed as Nexium®) received approval from the FDA in 2001.

Ibuprofen, Ketoprofen, and Naproxen

Next we will consider the widely used nonsteroidal anti-inflammatory drugs (NSAIDs), which include ibuprofen, ketoprofen, and naproxen among others. The anti-inflammatory, analgesic, and antipyretic properties of NSAIDs result from their inhibition of the enzyme cyclooxygenase (COX). COX enzymes

are involved in the biosynthesis of prostaglandins— biological small molecules that mediate a variety of processes such as inflammation and platelet aggregation. The various members of the "profen" class bear similar structural features, as one might expect given that these drugs target the same enzyme (Figure 3.15). Each of these molecules contains an aromatic ring system attached to the alpha carbon of propanoic acid, forming a single chirality center.

Of the two enantiomeric forms of these NSAIDs, only the *S* form is an effective inhibitor of COX enzymes. In the case of ibuprofen however, the inactive *R* enantiomer is converted in the body into the active *S* form by a metabolic process (fortuitously, the active *S* form is not converted to the inactive *R* form). This bioconversion would seem to mitigate any advantage of a single-enantiomer form of the drug—the *R* form is essentially a "pro-drug" that is converted in the body into the active drug species. Another factor to consider however is the possibility of adverse drug effects that might be associated with (*R*)-ibuprofen prior to its conversion to the active form. As a class, NSAIDs in fact do show a relatively high incidence of adverse effects, most commonly affecting the gastrointestinal tract and less commonly

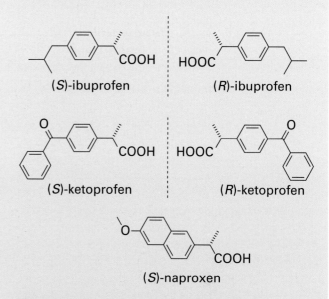

Figure 3.15 The *R* and *S* forms of the common nonsteroidal anti-inflammatory (NSAID) drugs ibuprofen and ketoprofen which have been developed both as racemic mixtures and as the pure *S* enantiomer. The NSAID (*S*)-naproxen was developed only in single-enantiomer form.

but more seriously involving the liver and kidneys. It also turns out that the bioconversion of (R)-ibuprofen to (S)-ibuprofen occurs at different rates in different individuals, a not inconsequential factor given that rapid drug action is desirable in an analgesic. For these reasons, (S)-ibuprofen was developed for use in single-enantiomer form and these products are now sold in some European countries.

Unlike ibuprofen, the R form of the NSAID keto-profen is not converted significantly into the active S form in the body. The rationale for a single-enantiomer form of ketoprofen is therefore more clear, since (R)-ketoprofen provides no particular therapeutic benefit to the patient. The active S enantiomer of ketoprofen has indeed been developed as a single-enantiomer drug (called dexketoprofen) and has the advantages

of requiring a lower dose and having more rapid onset of action as compared to the racemic form.

Our final example, the NSAID naproxen, was developed from the beginning in a single-enantiomer form, (S)-naproxen, and has never been approved for use as a racemic mixture. The original manufacturing process for (S)-naproxen involved the synthesis of racemic naproxen, which was then "resolved" (separated) into its two enantiomeric forms. In this industrial process, the actual production of racemic naproxen accounted for just one-third of the total manufacturing costs, the other two-thirds were associated with the laborious separation of naproxen enantiomers. Subsequent improvements in the resolution process have reduced overall manufacturing costs significantly however.

3.14 Exercises

Problem 3.1 Identify the chirality centers present in the following molecules. Which of the molecules are chiral and which are achiral? Which are meso compounds?

(a)

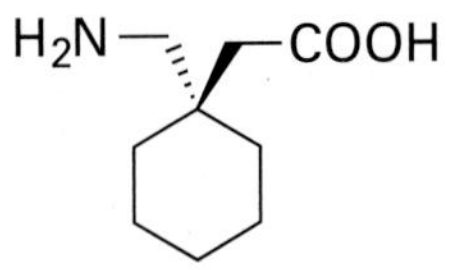

(b)

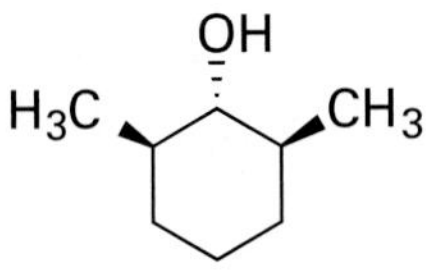

(c)

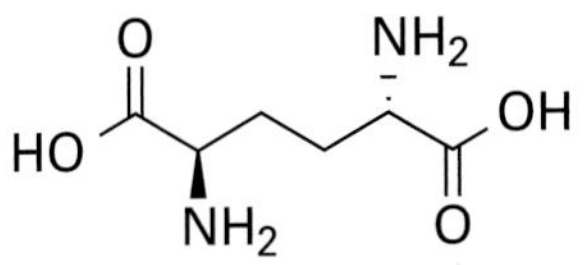

(d)

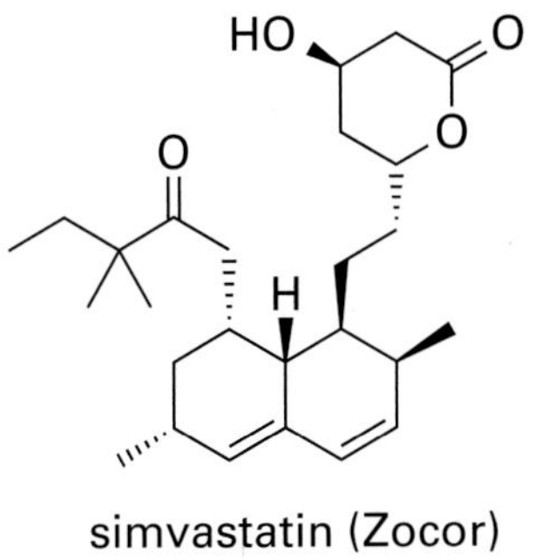

simvastatin (Zocor)

Problem 3.2 Identify the chirality centers in the following drug molecules and assign the configuration of each center as *R* or *S*.

(a)

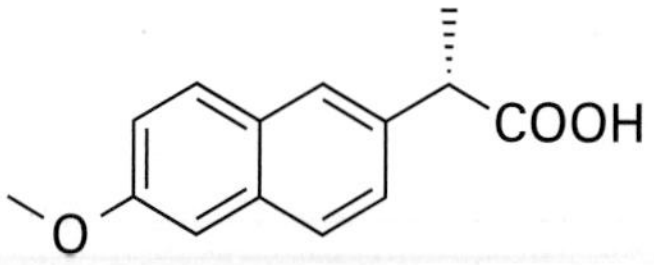

naproxen

(b)

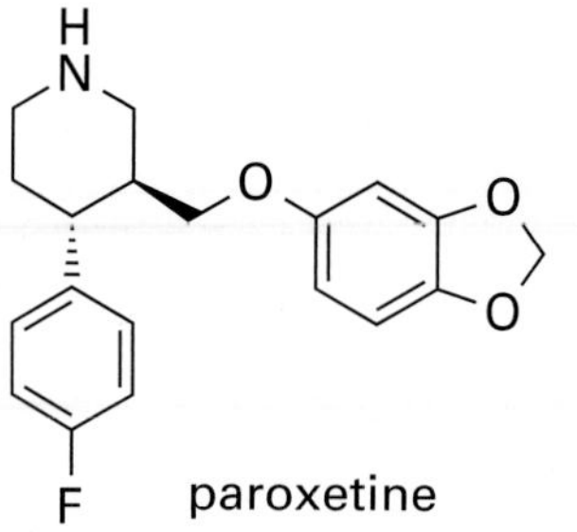

paroxetine

(c)

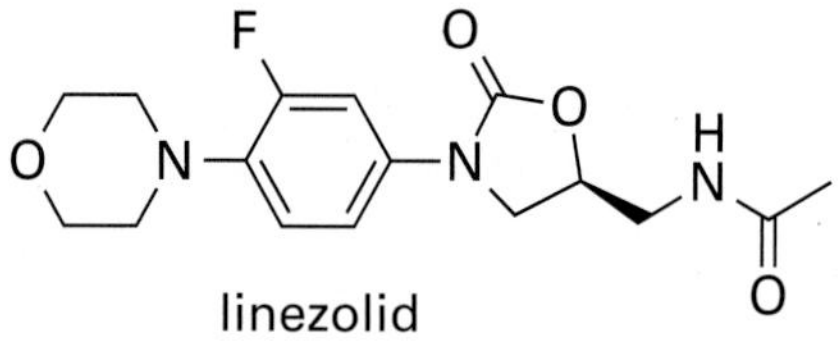

linezolid

(d)

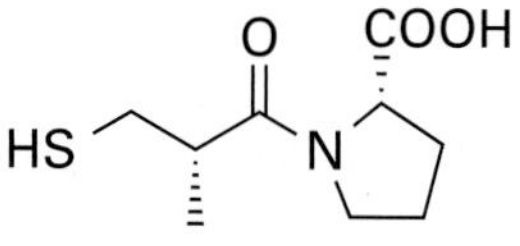

captopril

Problem 3.3 For each of the molecules shown below, draw the complete set of unique stereoisomers. Label the enantiomeric and diasteromeric relationships and identify any meso compounds.

(a)

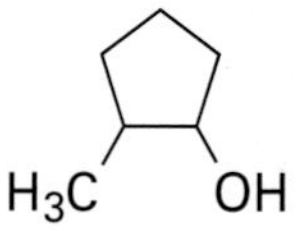

(b)

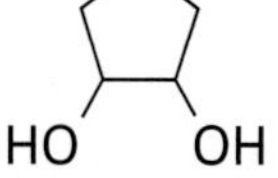

(c)

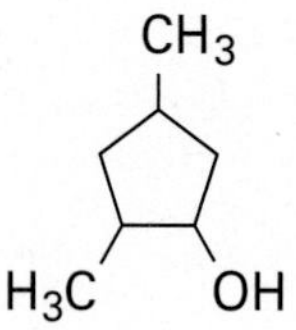

Problem 3.4 Determine whether each pair of molecules shown below are identical, enantiomers, diastereomers, or none of the above.

(a)

(b)

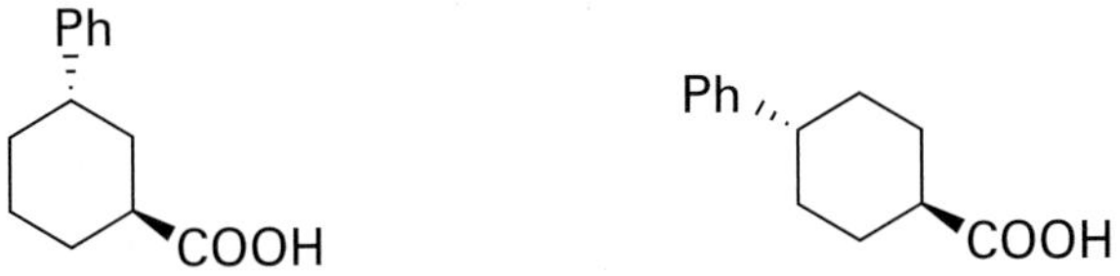

(c)

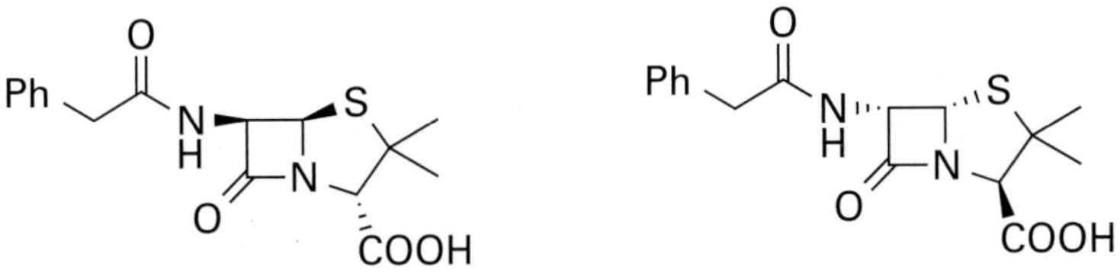

(d)

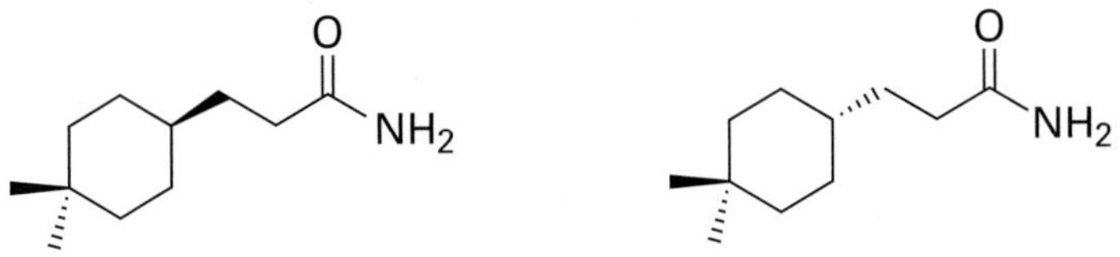

(e)

(f)

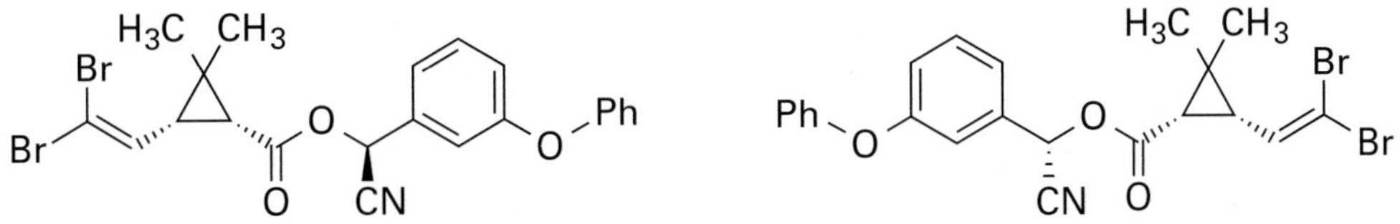

Problem 3.5 Which of the following compounds (**a**)–(**d**) are meso compounds?

(a)

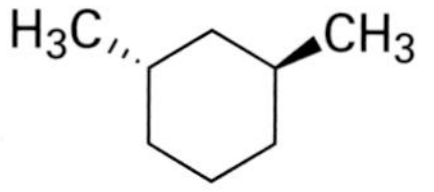

(b)

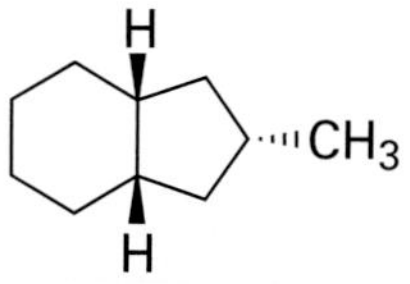

(c)

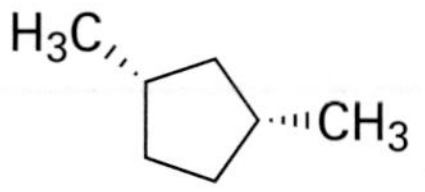

(d)

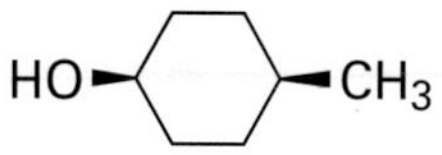

Chapter 4

Conformations of Organic Molecules

Adam Renslo

CHAPTER OUTLINE

4.1 Introduction

4.2 Newman Projections and Dihedral Angles

4.3 Conformations and Energies of Ethane—Torsional Strain

4.4 Conformations and Energies of Larger Acyclic Molecules—Steric Strain

4.5 Conformations of Small Rings

Box 4.1—The three major types of strain in organic molecules

4.6 Conformations of Cyclohexane and Related Six-Membered Rings

Box 4.2—Drawing chair conformations

4.7 Estimating the Conformational Preferences of Substituted Cyclohexanes

4.8 Conformationally Constrained Ring Systems

Box 4.3—Conformational constraint in opiate analgesics

4.9 Summary

4.10 *Case Study*—Neuraminidase Inhibitors and the Influenza Virus

4.11 Exercises

4.1 Introduction

In this chapter we will consider the **conformations**, or three-dimensional shapes, that organic molecules can adopt via *rotations* about single bonds in their structures. These rotations occur rapidly at physiological temperatures and so most molecules can readily adopt several distinct conformations that are in equilibrium with each other. These various conformations will have different free energies, which will determine the relative abundance of the different conformations. Two energetic extremes in the conformations of ethane are shown below, with the **staggered** conformation being lowest in energy (most favored) and the **eclipsed** conformation highest in energy (Figure 4.1). When a drug molecule interacts with its biological target, it must adopt a conformation (shape) that is compatible with binding to the target. The conformation of organic molecules is therefore a topic of great relevance to the action of drug molecules.

It is important at this stage to clarify the distinction between the terms configuration and conformation. As we learned in Chapter 3, configuration relates to the connectivity of atoms. A molecule might exist with either the *S* or *R* configuration at a chirality center but these two possibilities represent different molecules—they cannot interconvert without breaking and reforming chemical bonds. In contrast, two different conformations (or **conformers**) of a given molecule may have different shapes but they are still the same molecule—their interconversion requires only rotations about certain bonds. These rotations usually occur rapidly on the human timescale and so many different conformers are in equilibrium. To study the conformations of organic molecules then, we must imagine freezing time so that the different conformers can be compared and analyzed. This is what we will learn to do in this chapter.

staggered conformation of ethane

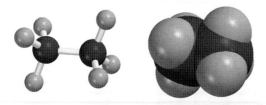

eclipsed conformation of ethane

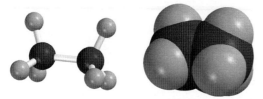

Figure 4.1 Staggered and eclipsed conformations of ethane represented as stick (left) and space-filling models (right). (Reproduced, with permission, from Carey FA, Giuliano RM. *Organic Chemistry*. 9th ed. New York: McGraw-Hill Education; 2014.)

4.2 Newman Projections and Dihedral Angles

To study the conformations of a simple organic molecule like ethane it is helpful to visualize rotations about single C–C bonds. Traditional structural drawings are less than ideal in this regard because they depict bonds from the side. An end-on view down the axis of a bond as it rotates provides a much better picture of what is happening. Consider the three different drawings of ethane below (Figure 4.2). All three drawings illustrate a "staggered" conformation but the Newman projection provides the clearest view of how the C–H bonds on the respective carbon atoms are staggered. A Newman projection represents a view looking exactly down the C–C bond axis. The carbon "in front" from this perspective appears with three C–H bonds separated by 120° (i.e., at 2, 6, and 10 o'clock). The carbon "behind" is shown as a circle with C–H bonds emanating from it and separated by 120° from one another. The angle of rotation between two specific bonds on the neighboring atoms is referred to as a **dihedral angle**. We can measure dihedral angles of 60° and 180° in the staggered conformation of ethane, depending on which specific C–H bonds are being compared.

It is important to note that the staggered conformation of ethane is only one of many possible conformations. These conformations may have similar or quite different energies depending on various factors, as we

(a) wedge-and-dash

(b) sawhorse

(c) Newman projection

Figure 4.2 Three representations of the staggered conformation of ethane. The Newman projection (c) provides the clearest indication of dihedral angles between neighboring C–H bonds. (Reproduced, with permission, from Carey FA, Giuliano RM. *Organic Chemistry*. 9th ed. New York: McGraw-Hill Education; 2014.)

will see. A useful way of visualizing the relative energies of different conformers is to plot the dihedral angle between two bonds against the corresponding potential energy. Such a plot is referred to as a potential energy diagram and typically takes the form of a series of peaks and valleys of varying complexity depending on the complexity of the molecule being studied. In the next two sections we will employ Newman projections and potential energy diagrams to understand the relative energies of the major conformers of ethane and butane.

4.3 Conformations and Energies of Ethane—Torsional Strain

The staggered conformation of ethane is the most stable and thus the most populated conformation. If you were able to take a snapshot of a collection of ethane molecules, the vast majority would be observed in staggered or nearly staggered conformations. In the staggered conformation of ethane, each C–H bond possesses a dihedral angle of 60° with respect to the nearest two C–H bonds on the neighboring carbon. On the opposite extreme one can imagine a conformation in which all dihedral angles between nearest C–H bonds is 0°. Viewed in a Newman projection down the C–C bond axis, each C–H bond would block, or eclipse, a C–H bond on the carbon atom immediately behind it. Accordingly this conformation is referred to as the "eclipsed" conformation, and is the least stable conformation of ethane (Figure 4.3). Our hypothetical snapshot of ethane molecules would have very few molecules in eclipsed conformations.

The staggered conformation of ethane is lower in energy than the eclipsed conformation by about 3 kcal/mole (~12 kJ/mol). The reason(s) for the special stability of staggered conformations has been surprisingly difficult to work out, with favorable orbital-orbital interactions and repulsive interactions both playing roles. Historically, chemists have used the term **torsional strain** to describe the preference for staggered conformations and this description is at least intuitively satisfying. Thus torsional strain can be thought of as the excess enthalpy required to adopt an eclipsed conformation starting from a staggered one.

Now let us examine a potential energy diagram describing all possible conformations of ethane. We will start with an eclipsed conformation and arbitrarily select two eclipsed C–H bonds with a dihedral angle of zero (the bonds to red hydrogen atoms in Figure 4.4). We then

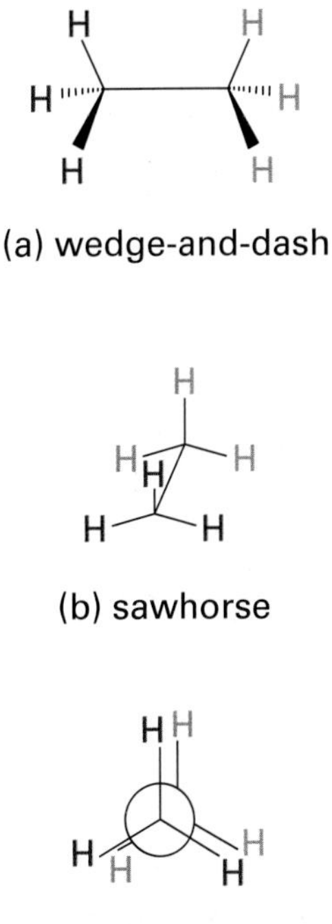

(a) wedge-and-dash

(b) sawhorse

(c) Newman projection

Figure 4.3 Three representations of the eclipsed conformation of ethane. (Reproduced, with permission, from Carey FA, Giuliano RM. *Organic Chemistry*. 9th ed. New York: McGraw-Hill Education; 2014.)

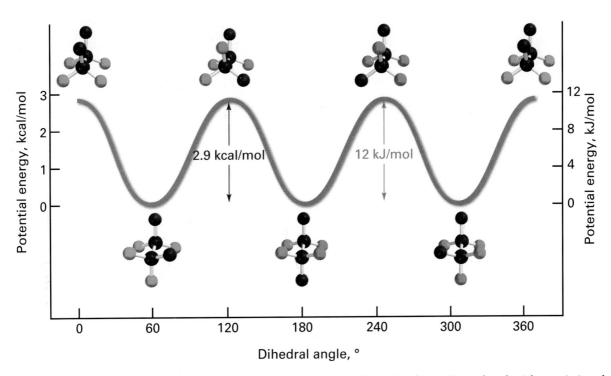

Figure 4.4 Potential energy diagram for a complete rotation about the C–C bond in ethane. (Reproduced, with permission, from Carey FA, Giuliano RM. *Organic Chemistry*. 9th ed. New York: McGraw-Hill Education; 2014.)

perform a full 360° rotation of the carbon atom in front, while holding the other carbon atom static (i.e., we examine all possible dihedral angles). Each time the ethane molecule adopts a staggered conformation we observe an energy minimum, while each time an eclipsed conformation is produced an energy maximum is observed (Figure 4.4). Note that with three C–H bonds on each carbon we have three minima and three maxima in a full rotation. Note also that because all bonds in question are the same (C–H bonds), each of the three minima and each of the three maxima are of equal energy (such states of equivalent energy are said to be degenerate). To summarize, a rotation of 360° about the C–C bond in ethane produces three eclipsed conformations, three staggered conformations, and many additional conformations that are somewhere between eclipsed and staggered, both geometrically and energetically.

4.4 Conformations and Energies of Larger Acyclic Molecules— Steric Strain

As we consider molecules more complex than ethane, additional factors begin to influence the relative energies of different conformers. To illustrate this we will next consider conformations of *n*-butane (C_4H_{10}), the molecule resulting from the addition of one methyl group to each carbon atom in ethane. While *n*-butane possesses three C–C bonds, each of which is free to rotate, we will focus our conformational analysis on the central (C2–C3) bond. As with our analysis of ethane, we imagine looking down the C2–C3 bond axis of *n*-butane using Newman projections (Figure 4.5). As before, a rotation of 360° will produce three eclipsed and three staggered conformers, along with many more conformers in between. The difference in the case of *n*-butane is that the C1 and C4 methyl groups will also interact through space, producing what is commonly referred to as **steric strain**. Not surprisingly, this strain will be greatest when the two methyl groups are nearest each other, which occurs when the C1–C2 and C3–C4 bonds are eclipsed (a dihedral angle of 0°). This particular conformer is denoted **syn** and is the highest energy conformation of *n*-butane because both torsional and steric strain are maximal (all bonds are eclipsed and the C1 and C4 methyl groups are nearest each other in space).

Other notable conformations of *n*-butane include the **gauche** and **anti** conformers, which can be produced by rotations of 60° or 180°, respectively, starting from a syn conformer (Figures 4.5 and 4.6). We expect that the anti conformer should be the most preferred conformer since the C1–C2 and C3–C4 bonds are staggered and the C1 and C4 methyl groups are maximally separated in

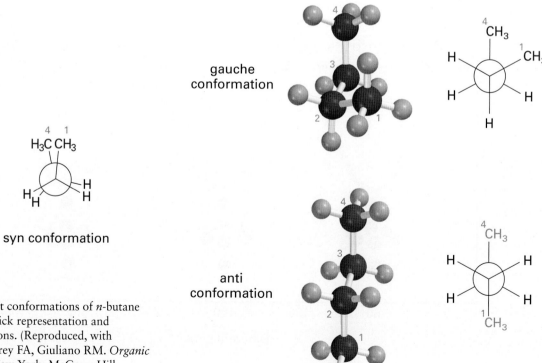

Figure 4.5 Important conformations of *n*-butane shown in ball-and-stick representation and as Newman projections. (Reproduced, with permission, from Carey FA, Giuliano RM. *Organic Chemistry*. 9th ed. New York: McGraw-Hill Education; 2014.)

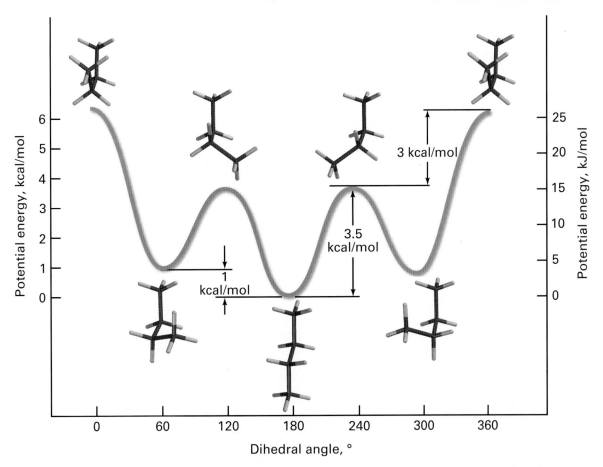

Figure 4.6 Potential energy diagram for a complete rotation about the C–C bond in *n*-butane. (Reproduced, with permission, from Carey FA, Giuliano RM. *Organic Chemistry*. 9th ed. New York: McGraw-Hill Education; 2014.)

space. Two energetically equivalent gauche conformers are produced by rotations of 60° clockwise or counterclockwise starting from the syn conformer. The gauche conformers are staggered like the anti conformer, but higher in energy since the C1 and C4 methyl groups are in closer proximity in the gauche conformation. Another way of saying this is that torsional strain is similar in the gauche and anti conformations but steric strain is greater in the gauche. A final conformer worth considering is that obtained via a 120° rotation from syn. This conformer will be eclipsed like the syn conformer but will be lower in energy since the C1 and C4 methyl groups are better separated (steric strain is reduced relative to syn).

The relative energies of *n*-butane conformers can be visualized with a potential energy diagram (Figure 4.6). Note that the combined effects of torsional and steric strain results in a more complex energy diagram than was the case with ethane. You may also note that the effects of steric strain become most significant at small dihedral angles (i.e., as one approaches the syn conformation). Thus, steric strain is primarily responsible for

the ~3 kcal/mol potential energy difference between the syn conformation and the other eclipsed conformations. In contrast, steric strain accounts for only a ~1kcal/mol potential energy difference between the gauche and anti conformations.

The effects of steric strain will of course be more significant as the interacting groups become larger or more numerous. For example, as one, two, or three methyl groups are added to the same carbon atom in ethane, the energetic barrier to rotation increases accordingly (Table 4.1). As halogen atoms of increasing size (F, Cl, Br, I) are added to ethane, we might well expect rotational barriers to increase and this is indeed the case as one moves from H to F to Cl. However, Cl and Br analogs surprisingly have similar rotational barriers despite the larger size of a Br atom compared to Cl. The explanation for this is that the C–Br bond is longer than the C–Cl bond and so the steric effects of the larger atom are offset by a longer bond. In the case of iodine the greater bond length more than compensates for the greater size and rotational barriers actually decrease. Note as well that

Table 4.1 Rotational Energy Barriers about the C–X Bond in CH_3–X.

Compound (CH_3–X)	Rotational barrier (kcal/mol)
CH_3–CH_3	2.9
CH_3–CH_2CH_3	3.4
CH_3–$CH(CH_3)_2$	3.9
CH_3–$C(CH_3)_3$	4.7
CH_3–CH_2F	3.3
CH_3–CH_2Cl	3.7
CH_3–CH_2Br	3.7
CH_3–CH_2I	3.2
CH_3–NH_2	2.0
CH_3–OH	1.1

methylamine (CH_3NH_2) and methanol (CH_3OH) have rotational barriers even lower than for ethane. This can be accounted for by a reduction in torsional strain due to a smaller number of interacting bonds (only two N–H bonds in methylamine and a single O–H bond in methanol). The lone pair electrons present on N and O contribute very little to the torsional strain of these molecules.

In summary, torsional strain and steric strain are key factors in determining the conformational preferences of small molecules. In the coming sections we will see how these same types of strain factor in the conformations of cyclic molecules and larger drug-sized molecules.

4.5 Conformations of Small Rings

Before we consider the conformations of cyclic molecules we must consider a third source of strain in small molecules. **Angle strain** is most common in cyclic molecules and results when a small ring size and/or the adoption of a particular conformation results in bond angles that are smaller (or larger) than the optimal value. Consider, for example, the case of cyclic hydrocarbons ranging between three and six carbon atoms (Table 4.2). Recall that for tetrahedral, sp^3 hybridized carbon, the preferred bond angle is ~109.5°. It should be obvious that C–C bond angles in cyclopropane and cyclobutane must be significantly smaller than the optimal value. Indeed, we find that cyclopropane and cyclobutane rings possess significantly greater angle strain than cyclopentane or cyclohexane, where bond angles can be very close to the ideal 109.5°.

Now let us consider the three-dimensional conformations of three, four, and five-membered ring systems. As illustrated below, the carbon framework of a cyclopropane ring is essentially flat, with all three carbon atoms lying in the same plane and rotation about the three C–C bonds effectively precluded.

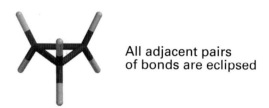

All adjacent pairs of bonds are eclipsed

(Reproduced, with permission, from Carey FA, Giuliano RM. *Organic Chemistry.* 9th ed. New York: McGraw-Hill Education; 2014.)

One consequence of this arrangement is that all C–H bonds in cyclopropane are eclipsed with respect to the C–H bonds on neighboring carbons. Thus cyclopropane effectively exists in a single conformation possessing severe angle strain and near-maximal torsional strain. Nevertheless, the cyclopropane ring is found in the structures of some drugs and is an example of

Table 4.2 Heats of Combustion (−$\Delta H°$) and Estimated Angle Strain for Cycloalkanes.

Cycloalkane	Number of CH_2 groups	−$\Delta H°$ (kcal/mol)	−$\Delta H°$ per CH_2 (kcal/mol)	Angle strain per CH_2 (kcal/mol)
Cyclopropane	3	499.8	166.6	10.6
Cyclobutane	4	650.3	162.7	6.7
Cyclopentane	5	786.6	157.3	1.3
Cyclohexane	6	936.8	156.0	0.0
Cycloheptane	7	1099.2	157.0	1.0
Cyclooctane	8	1258.8	157.3	1.3
Cyclotetradecane	14	2184.2	156.0	0.0

Source: Data from Carey FA, Giuliano RM. *Organic Chemistry.* 9th ed. New York: McGraw-Hill Education; 2014.

a kinetically stable ring system that harbors significant angle and torsional strain.

The case of cyclobutane is more interesting since some degree of rotation about C–C bonds is possible in the larger four-membered ring. The flat, fully eclipsed conformation of cyclobutane represents a high-energy extreme in which angle strain and torsional strain are maximal. Lower energy conformers of cyclobutane are those in which the carbocyclic ring is "puckered" slightly, which can be accomplished via small rotations about C–C bonds in the ring (as illustrated below). The result of these rotations is that the eclipsed C–H bonds move into partially staggered arrangements that reduce torsional strain. This analysis reveals dihedral angles smaller than the 60° value of staggered ethane, but still sufficient to relieve some of the torsional strain.

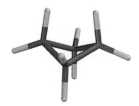

(Reproduced, with permission, from Carey FA, Giuliano RM. *Organic Chemistry*. 9th ed. New York: McGraw-Hill Education; 2014.)

Much more significant bond rotation is possible in the cyclopentane ring and so more effective staggering of the C–C bonds is possible. These partially staggered C–H bonds can be visualized with molecular models, or even with Newman projections, which are useful for analyzing cyclic molecules as well as acyclic ones. The puckered conformation of cyclopentane resembles an unsealed envelope with the flap lifted up (Figure 4.7(b)). Of the five C–C bonds in cyclopentane, four can adopt significantly staggered conformations but one C–C bond remains mostly eclipsed. As we will see in the next section, the cyclohexane ring is able to adopt a low-energy conformation in which all six C–C bonds are perfectly staggered and torsional strain is minimized.

The discussion above has focused on *unsubstituted* rings of three to five carbon atoms and the angle strain and torsional strain present in these rings. In the case of *substituted* cycloalkanes, steric interactions too impact conformational preferences. The effects of ring substitution on cyclohexane conformation will be discussed in great detail in Section 4.7 but it is worthwhile remembering that the introduction of substituents will have similar effects on the conformations of smaller ring systems as well. As an exercise, you might consider which conformations of cyclopentane (Figure 4.7) would be preferred if one or more methyl groups were added at various positions in the cyclopentane ring. The three major types of strain discussed in this and the previous two sections are summarized in Box 4.1.

Box 4.1 The three major types of strain in organic molecules.

As we have seen, three types of strain affect the conformational preferences of organic molecules. It is worth reviewing these here and making sure the distinctions between them are clear in your mind.

Torsional strain—As the name implies, torsional strain has to do with twisting (rotation) about single bonds. This strain is minimized when the bonds emanating from neighboring atoms are staggered, with an ideal dihedral angle of 60°. Torsional strain is maximized when the emanating bonds are eclipsed (dihedral angle of 0°).

Steric strain—Steric strain results when two substituents interact unfavorably through space. This can occur in both acyclic and cyclic molecules. Steric strain can be relieved by the adoption of conformations that increase the distance between the interacting substituents.

Angle strain—Angle strain is produced when bond angles deviate from the ideal value, as in three- and four-membered rings. Angle strain is also present in some larger ring systems, where severe torsional or steric strain is partially relieved by adoption of nonideal bond angles (see Table 4.2).

Figure 4.7 Representations of the (a) planar, (b) envelope, and (c) half-chair conformations of cyclopentane. (Reproduced, with permission, from Carey FA, Giuliano RM. *Organic Chemistry*. 9th ed. New York: McGraw-Hill Education; 2014.)

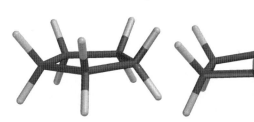

(a) planar

(b) envelope

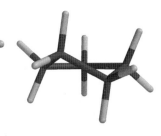

(c) half-chair

Figure 4.8 Representations of the chair conformation of cyclohexane as (a) ball-and-stick or (b) space-filling model. Hydrogen atoms located in equatorial positions are colored green while those in axial positions are colored red. (Reproduced, with permission, from Carey FA, Giuliano RM. *Organic Chemistry.* 9th ed. New York: McGraw-Hill Education; 2014.)

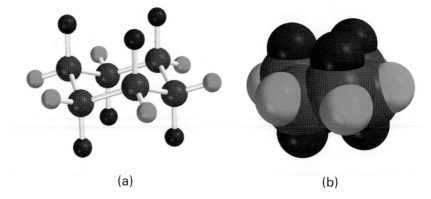

(a)   (b)

4.6 Conformations of Cyclohexane and Related Six-Membered Rings

The cyclohexane ring is able to adopt a specific conformation in which torsional strain, steric strain, and angle strain are all minimized. This conformation, called the **chair** conformation, possesses ideal 109.5° bond angles and six perfectly staggered C–C bonds. The chair conformation is shown above (Figure 4.8) but is best visualized with a molecular model in hand or on screen. Rotating the model, one is able to look down each C–C bond in turn and see the staggered orientation of all C–H bonds. Also evident from such inspection is that the C–H bonds in cyclohexane (of which there are 12 in total) project outward from the ring in one of two general orientations. Six of the C–H bonds are directed axially, with three above and three below the plane of the ring. The other six C–H bonds project equatorially from the sides of the ring. Thus, in examining the chair conformation of cyclohexane one can say that the ring substituents can adopt either an **axial** or **equatorial** position.

There are in fact two distinct chair conformations of cyclohexane, which interconvert rapidly via rotations about the C–C bonds that make up the ring. The two chair conformers are of equal energy in the case of unsubstituted cyclohexane, but are often of different energies in the case of substituted cyclohexanes. An interesting consequence of chair-to-chair interconversion is that all axial substituents move into equatorial positions and all equatorial groups in turn become axial (Figure 4.9). The act of interconverting chair conformers is commonly referred to as a "ring flip." Performing this operation on a physical molecular model is instructive as it makes clear that bond rotations alone are sufficient to interconvert chair conformations; no breaking of bonds need, nor should, occur (although the "bonds" of your plastic model may sometimes disconnect when you attempt a ring flip). Since models will not always be available to help in your analysis, it is also important to become adept at drawing chair conformations on the page (see Box 4.2 for some guidance).

In performing ring flips with models of cyclohexane one is likely to inadvertently produce other important conformations. Two of these are the **boat** and **twist-boat**. The boat conformation is higher in energy than the chair because two of its C–C bonds are eclipsed, as can be readily seen in the figure (Figure 4.10). The twist-boat conformation alleviates some of this torsional strain, as it has slightly more staggered conformations about the C–C bonds.

The relative energies of chair, boat, and twist-boat conformations can be compared using a potential energy diagram (Figure 4.11). Note first that the two degenerate chair conformations represent "global" energy minima whereas the degenerate twist-boat conformations occupy "local" energy minima ~5.5 kcal/mol higher in

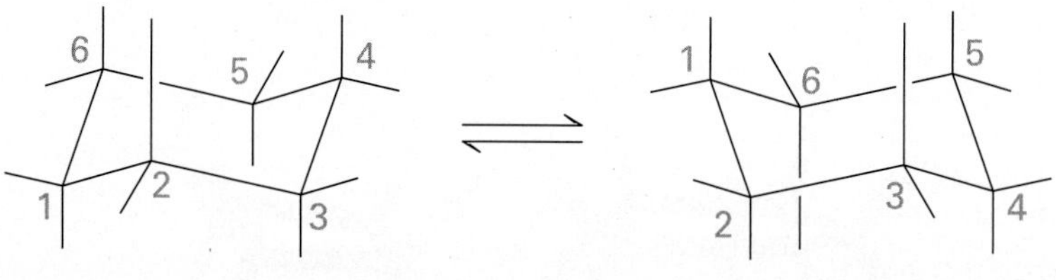

Figure 4.9 Interconversion of the chair conformation of cyclohexane. Note the atom numbering and that axial substituents become equatorial and vice versa upon chair-chair interconversion. (Reproduced, with permission, from Carey FA, Giuliano RM. *Organic Chemistry.* 9th ed. New York: McGraw-Hill Education; 2014.)

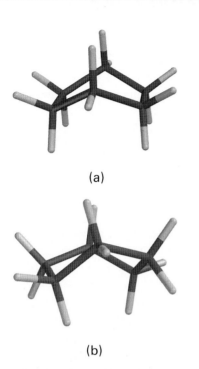

(a)

(b)

Figure 4.10 Additional cyclohexane conformations called (a) boat and (b) twist-boat. (Reproduced, with permission, from Carey FA, Giuliano RM. *Organic Chemistry*. 9th ed. New York: McGraw-Hill Education; 2014.)

energy. The boat conformation is higher in energy than the twist-boat due to greater torsional strain as noted above and also due to steric strain between the hydrogen atoms at the "bow" and "stern" of the boat. Note also from the energy diagram that the twist-boat conformers are intermediates on the path from one chair conformer to the other while the boat represents a transition state (energy maximum) between the two twist-boat intermediates. The energetic peak lying between chair and twist-boat conformers represents a transition state possessing a partially flattened ring system (half-chair), with more substantial torsional strain than either the chair or twist-boat conformers. The difference in energy between chair and twist-boat conformers is significant, translating to a ~10,000:1 chair:twist-boat ratio at room temperature.

The discussion so far has focused on cyclohexane itself, but six-membered heterocycles containing other atoms (nitrogen, oxygen, sulfur, etc.) will exhibit a similar preference for chair conformations. Oxygen and sulfur atoms in a heterocyclic ring will project one lone pair of electrons axially and one lone pair equatorially, just as saturated carbon atoms project one C–H bond in each orientation. An *sp*³ hybridized nitrogen atom in a heterocyclic ring will also have axial and equatorial substituents,

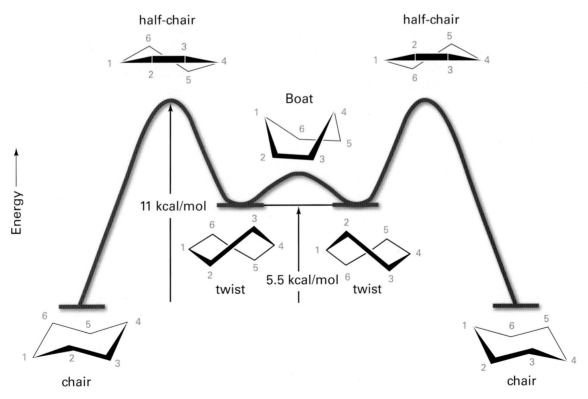

Figure 4.11 Potential energy diagram for conformations of cyclohexane. (Reproduced, with permission, from Carey FA, Giuliano RM. *Organic Chemistry*. 9th ed. New York: McGraw-Hill Education; 2014.)

one of which will be a lone pair of electrons. Just as with carbocyclic (all-carbon) rings, heterocyclic rings can undergo ring flips to produce two chair conformations, and can also adopt boat and twist-boat conformations.

4.7 Estimating the Conformational Preferences of Substituted Cyclohexanes

We will now consider conformations of carbocyclic or heterocyclic rings that bear substituents larger than hydrogen at one or more positions on the ring. Such substituted ring systems are very common in drug structures and so it is important to be able to predict their conformations. We will consider conformations of molecules in isolation but keep in mind that when an actual drug binds its biological target it may adopt a conformation distinct from the preferred low-energy conformation in solution. Usually it is preferable that the drug-bound conformation be close in energy to the overall minimum energy conformation of the free drug. However, the properties of drug binding sites can be quite different from that of aqueous solution, leading to different bound and free conformations in many cases.

To start, let us make a small modification to the cyclohexane ring—the introduction of a single methyl substituent—and then look at the effects of this modification on the two possible chair conformations. Recall that following a ring flip all equatorial substituents move into axial positions and vice versa. When all substituents are hydrogen, the two chair conformations are equivalent in energy but the same is not true of methylcyclohexane, as illustrated below.

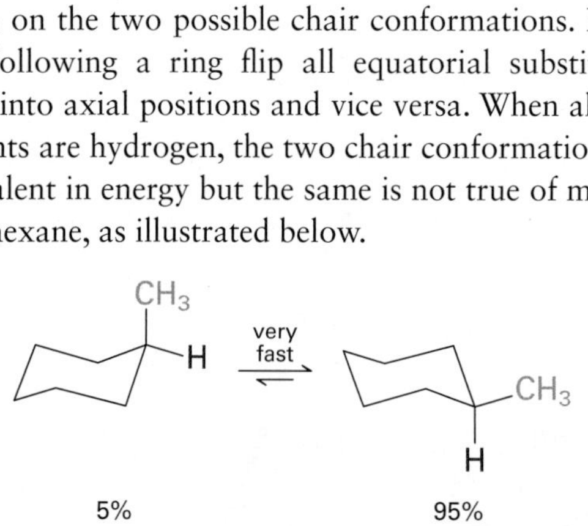

5%   95%

The chair conformation in which the methyl is in an axial position will be higher in energy than the chair conformation with an equatorial methyl group. Why should this be so? Torsional strain is similar in the two conformations since all C–C bonds in the ring remain staggered. The difference lies in the amount of steric strain experienced in the different conformations. When in the axial position the methyl group is in proximity to the other two axial substituents, both of which are hydrogen in this case. A ring flip moves the methyl group into an equatorial position, relieving the steric strain. By

inspection of a molecular model it should be clear that the methyl group in methylcyclohexane is further away from other ring hydrogen atoms when in an equatorial position. The difference in energy for these two chair conformations amounts to ~1.8 kcal/mol, translating to an equatorial:axial conformer ratio of ~20:1 at room temperature. The specific strain experienced by axial substituents is sometimes referred to as 1,3-diaxial strain but is simply another example of steric strain resulting from unfavorable through-space interactions.

The magnitude of 1,3-diaxial strain will be correlated with both the number and nature of the interacting groups. Larger groups will generally experience greater strain and the shape and electronic nature of the substituent are also important factors. Consider the table of conformation free energies ($-\Delta G°$) provided below (Table 4.3). The $-\Delta G°$ values presented represent the difference in free energy between chair conformations of substituted cyclohexane rings. You can also think of these values as the energetic "penalty" associated with placing a certain substituent in an axial rather than equatorial position. Hence, branched substituents like isopropyl and *tert*-butyl experience greater steric strain than a methyl group when in an axial position. Despite their larger size, halogen atoms like Cl, Br, and I experience less steric strain than methyl. This is a consequence of the longer carbon-halogen bond length, which alleviates some of the 1,3-diaxial strain. Linear *sp*-hybridized substituents like cyano ($-C\equiv N$) and alkynyl ($-C\equiv CH$) also experience little steric strain when in an axial position. The lone pairs on oxygen substituents like $-OH$ and $-OMe$ produce less steric strain than a hydrogen atom, explaining why $-OH$ and $-OMe$ groups pay a smaller penalty than a methyl group.

While the $-\Delta G°$ values in Table 4.3 were generated for *mono-substituted* cyclohexanes, we can use these values to estimate the conformational preferences of more highly substituted cyclohexanes and six-membered aliphatic heterocycles. To do this we must first draw the substituted cyclohexane in the two possible chair conformations. We start by drawing the carbon skeleton and then introduce the substituents, being careful to place them correctly in axial or equatorial orientations (see Box 4.2 for guidance). Typically one will be converting a wedge-and-dash type drawing into a conformational representation, as shown below for the two chair conformers of a substituted cyclohexane (Figure 4.12). To ensure that the substituents are properly positioned on your chair drawings, it is a good idea to number the carbon atoms in the various drawings (numbering schemes can be arbitrary as long as they are consistent between drawings).

At this point it is a good idea to review Figure 4.12 carefully. You should be able to see that for each chair

Table 4.3 Conformational Free Energies for Cyclohexane Substituents ($-\Delta G°$).

Substituent	$-\Delta G°$ (kcal/mol)	Substituent	$-\Delta G°$ (kcal/mol)
–F	0.26	–C≡CH	0.5
–Cl	0.53	–C≡N	0.2
–Br	0.48	–C_6H_5 (Ph)	2.9
–I	0.47	–OC(=O)CH_3 (–OAc)	0.71
–CH_3 (Me)	1.8	–C(O)OH	1.35
–CH_2CH_3 (Et)	1.8	–C(O)OCH_2CH_3	1.15
–CH(CH_3)$_2$ (i-Pr)	2.1	–OH	0.6
–C(CH_3)$_3$ (t-Bu)	>4.5	–OCH_3	0.6
–CH=CH_2	1.7	–NO_2	1.16

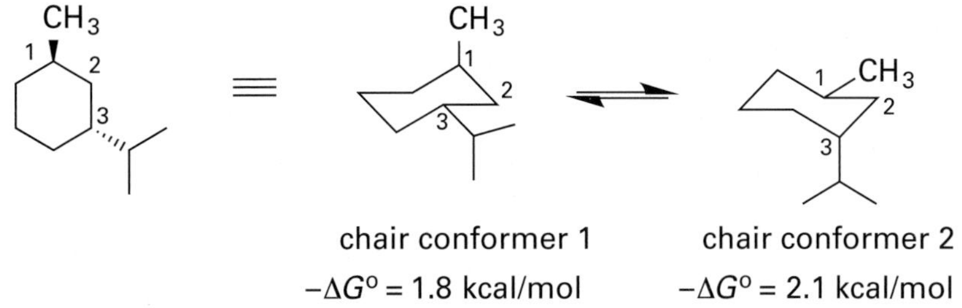

Figure 4.12 Wedge-and-dash and chair conformers of a substituted cyclohexane, labeled with an arbitrary but consistent atom numbering scheme.

chair conformer 1
$-\Delta G° = 1.8$ kcal/mol

chair conformer 2
$-\Delta G° = 2.1$ kcal/mol

conformer, the C1 methyl and C3 isopropyl groups move between axial and equatorial positions following the ring flip. Another important point is that the C1 methyl group is pointing "up" and the C3 isopropyl "down" in both chair conformers, just as in the original wedge-and-dash representation. In other words, performing a ring flip does not change the configuration at C1 or C3, it only affects whether the substituent is in an axial or equatorial position. One good way to double-check your work is to assign the configuration of stereocenters as R or S in your wedge-and-dash and chair conformational drawings (configurations should not change).

Having correctly drawn the two chair conformations, we will now consider their relative energies. We see that conformer 1 has a methyl group in an axial position while conformer 2 has a larger, isopropyl group in an axial position. According to the $-\Delta G°$ values in Table 4.3, conformer 1 should be favored over conformer 2

by ~0.3 kcal/mol (the difference in the energetic penalty for an axial methyl vs. an axial isopropyl group, or $2.1-1.8 = 0.3$ kcal/mol). In this case the conformers are relatively close in energy and both will be significantly represented. Next, let us consider the conformations of a diastereomer of this same molecule, with a different configuration at C–3 (Figure 4.13). In this case, both the methyl and isopropyl groups are axial in conformer 1 while both are equatorial in conformer 2. Accordingly, conformer 2 pays no energetic penalty for axial substituents while conformer 1 pays two penalties ($1.8 + 2.1 = 3.9$ kcal/mol). The difference in energy between conformers 1 and 2 is thus ~3.9 kcal/mol and conformer 2 will be the predominant conformation of this molecule. This same approach can be used for even more highly substituted cyclohexanes and also for unsaturated cyclohexenes, when their chair-like conformers are drawn as shown in Box 4.2.

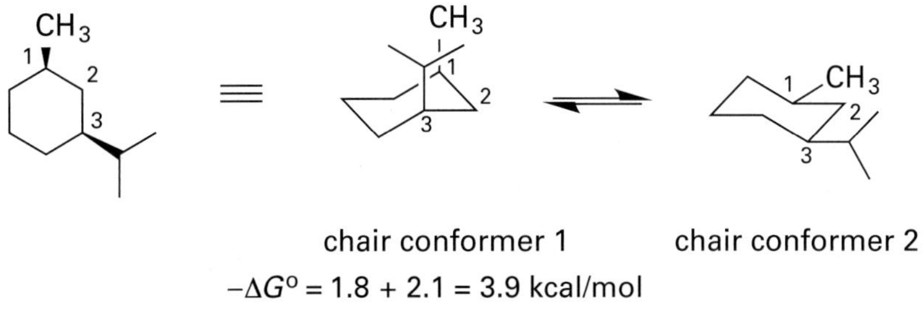

Figure 4.13 Wedge-and-dash and chair conformers of a substituted cyclohexane, a diastereomer of the molecule in Figure 4.12. Chair conformer 2 pays no energetic penalty for axial substituents and is therefore ~3.9 kcal/mol lower in energy than conformer 1.

chair conformer 1
$-\Delta G° = 1.8 + 2.1 = 3.9$ kcal/mol

chair conformer 2

Box 4.2 Drawing chair conformations.

The chair conformation of cyclohexane is represented on paper as shown in Figure 4.9 and is intended to present the molecule as viewed from the side and slightly above the plane of the ring. Again, the use of a model will be helpful in making the connection between two- and three-dimensional representations. Note that the axial bonds (shown in red) are joined to the ring by vertical lines while equatorial bonds (shown in blue) are joined to the ring at oblique angles. As illustrated below, it is usually easiest to start by drawing all the axial bonds, and then the equatorial bonds. Equatorial bonds are more difficult to draw accurately but this task is made easier by remembering that each equatorial bond should be parallel to two of the C–C bonds within the cyclohexane ring, as illustrated.

(1) Begin with the chair conformation of cyclohexane.

(2) Draw the axial bonds before the equatorial ones, alternating their direction on adjacent atoms. Always start by placing an axial bond "up" on the uppermost carbon or "down" on the lowest carbon.

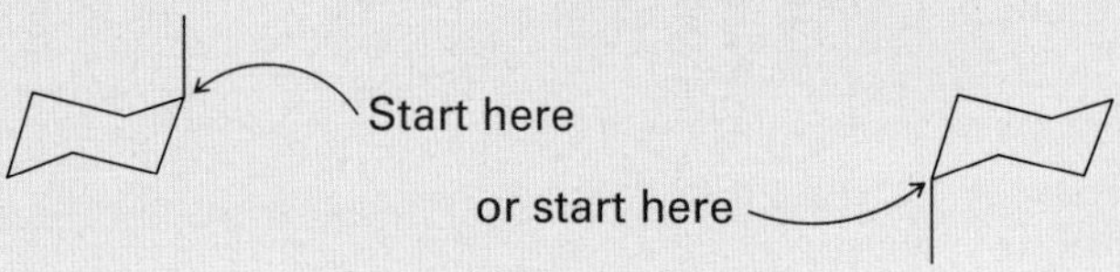

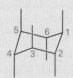 Start here

or start here

Then alternate to give

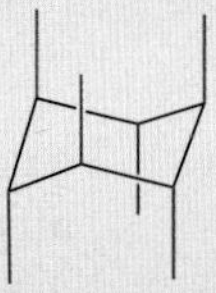

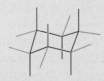 in which all the axial bonds are parallel to one another

(3) Place the equatorial bonds so as to approximate a tetrahedral arrangement of the bonds to each carbon. The equatorial bond of each carbon should be parallel to the ring bonds of its two nearest neighbor carbons.

Place equatorial bond at C1 so that it is parallel to the bonds between C2 and C3 and between C5 and C6.

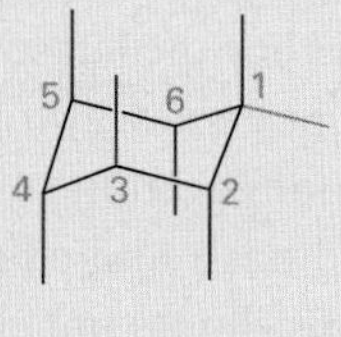

Following this pattern gives the complete set of equatorial bonds.

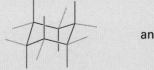

(4) Practice drawing cyclohexane chairs oriented in either direction.

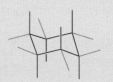   and

(Reproduced, with permission, from Carey FA, Giuliano RM. *Organic Chemistry.* 9th ed. New York: McGraw-Hill Education; 2014.)

Six-membered rings containing a double bond can also be drawn as chair-like representations, as illustrated below. The convention is to show the molecule as if viewed in the plane of the double bond. Substituents directly attached to the double bond can be shown but are typically omitted since the point of these drawings is to evaluate the positions of substituents on the saturated ring atoms. The axial and equatorial positions are shown in the diagram below. As with saturated ring systems, a ring flip produces a second chair-like conformation in which all equatorial positions become axial and vice versa.

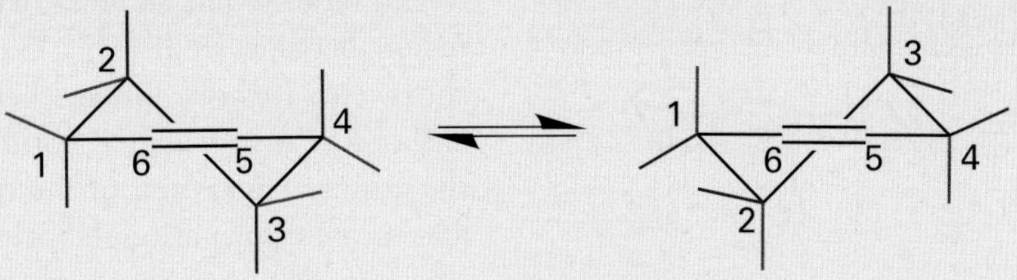

4.8 Conformationally Constrained Ring Systems

In the previous sections, we saw that the size and nature of substituents on a C–C bond or cyclic ring system will determine which conformation(s) are preferred. We can say that the presence of certain (usually large) groups limits or *constrains* the number of possible conformations. Such **conformational constraint** is important in drug design since it is one way that specific conformations (say, the one that best binds a drug target) can be favored over others. We will now discuss other types of conformational constraint that result from the joining of two rings together in various ways (Figure 4.14).

The first way that two rings can be joined together is via a single atom, resulting in a **spirocyclic** ring system (as in buspirone). The spirocyclic ring connection does not usually produce significant conformational constraint, since the effect is like having two identical or similar substituents at a particular ring atom. To see this, try building a model of the spirocyclic ring system in buspirone and comparing its conformational flexibility to that of simple five- or six-membered ring systems.

A second way to join rings is via bonds on immediately adjacent atoms. This results in a **fused** ring system, as illustrated for trovafloxacin. Ring fusion can have a significant effect on conformational flexibility, as we will see in our discussion of decalin to follow. The third possibility for joining rings involves bonds on nonadjacent atoms. This produces a **bridged** ring system with usually quite significant effects on conformational flexibility. To see this, build a model of the bridged ring system in varenicline and compare its conformational flexibility to the molecule that lacks the CH_2 "bridge."

We will discuss ring fusion in more detail since it is a common motif in bioactive molecules and drugs. A simple example is decalin, formed by fusing two cyclohexane rings together. Decalin can exist in two diastereomeric forms called *trans-* or *cis*-decalin depending on just how the two rings are connected (Figure 4.15). As with cyclohexane, decalin exists primarily in chair-like conformations, where torsional strain is minimal and all C–C bonds are staggered. A key difference is that in *trans*-decalin, all C–C bonds at the ring fusion are

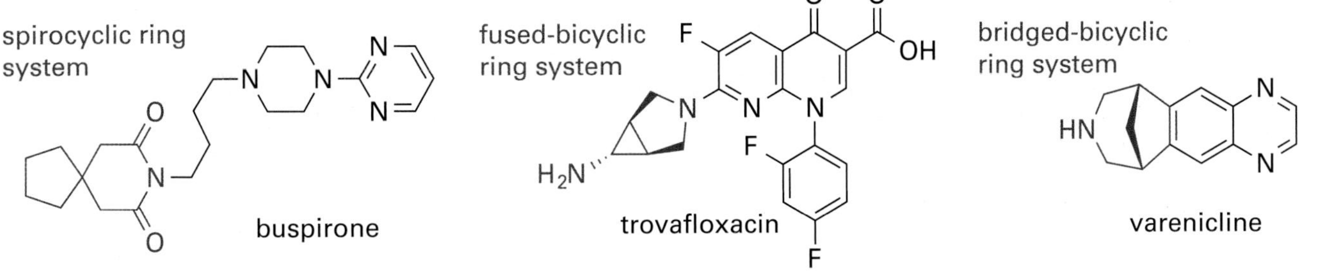

Figure 4.14 Examples of conformational constraint in drug molecules.

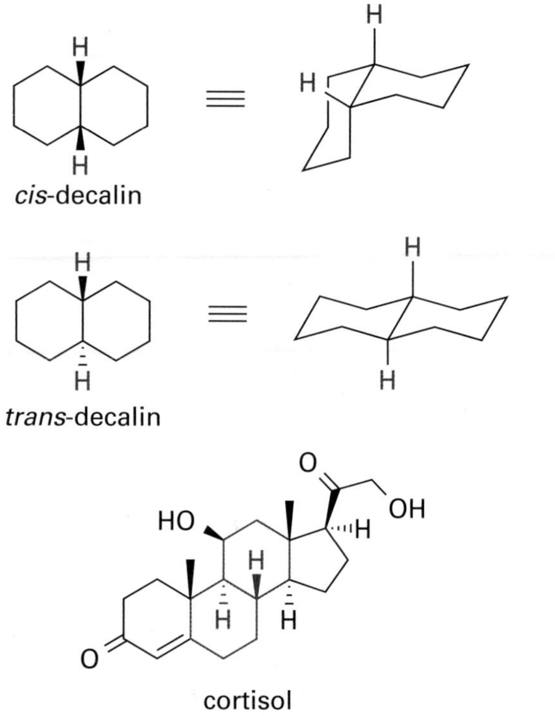

Figure 4.15 Structures and chair drawings of *cis-* and *trans-*decalin. Only *cis-*decalin is able to undergo chair-chair interconversion. The more rigid *trans-*decalin ring system forms the backbone of many steroid hormones, including cortisol.

equatorially positioned whereas both axial and equatorial C–C bonds make up the fusion in *cis-*decalin. This may seem a minor point, but the resulting conformational effects are quite dramatic. Most notable is that only *cis-*decalin is capable of chair-chair interconversion. For the same transformation to occur in *trans-*decalin would require that all equatorial C–C bonds at the ring fusion become axial. This is not possible because the short (two carbon) linkage between the resulting axial carbons is insufficient to bridge the distance between the atoms. Thus, each of the two rings in *trans-*decalin acts as a conformational "lock" on the others ability to ring flip. To convince yourself that this is true, build a model of *trans-*decalin and attempt a chair-chair interconversion. What happens? Does your model survive the attempted ring-flip intact?

An important consequence of this conformational inflexibility is that the *trans-*decalin ring system is exceptionally rigid. This is perhaps why nature employs the *trans-*decalin ring system at the core of many steroid hormones (e.g., cortisol, Figure 4.15). The *trans-*decalin ring in steroids provides a rigid scaffold upon which functional groups are precisely displayed to interact with their specific hormone receptors. Additional examples of conformational constraint in bioactive molecules are described in Box 4.3.

Box 4.3 Conformational constraint in opiate analgesics.

The example of naturally occurring and synthetic opiate analgesics provides a contrast in different approaches to achieving conformational constraint. The ring fusions and bridged-bicycles embedded in the structure of morphine (and its methyl ether, codeine) lend a highly rigid and spherical aspect to these structures. A *cis-*decalin core (shown in blue) is bridged by a three-atom linkage (in green) containing a basic amine. The molecule is further rigidified by fusions to aryl and tetrahydrofuran rings. The result is a T-shaped arrangement in which the aromatic ring lies perpendicular to the aliphatic core of the

molecule. This molecular architecture is mimicked by many synthetic analgesics, such as fentanyl, where conformational constraint is achieved by a very different approach. In fentanyl, the hindered secondary amide restricts free rotation of the aromatic and piperidine rings, forcing these groups into an orthogonal orientation that mimics the T-shaped conformation of morphine. Thus, the desired pharmacological outcome (analgesia resulting from agonism of opioid receptors) is accomplished by different means in the case of naturally occurring opiates like morphine and synthetic ones like fentanyl.

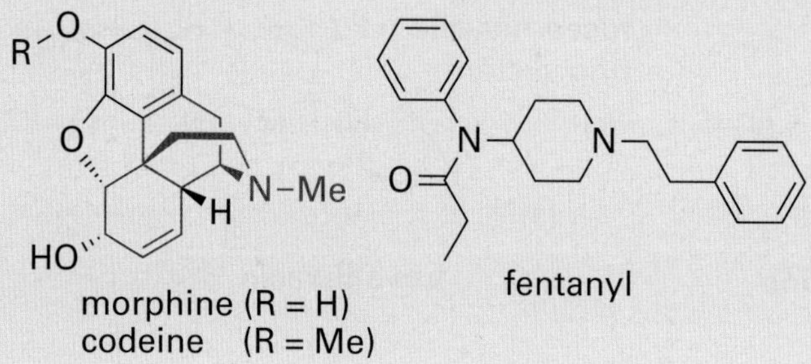

morphine (R = H)
codeine   (R = Me)

fentanyl

4.9 Summary

Section 4.1 Rotations about single bonds in molecules result in different interconverting shapes or **conformations**. Specific conformations (also called **conformers**) may be different in shape and energy but their interconversion does not involve breaking bonds, only rotations about bonds.

Section 4.2 **Newman projections** are a convenient way to visualize rotations about specific bonds and the different conformations that result. The angle formed between two specific bonds on adjacent atoms, as viewed in Newman projection, is called a **dihedral angle**.

Section 4.3 Rotation about the C–C bond in ethane produces two extreme conformations, **staggered** and **eclipsed**. Staggered conformations (60° dihedral) are preferred over eclipsed conformations (0° dihedral). **Torsional strain** refers to the excess energy required to adopt an eclipsed conformation.

Section 4.4 Larger acyclic molecules like *n*-butane have more complex potential energy diagrams than ethane due to the effects of **steric strain** combined with torsional strain. Steric strain results from unfavorable through-space interactions between atoms.

Section 4.5 **Angle strain** is the excess energy resulting from the adoption of bond angles smaller or larger than the preferred values. Small rings of three to four atoms experience severe angle strain and torsional strain due to their necessarily flat or nearly flat conformations. Five-membered rings have much less angle strain and can alleviate torsional strain by forming puckered conformations.

Section 4.6 Cyclohexane and related six-membered heterocyclic rings exist in an especially stable conformation known as the **chair**, in which torsional strain and angle strain are both negligible. Other conformations available to these rings include the **boat** and **twist-boat** which are significantly higher in energy but are intermediates in the interconversion of chair conformations.

Section 4.7 The introduction of non-hydrogen substituents on six-membered ring atoms introduces steric strain that in turn impacts the conformational preferences of the ring system. Typically one chair form is preferred over the other and the low-energy conformer can be predicted using tables of conformational free energies for axial substituents.

Section 4.8 The presence of ring fusions or bridged ring systems typically introduces constraints on the conformational flexibility of molecules. Free rotation about single bonds can be constrained by the introduction of bulky substituents proximal to the bond undergoing rotation.

4.10 Case Study—Neuraminidase Inhibitors and the Influenza Virus

The influenza pandemic of 1918 caused the deaths of many tens of millions of people worldwide. Later pandemics in 1957 and 1968 were only somewhat less catastrophic, causing around a million deaths. In more recent years, the emergence of the influenza variant H5N1 ("bird flu") has highlighted the potential for future pandemics, and the need for effective therapeutics to treat influenza. The influenza virus is composed of a protein "envelope" surrounding a payload of viral RNA that encodes for around a dozen viral proteins. One of these proteins is the pH-activated proton channel M2 that we discussed earlier (Chapter 2, Box 2.1) and is inhibited by the anti-influenza drug amantadine. Amantadine and a close analog were the only options for treating flu prior to the approval in the late 1990s of the neuraminidase inhibitor oseltamivir (Tamiflu®), the topic of this case study (Figure 4.16).

Hemagglutinin and neuraminidase comprise the main components of the viral envelope. Hemagglutinin is a glycoprotein that recognizes sialic acid groups displayed on host cells, and thus plays an important role in viral infection. Neuraminidase is an enzyme that removes sialic acid from the surface of the host cell and virus particle, thus facilitating egress of newly formed viral particles. Enzymatically speaking, neuraminidase is a glycoside hydrolase—an enzyme that cleaves the glycosidic C–O bonds between sialic acid and other sugars in glycoproteins. Neuraminidase inhibitors such as oseltamivir and zanamivir were conceived as transition-state analogs—structural mimics of the transition-state intermediate formed during glycan hydrolysis in the active site of neuraminidase.

The glycolysis reaction performed by neuraminidase involves breaking the glycosidic C–OR bond and forming a new C–OH bond (Figure 4.17). The reaction proceeds through a carbocation intermediate in which the positive charge is stabilized by the neighboring oxygen atom. This intermediate has significant double bond character, resulting in partial flattening of the six-membered ring, as shown. Neuraminidase accelerates the glycolysis reaction by binding to the flattened transition-state intermediate with greater affinity than either the substrate or product (both of which have chair-like conformations). For example, binding will be tighter when the carboxylate side chain lies in the same plane as the six-membered ring (as in the transition-state intermediate) and weaker when it is in an axial position (as in substrate and product). This is why in the drugs oseltamivir and zanamivir the carboxylate side chain is made to project from an sp^2-hybridized carbon atom and thus lie in the plane of the ring. These drugs are designed to conformationally mimic the transition-state intermediate. Unlike the transition-state intermediate however, the drug molecules cannot undergo further reaction, and instead remain tightly bound within the active site, inhibiting the enzyme.

Comparing the structures of oseltamivir and zanamivir to sialic acid reveals some additional changes made by the medicinal chemists who developed these compounds. Both oseltamivir and zanamivir retain the carboxylate and N-acetyl (–NHAc) side chains of sialic acid, which were found to be optimal substituents at their respective positions. The hydroxyl substituent of sialic acid however was

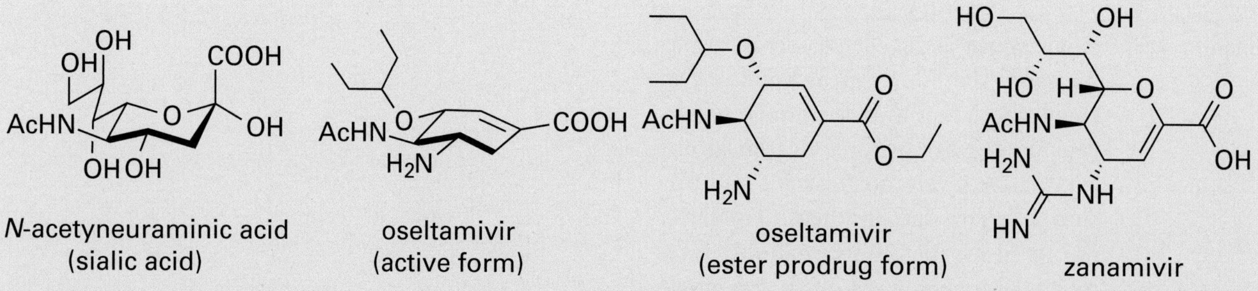

N-acetyneuraminic acid (sialic acid)

oseltamivir (active form)

oseltamivir (ester prodrug form)

zanamivir

Figure 4.16 Chemical structures of sialic acid, the neuraminidase inhibitors oseltamivir (in active and prodrug forms), and zanamivir. The active form of oseltamivir is shown in its chair-like conformation.

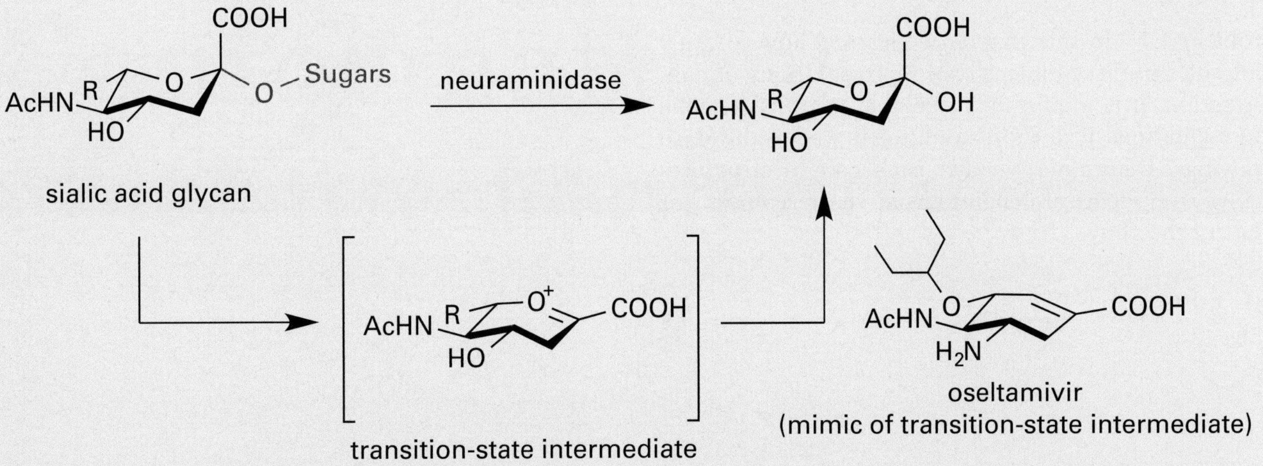

Figure 4.17 Partial structure of a sialic acid glycan with the glycosidic bond shown in blue. Neuraminidase accelerates glycosidic bond cleavage by binding to the transition-state intermediate with higher affinity than to the glycan substrate or glycolysis product. Drugs like oseltamivir were designed to mimic the transition-state intermediate and thereby inhibit the enzyme.

replaced with a primary amine or guanidine function in oseltamivir and zanamivir, respectively. These basic groups afford a stronger interaction with neuraminidase; the X-ray crystal structure of oseltamivir bound to neuraminidase reveals an ionic/hydrogen bonding interaction between the amine function and Glu119 and Asp151. A notable difference between the two drug structures is that zanamivir retains the glycerol (trihydroxypropyl) side chain of sialic acid whereas oseltamivir bears a much more hydrophobic 3-pentyloxy group at the same position. Interestingly, the pentyloxy group appears to interact with the hydrophobic π face of an Asp-Arg hydrogen bonding pair in neuraminidase. Recall that Asp-Arg pairs are known to stack on the hydrophobic face of Tyr and Phe side chains in protein structures (Chapter 2, Figure 2.11). A similar motif is apparently behind the ability of neuraminidase to recognize both hydrophilic and hydrophobic side chains on sialic acid -inspired inhibitors.

4.11 Exercises

Problem 4.1 In this chapter we learned how to draw molecules in three-dimensional representations of conformation. It is important to be able to translate such representations into more traditional wedge-and-dash drawings. Determine whether each pair of structures below are identical, enantiomers, diastereomers, or none of the above.

(a)

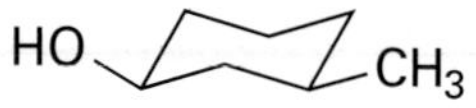

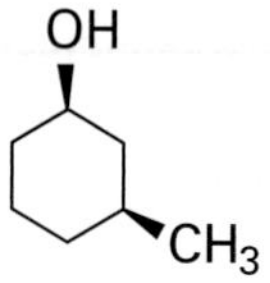

(b)

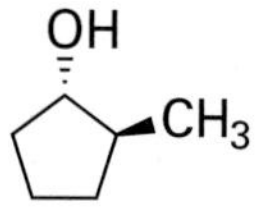

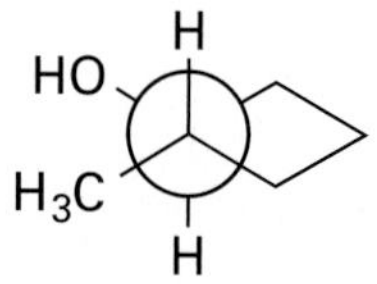

(c)

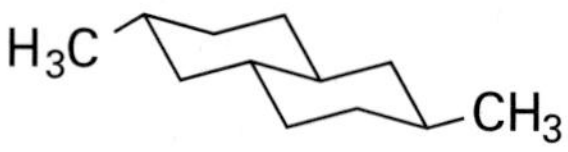

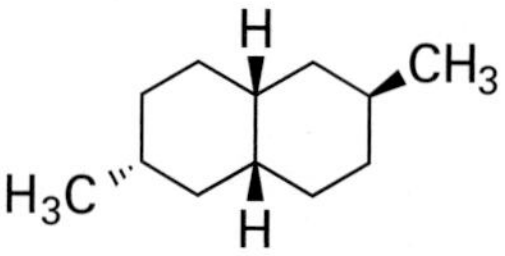

(d)

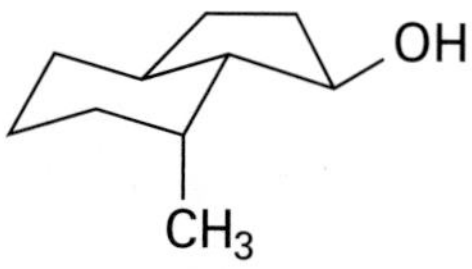

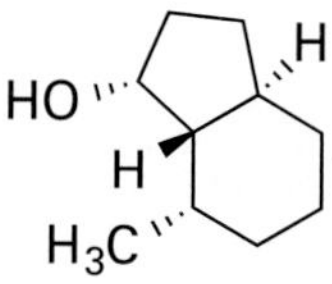

(e)

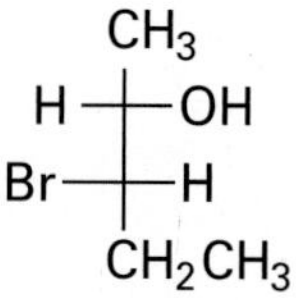

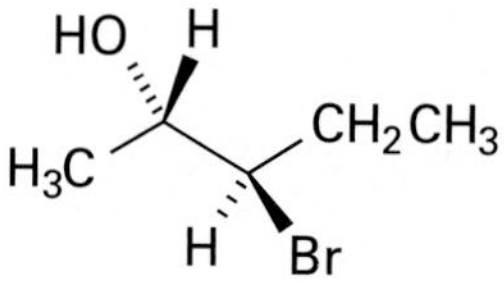

(f)

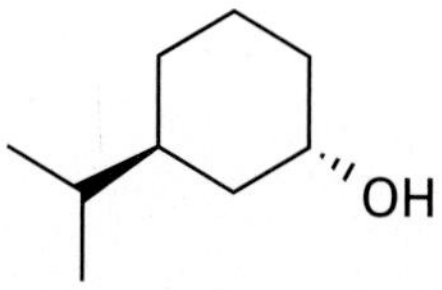

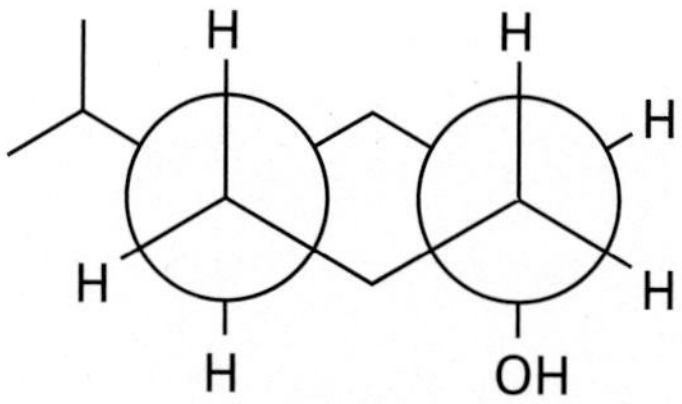

(g)

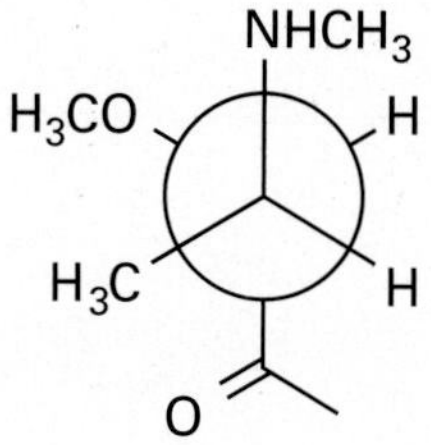

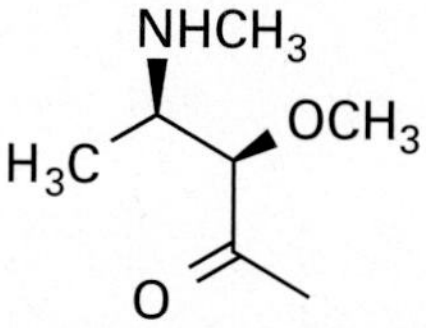

Problem 4.2   For each pair of conformers shown below, which do you predict would be lower in energy and why?

(a)

(b)

(c)

Problem 4.3   For each molecule below, draw the two possible chair conformations and estimate the difference in energy between the conformations using the $-\Delta G°$ values from Table 4.3.

(a)

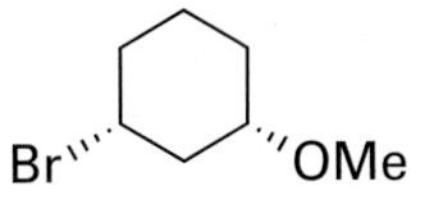

(b)

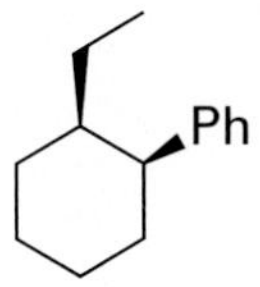

(c)

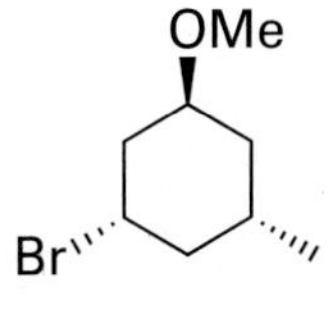

(d)

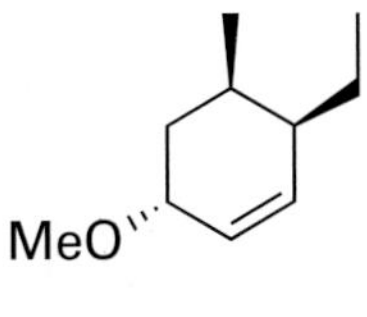

(e)

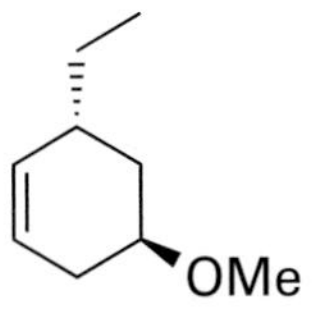

Chapter 5

Acid-Base Chemistry of Organic Molecules

Susan Miller

CHAPTER OUTLINE

5.1 Introduction

5.2 Three Theories of Acids and Bases

5.3 Self-Ionization of Water and the pH Scale

5.4 Avoiding Confusion—Use of "Acid" and "Base" and Related Terms

5.5 The Acid Dissociation Constant K_a and pK_a as a Measure of Acid Strength

5.6 Electronegativity and Size of Atoms and Acid/Base Strength

5.7 Atom Hybridization and Acid/Base Strength

5.8 Resonance Electronic Effects on Acid/Base Strength

5.9 Inductive Electronic Effects of Substituents on Acid/Base Strength

5.10 Combined Inductive and Resonance Effects on Acid/Base Strength

5.11 Proximity and Through-Space Effects on Acid/Base Strength

5.12 The Henderson–Hasselbalch Relationship and Acid/Base Equilibria as a Function of pH

5.13 Summary

5.14 *Case Study*—Discovery of Tagamet

5.15 Exercises

5.1 Introduction

While carbon (C) and hydrogen (H) form the foundation of organic molecules, the rich diversity and specificity of interactions between biological and drug molecules arises from the presence of heteroatoms (N, O, S, P, halides) when they combine with C and H to form various functional groups. One property of many heteroatom containing molecules is a certain acidity or basicity at physiological conditions that can contribute to the reactivity and physiochemical properties of the molecule. Although drug molecules are often designed to have little or no chemical reactivity as administered, once absorbed they are metabolized (i.e., undergo chemical conversions catalyzed by the enzymes of drug metabolism) to give products with new functional groups having enhanced reactivity, potentially leading to adverse side effects. In addition to influencing reactivity, acid/base properties and the charge state of a drug

molecule contribute significantly to its relative solubility in water (as found in the interior of cells and in bodily fluids) versus nonpolar media (as found in the lipid membranes of cells). This differential solubility impacts the absorption of the drug and hence the amount that needs to be administered to achieve the desired effect. In this chapter, we review the principal models of acid and base behavior and discuss the relationship of structure and bonding to the acidity of different types of "X–H" bonds (C–H, N–H, O–H, S–H) and the basicity of the lone pairs of electrons on the corresponding "X" atoms (:N, :O, :S).

5.2 Three Theories of Acids and Bases

In the late 1800s, Arrhenius proposed a theory of acids and bases based on observations of "what happens" when a substance is dissolved in pure water. The key observation was that some substances cause an increase in the hydrogen ion concentration, [H⁺], when dissolved in water and others cause an increase in the hydroxide concentration, [OH⁻]. On this basis, Arrhenius defined an acid as a compound that dissociates in water to give H⁺ and an anion (e.g., HCl → H⁺ + Cl⁻), and a base as a compound that dissociates in water to give a cation and OH⁻ (e.g., KOH → K⁺ + OH⁻). Although the noted changes in [H⁺] and [OH⁻] can be a useful description of acid/base behavior for certain systems, the model is limited in the scope of acids/bases and solvents (water only) that can be described.

A more general theory of acids and bases that focuses specifically on "who has the proton" was proposed separately in 1923 by Brønsted in Denmark and by Lowry in England. In this model, the proton never exists in solution as an isolated ion because it is energetically too unstable. Instead it is always covalently bonded to another atom, but can be transferred between lone pairs of electrons on two different atoms. In this *proton transfer* reaction, the proton donor is the Brønsted–Lowry acid and the proton acceptor, that is, the atom (or atom within a molecule) that takes the proton from the acid, is the Brønsted–Lowry base (Figure 5.1). The Brønsted–Lowry model of acids and bases is the foundation for our discussions in this chapter.

In a typical Brønsted–Lowry acid-base reaction (Figure 5.1) the initial acid (HA) is converted to its **conjugate base** (:A⁻), and the initial base (B:) is concomitantly converted to its **conjugate acid** (BH⁺). Significantly, this approach to acid/base chemistry focuses attention on the molecular structures of the two bases that transfer H⁺ between them (B: and :A⁻ in Figure 5.1) allowing a direct comparison of the relationship of structure to basicity. Furthermore, since the acid and base forms of the same molecule (e.g., H–A and :A⁻) differ by only a single proton (H⁺), analysis of trends in acidity or basicity as a function of molecular structure provides significant insight into the relationship of structure to reactivity.

The Brønsted–Lowry definition is much broader in scope and works for different solvents, since H⁺ can be transferred between bases in any solvent. However, the behavior that Arrhenius observed for bases and acids in water is also consistent with the Brønsted–Lowry

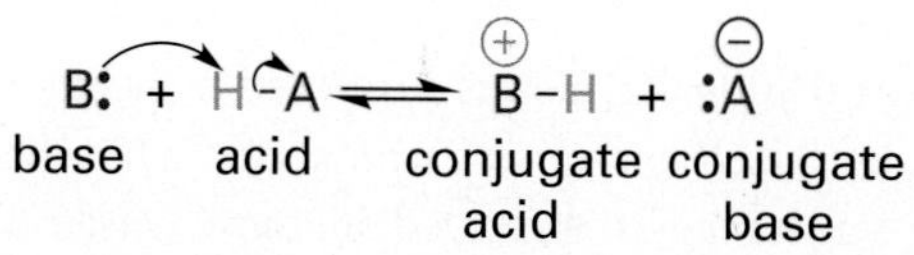

Figure 5.1 Proton transfer reaction between a Brønsted–Lowry acid and base.

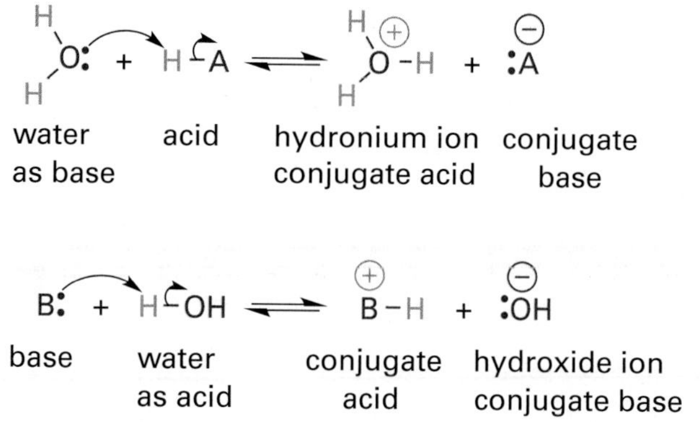

Figure 5.2 Reactions showing the relationship between the Brønsted–Lowry and Arrhenius definitions of acids and bases. Only those lone pair electrons involved in the acid-base reaction are shown explicitly.

definition, in the sense that water (H₂O) can act as either a base to accept a proton from another acid or as an acid to donate a proton to a base (Figure 5.2). Molecules like water that can act as both an acid and a base are called **amphoteric** molecules. Conceptually, the only difference between the models for the reaction of a neutral HA acid in water is that the proton is transferred to a water molecule to produce a hydronium ion rather than simply dissociating to H⁺. Note that only one of the two lone pairs on oxygen is shown in the acid-base reaction involving water (Figure 5.2). For simplicity's sake, we will generally show only the lone pair involved in the acid-base reaction in the schemes and tables of this chapter.

A completely separate notion of acids and bases was devised by G. N. Lewis in 1923 and formally proposed in 1938. Rather than focusing only on protons, Lewis' theory asks "who has the *electrons*?". Thus, a **Lewis acid** is an *electron acceptor* and a **Lewis base** is an *electron donor*. With this definition, any atom that has a positive charge, a partial positive charge, or an unfilled valence shell of electrons is considered a Lewis acid. Metal ions such as Zn²⁺, Ca²⁺, and Mg²⁺ are common positively charged Lewis acids of importance in biological systems. Carbons found in highly polar bonds such as in a carbonyl group (δ⁺ C=O δ⁻) are important Lewis acids involved in many important biological reactions. Since boron has only three valence shell electrons of its own, compounds like BF₃ are two electrons short of an octet, and thus are very strong Lewis acids (if not biologically relevant ones). Essentially any Brønsted base can also be considered a Lewis base since both utilize a lone pair of electrons to react with their corresponding acids (Figure 5.3).

Note that whereas a Brønsted acid gives up its proton to a different Brønsted base when they react, a Lewis

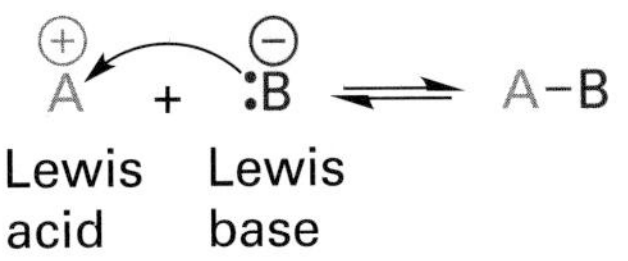

Lewis acid   Lewis base

Figure 5.3 Reaction illustrating Lewis theory definition of acids and bases.

acid combines (i.e., forms a bond) with a Lewis base when they react (Figure 5.3). The Lewis conception of acids and bases is very useful for discussions of chemical reactivity and we will return to it in Chapters 6 and 7.

5.3 Self-Ionization of Water and the pH Scale

The observation that pure water has low levels of H^+ and OH^- is easily understood by the Brønsted–Lowry theory. In this self-ionization behavior, one molecule of water acts as the proton donor (acid) and a second molecule acts as the proton acceptor (base) to generate hydroxide and a hydronium ion (H_3O^+).

$$H_2O: + H_2O \xrightleftharpoons{K_{eq}} H_3O^+ + :OH^- \quad K_{eq} = \frac{a_{H_3O^+} \cdot a_{:OH^-}}{a_{H_2O} \cdot a_{H_2O}}$$

As noted in the equation above, thermodynamic equilibrium constants (K_{eq}) are formally defined by the activities (a_i) of each species. However, for dilute solutions where the solvent is in vast excess, the activity of the solvent (water in this case) is unity ($a_{H_2O} = 1$) and the activities for the dilute ions are essentially equal to their molar concentrations ($a_{H_3O^+} \sim [H_3O^+]$, $a_{OH^-} \sim [:OH^-]$). As a result, the equilibrium dissociation constant for the self-ionization reaction of water (its acid dissociation constant) is simplified to

$$K_w = [H_3O^+][:OH^-]$$

At 25°C, $K_w = 10^{-14}$ M², and since the self-ionization reaction yields equal amounts of H_3O^+ and OH^-, both are present at 10^{-7} M in pure water. As other acids or bases are dissolved in and react with water, the concentrations of H_3O^+ and OH^- re-equilibrate such that their product always equals 10^{-14}. Thus when $[H_3O^+] = 1$ M, $[OH^-] = 10^{-14}$ M and vice versa. To simplify discussions of the relative acidity of aqueous solutions, we use the pH scale, where

$$pH = -\log_{10}[H_3O^+]$$

For pure water with $[H_3O^+] = 10^{-7}$ M, the pH = 7, which is also referred to as neutral pH because the

concentrations of H_3O^+ and OH^- ions are equal. Acidic solutions have higher concentrations of H_3O^+ ($[H_3O^+] > [OH^-]$) and pH values < 7, whereas basic solutions have lower concentrations of H_3O^+ ($[H_3O^+] < [OH^-]$) and pH values > 7.

5.4 Avoiding Confusion—Use of "Acid" and "Base" and Related Terms

In our descriptions of the three theories of acids and bases above, we found that the terms "acid" and "base" can mean several different things depending on the context in which they are used. An acid can be (1) a substance that increases the concentration of protons (hydronium ions), $[H_3O^+]$, when dissolved in pure water—Arrhenius acid; (2) a proton donor—Brønsted–Lowry acid; (3) an electron pair acceptor—Lewis acid. Conversely, a base can be (1) a substance that increases the concentration of hydroxide ions, $[OH^-]$, when dissolved in pure water—Arrhenius base; (2) a proton acceptor—Brønsted base; (3) an electron pair donor—Lewis base.

Two additional pairs of terms used in discussions of acids and bases, acidic/basic and acidity/basicity, may also bring confusion as they are used in more than one context. The most common contexts for each pair include:

The terms "acidic" and "basic" are typically used in four contexts. The first is to describe the property of a solution. Any solution where [acid] > [base] could be described as "acidic," and the converse situation where [base] > [acid] could be described as "basic." Aqueous solutions of pH lower than 7, where $[H_3O^+] > [OH^-]$, are acidic and those of pH higher than 7, where $[OH^-] > [H_3O^+]$, are basic. The second context is to describe the property of a compound. For example, any acid can also be called an acidic molecule or an acidic compound, and conversely, any base can also be called a basic molecule or a basic compound. The third context is to describe a property of a functional group. Functional groups that can act as a proton donor are acidic functional groups, while those that can act as a proton acceptor are basic functional groups. For example, the carboxylic acid group, which has the general formula RCOOH, is an acidic functional group, and an amine, which has the general formula R_3N: is a basic functional group. Finally, the fourth context is to describe the property of a specific X–H bond in a Brønsted–Lowry acid or a specific lone pair of electrons in a Brønsted–Lowry base. Using the same examples, the specific bond that is acidic in a carboxylic acid is the O–H bond and the specific pair of electrons that is basic in an amine is the N: lone pair.

The terms "acidity" and "basicity" are typically used in two contexts. The first is to describe how far the pH of an aqueous solution deviates from pH 7. The acidity of a solution varies from weak to strong as the pH decreases from 7 to 0, while the basicity of a solution varies from weak to strong as the pH increases from 7 to 14. The second context is to describe the relative strength of an acid or base, respectively. The more readily a Brønsted–Lowry acid gives up its proton, the greater is its acidity. The more attracted a Brønsted–Lowry base is to a proton, the stronger is its basicity.

5.5 The Acid Dissociation Constant K_a and pK_a as a Measure of Acid Strength

The relative strengths of acids are determined by comparisons of their acid dissociation constants. Although these have been measured in different solvents, the most commonly used and most relevant acid dissociation constants for discussing molecules in biological systems are those measured in water with concentrations expressed in units of moles per liter (M).

$$H_2O: + HA \underset{}{\overset{K_a}{\rightleftharpoons}} H_3O^+ + :A^- \quad K_a = \frac{[H_3O^+][:A^-]}{[HA]}$$

Although water is a reactant (Brønsted base) in this equilibrium, its concentration does not appear in the equation for the acid dissociation constant (K_a) for the same reason noted above for the self-ionization of water. Since the acid and base forms of a molecule (e.g., H–A and :A$^-$) only differ by a single proton (H$^+$), any structural features that make H–A a stronger acid must also make its conjugate base :A$^-$ a weaker base. Thus, we can evaluate trends in the strengths of acids and bases by considering how structural features affect *either* the acidity of H–A or the basicity of :A$^-$. For this reason, and to simplify comparisons of various kinds of acids and bases, we typically evaluate the strength of uncharged bases B: by determining an acid dissociation constant (K_a) *for the conjugate acid* BH$^+$ as it transfers its proton to water (as illustrated in the following equation). In this way both the acidity of H–A acids and the

basicitiy of B: bases can be compared on the same scale (K_a or pK_a as defined below).

$$H_2O: + HB^+ \underset{}{\overset{K_a}{\rightleftharpoons}} H_3O^+ + :B \quad K_a = \frac{[H_3O^+][:B]}{[HB^+]}$$

Very strong acids such as HI, HBr, and H$_2$SO$_4$ dissociate almost completely when dissolved in water, so their K_a values are all $\gg$ 1 M. (These cannot actually be measured in water but can be determined relative to water using other solvents.) On the other hand, functional groups in organic molecules are typically weak or very weak acids and have K_a values ranging from 10^{-1} down to 10^{-50} M. To simplify discussions of this large range of values, acid dissociation constants are expressed as pK_a (also called acidity constants) where

$$pK_a = -\log K_a$$

This is analogous to the use of pH to express hydronium ion concentrations, as discussed already. Using this scale, acids with a p$K_a < 0$ are very strong acids and the acidity of X–H bonds decreases as the pK_a increases above 0. Very weak acids with conjugate bases stronger than hydroxide ion do not dissociate to any significant extent in water and have K_a values $< K_w = 10^{-14}$ (p$K_a > 14$). (These also cannot be measured in water but are estimated relative to water using other solvents.)

Tables 5.1 and 5.2 list structures of acid and conjugate base forms of the most common HA and BH$^+$ type functional groups found in biological and drug-like molecules along with their pK_a values. The structures shown in the table have only a single functional group to underline the relationship of the specific structural features in these molecules to their relative acidity (and basicity). The acidic proton is colored blue in each example and the structural features contributing to the basicity of the X: atom (and corresponding acidity of the X–H bond) are colored red and range from a single atom in some cases to the whole molecule in others. The tables are organized by descending pK_a (very weakly to very strongly acidic) from top to bottom. The trend in the strength of the corresponding conjugate base is of course in the opposite direction, from very strong bases at the top to very weak ones at the bottom. Thus, when comparing two functional groups, the one with a higher pK_a value is the weaker acid and has the stronger conjugate base. We will refer back to these tables in later sections as we discuss how structural features of molecules and their substituents affect acidity and basicity.

Table 5.1 Acidity Constants (pK_a) of Selected HA Type Acids: C–H, N–H, O–H, S–H, H–X.

Acid name	Acid structure	pK_a	Conjugate base
Methane	H_3C-H	55–60	$H_3\text{-}C\text{:}^{\ominus}$
Benzene	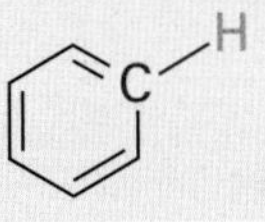	44	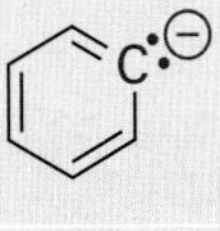
Ethylene		~44	
Methylamine	$H_3C\text{-}NH_2$	35–40	$H_3C\text{-}\overset{\ominus}{\ddot{N}}H$
Ethyne (acetylene)	$HC\equiv C-H$	~25	$HC\equiv C\text{:}^{\ominus}$
Aniline (Ar–NH_2)	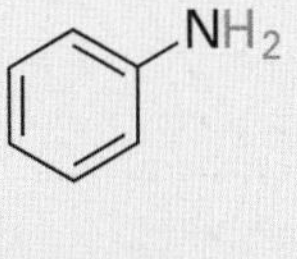	25	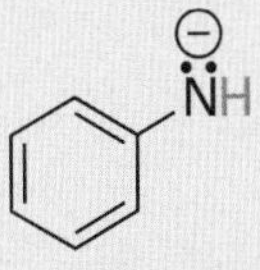
Ethyl acetate (ester α-C–H)	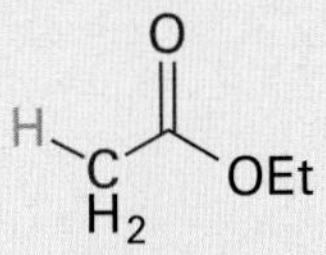	24–25	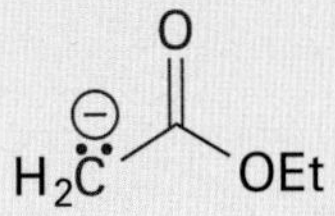
Acetamide (carboxamide)	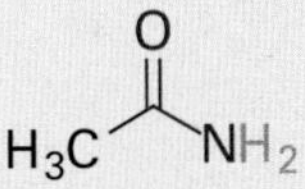	17–20	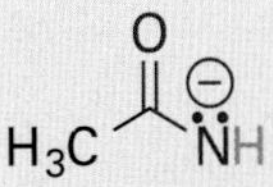
Methanol (alcohol)	H_3C-OH	15.2	$H_3C\text{-}O\text{:}^{\ominus}$ methoxide
Water	HOH	15.7	$H\ddot{O}^{\ominus}$ hydroxide
Sulfonamide	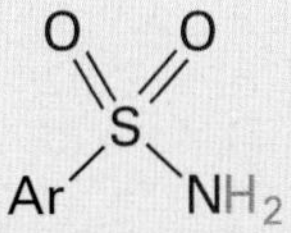	10–11	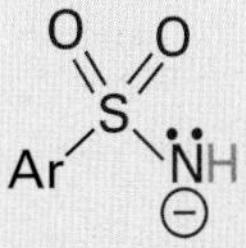
Phenol	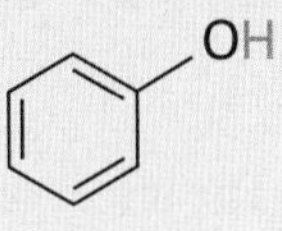	10	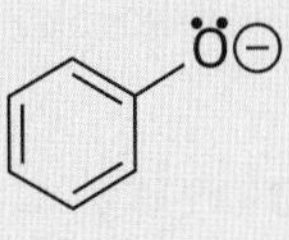 phenoxide or phenolate
Methanethiol	CH_3SH	~10	$CH_3\ddot{S}^{\ominus}$ thiolate
Diacetylimide	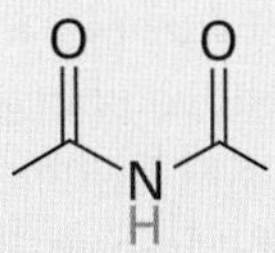	9–10	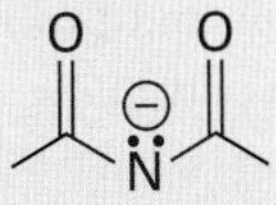

Table 5.1 Acidity Constants (pK_a) of Selected HA Type Acids: C–H, N–H, O–H, S–H, H–X. (*continued*)

Acid name	Acid structure	pK_a	Conjugate base
Pentane-2,4-dione (1,3-diketone)	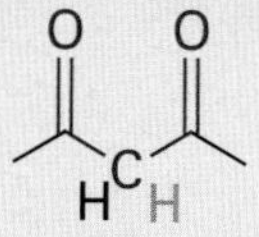	~9	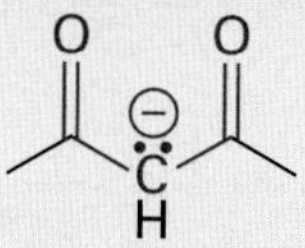
Hydrogen sulfide	H–SH	7.0	H–S:$^\ominus$
Thiophenol (Ar–SH) (aryl thiol)	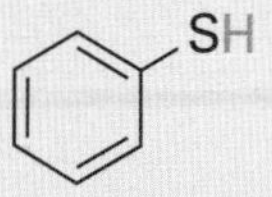	6.5	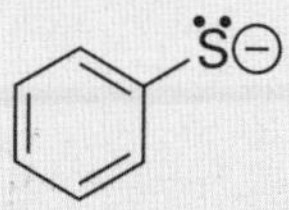 thiophenoxide or thiophenolate
Acetic acid (carboxylic acid)	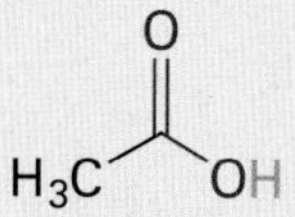	4.7	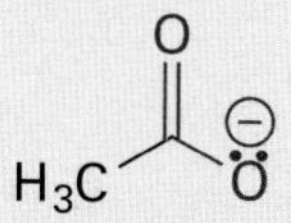 carboxylate
Hydrogen fluoride	H–F	3.1	:F$^\ominus$
Hydrogen sulfate ion	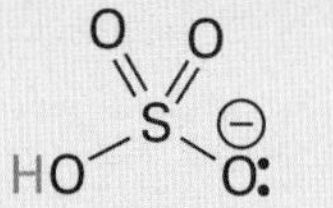	2.0	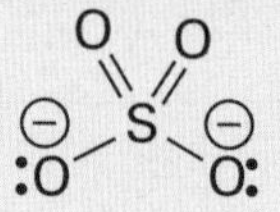
Methanesulfonic acid	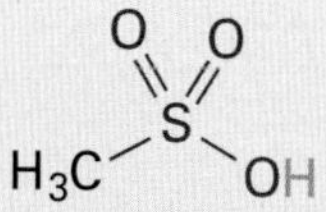	–2.6	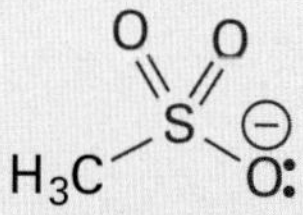 methanesulfonate ion
Hydrogen chloride	H–Cl	–3.9	:Cl$^\ominus$
Sulfuric acid	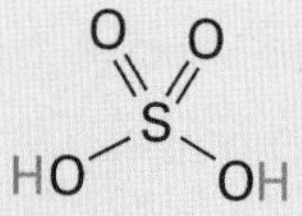	–4.8	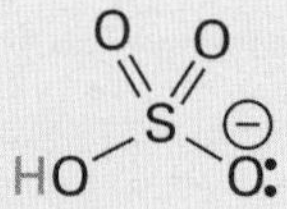
Hydrogen bromide	H–Br	–5.8	:Br$^\ominus$
Hydrogen iodide	H–I	–10.4	:I$^\ominus$

Only those lone pair electrons involved in the acid-base reaction are shown explicitly.

5.6 Electronegativity and Size of Atoms and Acid/Base Strength

Two intrinsic properties of atoms affect the strengths of X–H bonds independent of other structural features. The first of these is the *electronegativity* of X, which was introduced in Chapter 1 and can be compared for elements within the same period (i.e., row of the periodic table) that use the same valence shell electrons to form bonds (Table 5.3).

The effect of electronegativity on acidity can be seen in the acidities (pK_a values) of the simple compounds CH_4, NH_3, H_2O, and HF, based on elements from the second row of the periodic table (Figure 5.4).

As the electronegativity of the X: atom increases in this series, the polarity of the X–H bond increases so that the H carries a larger partial positive charge (δ^- X–H δ^+) and the equilibrium for proton transfer to water increases (the acid becomes stronger). Another way to look at this series is that as the X atom becomes more electronegative,

Table 5.2 Acidity Constants (pK_a) of Selected BH$^+$ Type Acids: +N–H, +O–H, +S–H.

Acid name	Acid structure	pK_a	Conjugate base
Guanidinium ion	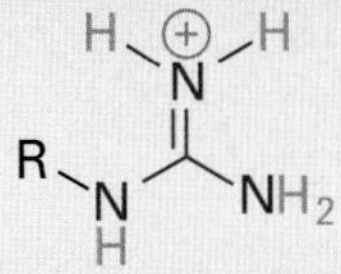	13.6	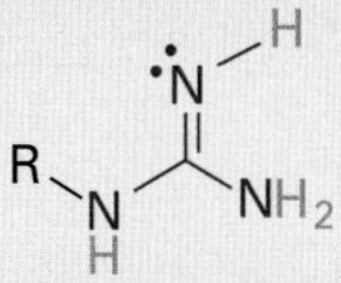 guanidine
Isopropyl ammonium ion	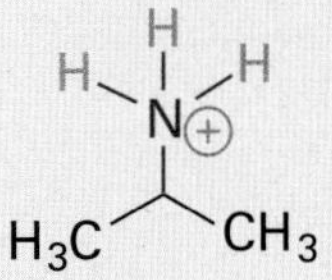	~11	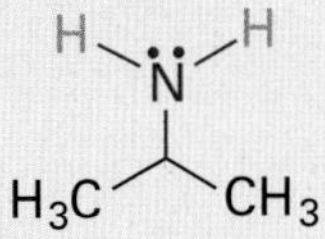
Methylammonium ion	$CH_3–\overset{+}{N}H_3$	10.6	$CH_3–\overset{..}{N}H_2$ methylamine
Isopropyl iminium ion	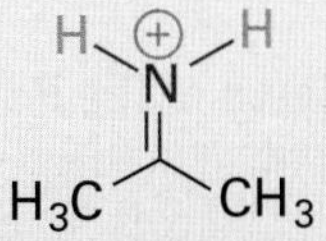	8–9	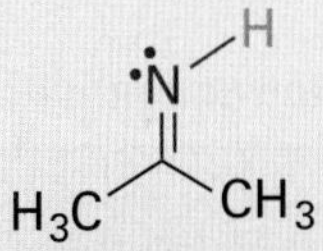 imine
Imidazolium ion	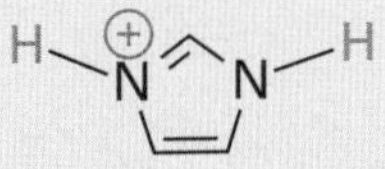	7	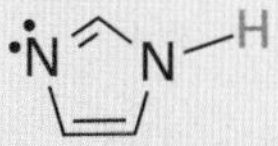 imidazole
Pyridinium ion	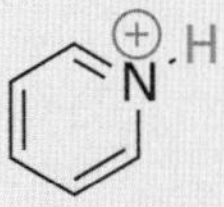	5.2	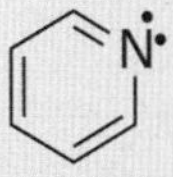 pyridine
Anilinium (Ar–NH$_3^+$) (aryl ammonium)	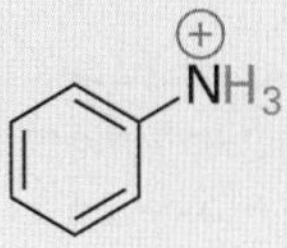	4.6	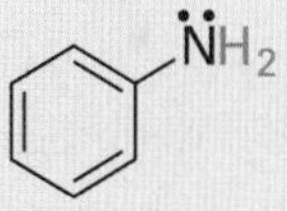
Protonated amide	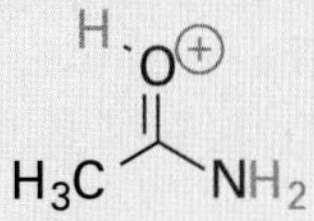	−1.4	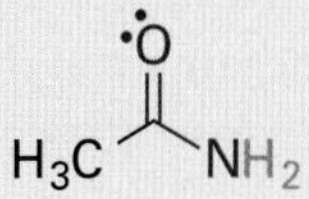
Hydronium	$H\overset{+}{O}H_2$	−1.74	$H\overset{..}{O}H$
Protonated methanol	$CH_3–\overset{+}{O}H_2$	−2	$CH_3–\overset{..}{O}H$
Protonated isopropyl alcohol	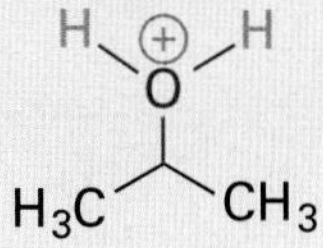	−3	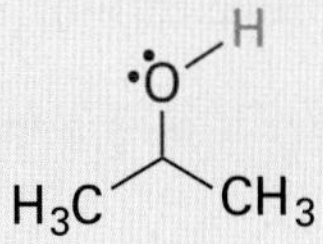
Dimethyloxonium ion	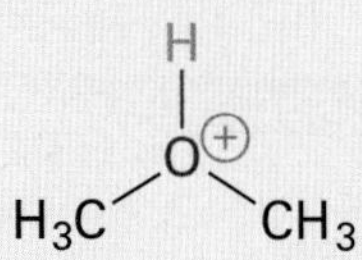	−4	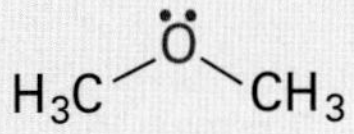 dimethylether

Table 5.2 Acidity Constants (pK_a) of Selected BH$^+$ Type Acids: +N–H, +O–H, +S–H. (*continued*)

Acid name	Acid structure	pK_a	Conjugate base
Protonated methyl acetate	(structure)	−6.5	(structure)
Protonated methanethiol	$CH_3–SH_2^{\oplus}$	−7	$CH_3–\ddot{S}H$
Protonated acetone	(structure)	−7.2	(structure)

Only those lone pair electrons involved in the acid-base reaction are shown explicitly.

Table 5.3 Electronegativities of Elements in the First Three Rows of the Periodic Table.

Period	Group number						
	1A	2A	3A	4A	5A	6A	7A
1	H 2.1						
2	Li 1.0	Be 1.5	B 2.0	C 2.5	N 3.0	O 3.5	F 4.0
3	Na 0.9	Mg 1.2	Al 1.5	Si 1.8	P 2.1	S 2.5	Cl 3.0

it can stabilize negative charge better and thus let go of a proton more easily. With regard to the conjugate base :X$^-$, we would say that the more electronegative the atom X, the weaker the base :X$^-$. So comparing across rows, increasing electronegativity of the X atom increases acidity of X–H and decreases basicity of :X$^-$.

The trend also holds for acids of the BH$^+$ type as seen in the following example where the more electronegative oxygen is much less basic than nitrogen in a similar context (Figure 5.5).

The negative pK_a value indicates that protonated methanol (CH$_3$OH$_2^+$) is quite a strong acid and

Figure 5.4 Example of effect of electronegativity on the acidity of X–H bonds in similar molecular contexts. (Reproduced, with permission, from Carey FA, Giuliano RM. *Organic Chemistry.* 9th ed. New York: McGraw-Hill Education; 2014.)

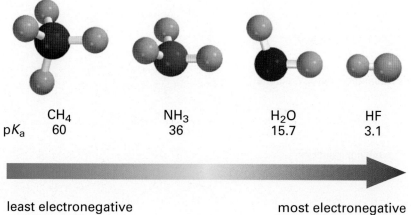

	CH$_4$	NH$_3$	H$_2$O	HF
pK_a	60	36	15.7	3.1

least electronegative
weakest acid

most electronegative
strongest acid

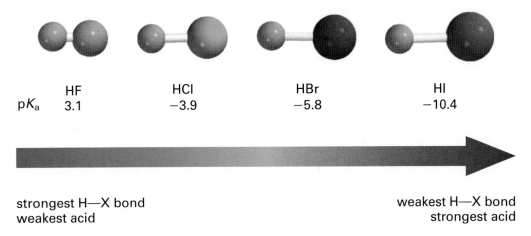

$$\overset{\oplus}{CH_3NH_3} \qquad \overset{\oplus}{CH_3OH_2}$$

$$pK_a = \quad 10.6 \qquad\qquad -2$$

Figure 5.5 Effects of electronegativity on the acidity of +X–H bonds in similar molecular contexts (elements in the same row of the periodic table).

$$\overset{\oplus}{CH_3OH_2} \qquad \overset{\oplus}{CH_3SH_2}$$

$$pK_a = \quad -2 \qquad\qquad -7$$

Figure 5.7 Example of the effects of atom size X on the acidity of +X–H bonds in similar molecular contexts (elements in the same column of the periodic table).

	HF	HCl	HBr	HI
pK_a	3.1	−3.9	−5.8	−10.4

strongest H—X bond
weakest acid

weakest H—X bond
strongest acid

Figure 5.6 Example of effect of the size of the X atom on the acidity of X–H bonds in similar molecular contexts.

therefore that *neutral* O: in methanol (CH₃OH) must be a very weak base. By contrast, the pK_a of methyl ammonium ion (CH₃NH₃⁺) indicates that it is a very weak acid and therefore that neutral N: in methylamine (CH₃NH₂) must be a reasonably strong base. Thus, the relative electronegativities of N and O correctly predict that neutral N: will be a better base than neutral O: and that CH₃OH₂⁺ is a stronger acid than CH₃NH₃⁺. Note however that such predictions will hold only when the atoms being compared are in the same *charge state*, as is the case in the comparisons shown in Figures 5.4 and 5.5.

The second intrinsic property of elements that influences the acidity of their X–H bonds is their size. Elements within the same group (i.e., column) in the periodic table have the same number of valence shell electrons, but increase in size as we move down the table. As the atomic size increases, the X–H bond becomes longer, which weakens the bond and increases its acidity (Figure 5.6).

From the point of view of the conjugate base :X⁻, the negative charge becomes increasingly spread out as the size (i.e., volume) of the X atom increases. In general, as the negative charge in the conjugate base becomes more spread out, it becomes better stabilized and thus basicity decreases. So comparing down columns, increasing size of the X atom increases acidity of X–H and decreases basicity of :X⁻. As illustrated below, this trend also holds for acids of the BH⁺ type (Figure 5.7).

5.7 Atom Hybridization and Acid/Base Strength

Acidic X–H bonds are always covalent single bonds (σ bonds) arising from overlap of an atomic orbital on the X atom and the 1s orbital of H. The most common X atoms in organic molecules will be C, N, or O atoms involved in single, double or triple bonds. As discussed in Chapter 1, the σ-bonding orbitals associated with individual C, N, and O atoms are frequently envisioned as hybrid orbitals with varying degrees of s and p character, depending on the type of hybridization (*sp*, *sp²*, or *sp³*). Experimentally, it is observed that as hybridization of the orbital involved in an X–H bond changes from $sp^3 \rightarrow sp^2 \rightarrow sp$, the X–H bond becomes more acidic. This effect is shown for a series of similar molecules with acidic N–H and O–H bonds in the table (Table 5.4).

The explanation for this trend is that as the hybridization of an atom changes from $sp^3 \rightarrow sp^2 \rightarrow sp$, the percentage of "s" character increases from 25% to 33% to 50%. Recall that s orbitals are spherical in shape such that the electrons surround and overlap with the positively charged nucleus. In contrast, p orbitals have a bilobed "dumbbell" shape with a node at the nucleus such that the electrons are distributed further away from the nucleus. Thus, with increasing s character of the bonding orbital on the X atom (C, N, O), electrons

Table 5.4 Effect of X Atom Hybridization on Acidities of C–H, N–H, and O–H Acids (R = Methyl).

		C–H	pK_a	N–H	pK_a	O–H	pK_a
weaker acids	sp^3	$H_3C-\overset{H}{\underset{H_2}{C}}$	~50	$R_2HC-\overset{\oplus}{\underset{H_2}{N}}^H$	10-11	$R_2HC-\overset{\oplus}{\underset{H}{O}}^H$	–2 to –3
	sp^2	$H_2C=\overset{H}{\underset{H}{C}}$	~44	$R_2C=\overset{\oplus}{\underset{H}{N}}^H$	~8	$R_2C=\overset{\oplus}{O}^H$	–7
stronger acids	sp	$HC\equiv C-H$	~25				

in the X–H σ bond interact more strongly with the positively charged nucleus of X and less so with the bound proton. This results in a weakening of the X–H bond strength and an increased acidity (lower pK_a).

5.8 Resonance Electronic Effects on Acid/Base Strength

In Chapter 1 we saw how resonance delocalization imparts partial double-bond character to amide bonds and affords special stabilization in aromatic ring systems like benzene. Not surprisingly, resonance delocalization of electrons plays a very important role in modulating the strengths of acids and bases as well. There are two major ways this can occur. The first is when lone pair electrons belonging to the basic X atom are delocalized and thus *withdrawn* into a larger π system (tending to make the X–H bond *more acidic* since :X⁻ is stabilized). The second case is when another atom *donates* electrons into a π system that involves the basic X atom (tending to make the X–H bond less acidic since :X⁻ is destabilized). We will see examples of both cases below, although the former scenario of electron withdrawal is more common than the latter.

As a first example of the effects of electron *withdrawal* through resonance delocalization, consider the trend in pK_a values for several O–H containing functional groups (Figure 5.8). Each of the O–H bonds is potentially

acidic, but the O atoms are attached in different molecular contexts allowing variable amounts of resonance electron delocalization and large differences in the relative acidities of the O–H bonds.

Moving from left to right in this series the acids become stronger and the conjugate bases become weaker (less basic) as the negative charge becomes more spread out. In the conjugate base of methanol (i.e., the methoxide anion, CH_3O^-), the negative charge remains localized on the O atom and hence the basicity is similar to the basicity observed in HO^- (pK_a for H_2O = 15.7).

Next in the series is phenol, the conjugate base of which is the phenoxide anion. The resonance hybrid structure of phenoxide (Figure 5.9) shows how the negative charge is distributed between the oxygen atom and the *para*- and *ortho*-carbon atoms by resonance delocalization. Since oxygen is more electronegative than carbon, the oxygen of phenoxide still carries the largest fraction of negative charge. However, the fractional charge on oxygen is much less in phenoxide as compared to methoxide and thus is less attractive to a proton (less basic). Comparing the pK_a values (and recalling that each ΔpK_a of 1 equals a 10-fold difference in relative basicity/acidity), the phenoxide anion is more than 100,000-fold less basic than the methoxide anion.

Next in our series is acetic acid (pK_a = 4.7), the conjugate base of which is the acetate anion (Figure 5.10). In acetate, the negative charge is delocalized onto two equally electronegative oxygen atoms, since the two

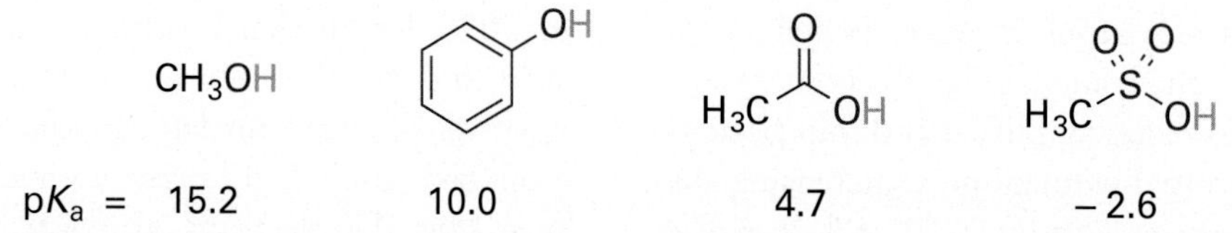

CH_3OH	phenol	$H_3C-\overset{O}{\overset{\|}{C}}-OH$	$H_3C-\overset{O\ \ O}{\underset{}{S}}-OH$
pK_a = 15.2	10.0	4.7	–2.6

Figure 5.8 Example of effect of increasing resonance delocalization in functional groups with the same type of acidic X–H bond. In this figure and those that follow, atoms directly involved in resonance delocalization are shown in red.

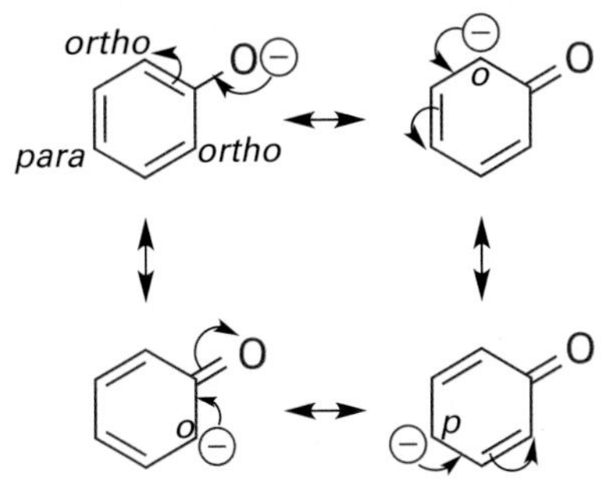

Figure 5.9 Resonance structures for phenoxide anion showing distribution of negative charge from O onto *ortho*- and *para*-carbon atoms of the phenyl ring.

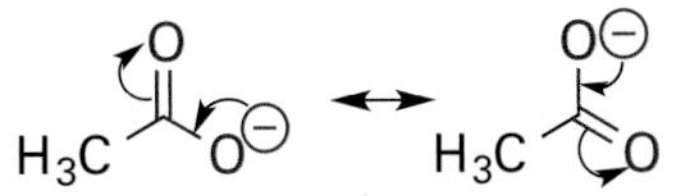

Figure 5.10 Resonance structures of acetate anion showing equal distribution of negative charge on the two oxygen atoms.

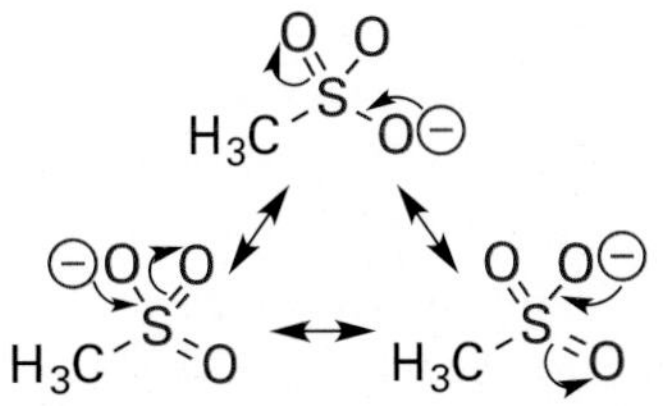

Figure 5.11 Resonance structures for methylsulfonate anion with the negative charge distributed equally among three oxygen atoms.

resonance structures are identical. Each oxygen atom carries only 50% of the negative charge, which further stabilizes the anion and weakens the attraction to a proton. Comparing pK_a values, this equal distribution of negative charge on two identical electronegative atoms makes the acetate anion more than 10 billion-fold less basic than methoxide anion and more than 100,000-fold less basic than phenoxide anion. This concept is extended further in the sulfonate anion (Figure 5.11) in

which the negative charge is distributed equally among three oxygen atoms. Partial charge on each oxygen atom is reduced to just ~33%, affording the least "proton-seeking" conjugate base in the series.

To summarize, delocalization of electrons such that the negative charge is spread out among many atoms lowers the fractional charge on the X atom, which lowers its basicity and increases the acidity of its conjugate acid (X–H). Likewise, delocalizing electrons onto more electronegative atoms like oxygen is more effective at lowering basicity than delocalization onto less electronegative atoms like carbon.

Consider now some similar trends in acids based on nitrogen, that is, N–H acids (Figure 5.12). Consistent with the difference in electronegativity between N and O, each of the N–H acids in Figure 5.12 is substantially weaker than the corresponding O–H acids in Figure 5.8. As with the oxygen acids, we see the same trend of increasing acidity of the N–H bond (and decreasing basicity of :N⁻) with increased resonance delocalization. Note, however, that the magnitude of change in acidity (and basicity) is significantly greater for the N–H acids. For example, we observe a much larger difference in acidity for aniline and methylamine (~13 pK_a units, or 10^{13}-fold) than we saw between phenol and methanol (5 pK_a units, or 10^5-fold). This difference between N and O bases can be understood in terms of electronegativity. Since N and C are closer in electronegativity than O and C (Table 5.3), the *ortho*- and *para*-carbon atoms in the aniline anion (PhNH⁻) share a larger proportion of the negative charge with N than the analogous carbon atoms in phenoxide share with O. Similarly, resonance delocalization in the acetamide anion results in >50% of the negative charge residing on the more electronegative O atom. This effect is greater than in the analogous case of acetate (Figure 5.10), where the charge is equally shared between the two oxygen atoms. Similar analyses can be extended to the other N–H acids in Figure 5.12 and for C–H type acids as well.

To summarize then, the stabilization of X⁻ anions by resonance delocalization leads to a weaker base and to more acidic X–H bonds. Moreover, these effects are

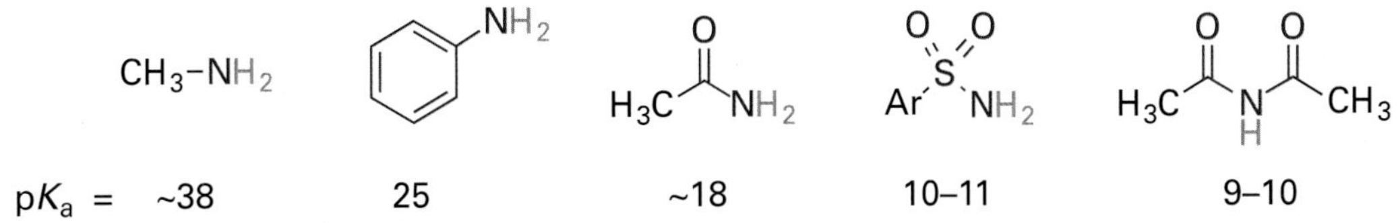

Figure 5.12 Comparison of acidities for neutral N–H acids shows same trend of increasing acidity with increasing electron delocalization, especially onto more electronegative atoms.

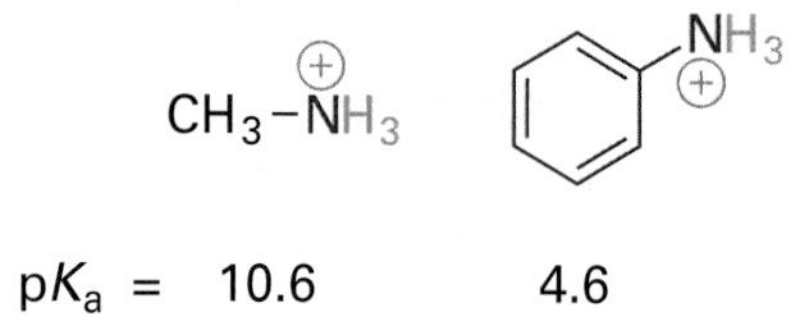

Figure 5.13 Example of increased acidity of +N–H acids with increasing resonance electron delocalization in the conjugate base.

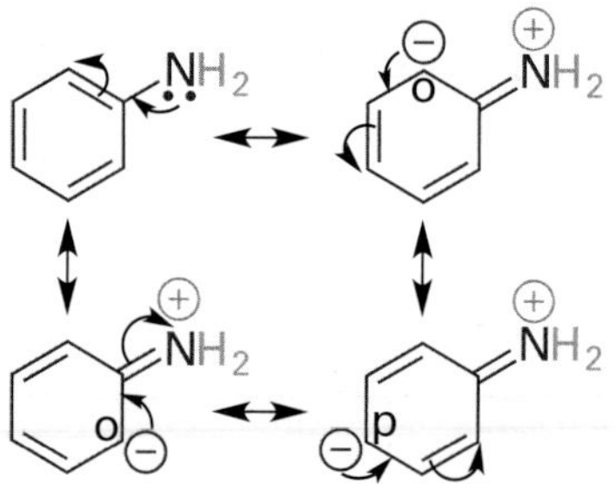

Figure 5.14 Resonance structures showing distribution of electron density among the N atom and the *ortho-* and *para*-carbon atoms of the phenyl ring.

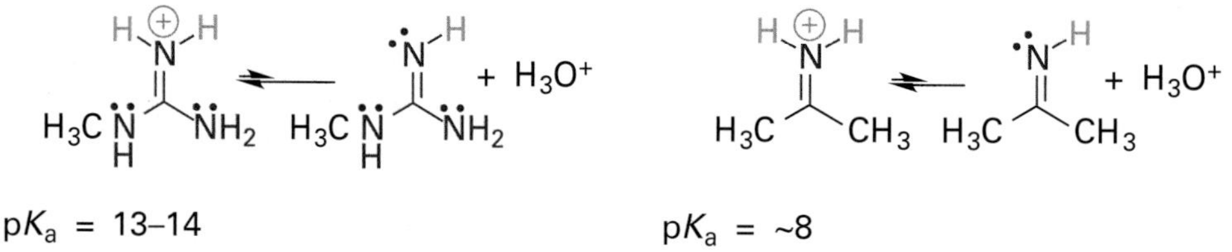

Figure 5.15 Acid-base reactions and pK_a values for the guanidinium ion (left) and an iminium ion (right).

stronger in cases where the charge can be shared by atoms of greater electronegativity than the X atom.

5.8.1 Resonance Delocalization in BH⁺ Type Acids

Now we will consider the effects of resonance delocalization of BH⁺ type acids and their neutral conjugate bases (B:). Comparing the pK_a values of two ammonium acids (R–NH$_3^+$) we see that the example where R = Ph is significantly more acidic than when R = Me (Figure 5.13). This suggests that the aromatic ring provides significant stabilization of the conjugate base, which in this case is the *neutral* molecule aniline. Inspection of a resonance hybrid of aniline shows how the lone pair electrons on nitrogen delocalize into the aromatic ring (Figure 5.14). With its electron density decreased, the N: atom in aniline is less basic than in methylamine and the

corresponding anilinium ion (C$_6$H$_5$NH$_3^+$) is more acidic than the methylammonium ion (CH$_3$NH$_3^+$).

In the examples above, we saw how delocalization of electrons from :X into a π system generally lowers the basicity of :X and makes the X–H bond more acidic. Now let's examine some cases where *resonance donation* of electrons into a π system raises the basicity of :X and reduces acidity of the X–H bond of interest.

To illustrate this effect we will first compare the acidities of the guanidinium and iminium ions, which are BH⁺ type acids (Figure 5.15). In both cases, the N–H σ bond of interest involves an sp^2 hybrid orbital on a nitrogen atom that is also involved in a C=N π bond. In the case of the iminium ion, the pK_a simply reflects the intrinsic basicity of sp^2-hybridized N. In the guanidinium ion, however, two N atoms are bound to carbon and each can contribute its lone pair electrons into the C=N π bond. The easiest way to see this is to examine a resonance hybrid structure of the guanidinium ion (Figure 5.16). As you can see, the effect of this resonance donation is to distribute the positive charge among all three nitrogen atoms. This greatly stabilizes the guanidinium ion, making it less prone to give up a proton and so much less acidic (pK_a = ~13–14) than the iminium ion. From the perspective of the conjugate bases, we might say that guanidine is a much stronger base than an imine because it can more readily stabilize the positive charge that comes with attaining a proton.

Another example of the same effect is apparent in a comparison of the relative acidities of the aromatic

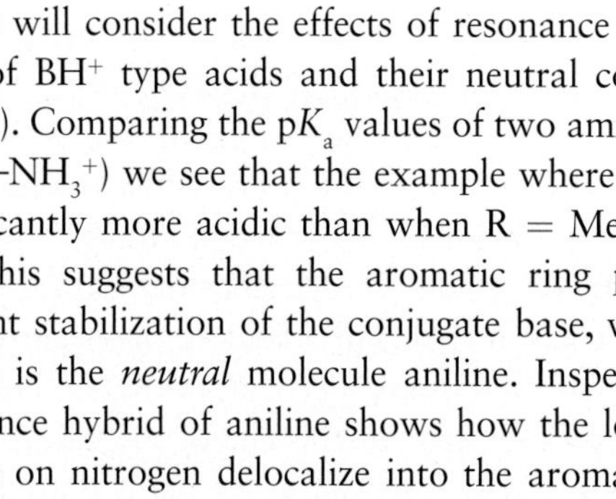

Figure 5.16 Resonance structures showing distribution of positive charge among all three N atoms of the guanidinium ion.

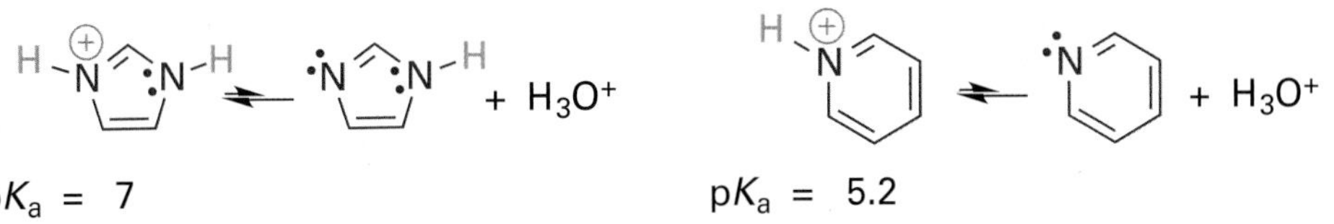

Figure 5.17 Acid-base reactions and pK_a values for the imidazolium ion (left) and the pyridinium ion (right).

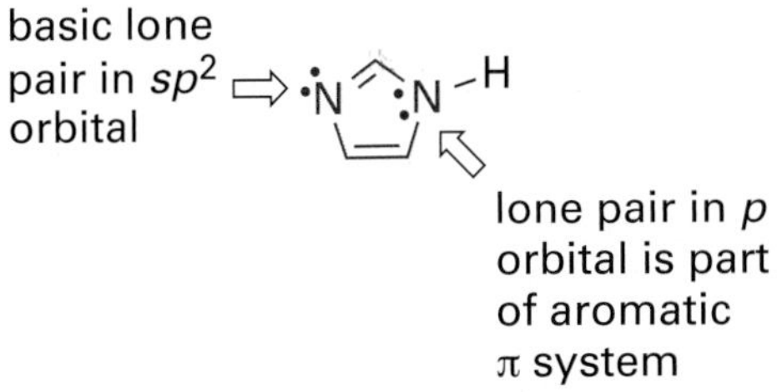

Figure 5.18 Lone pairs of electrons in different types of orbitals have different basicities. Lone pairs in sp^2-orbitals are basic and can be protonated. Lone pairs in *p*-orbitals that are part of an aromatic π system are not basic and do not become protonated.

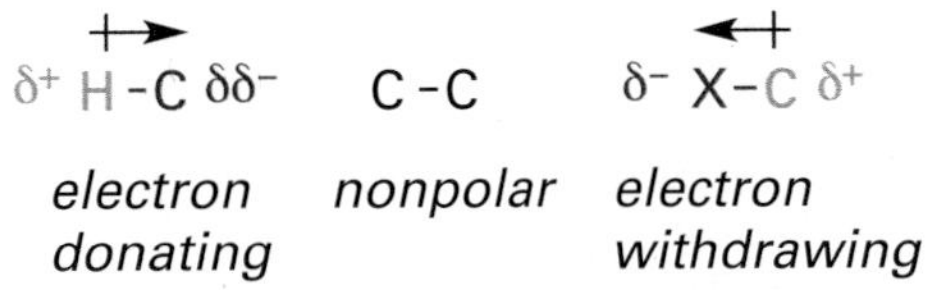

Figure 5.19 Polarized bonds between atoms with different electronegativities may be inductively electron donating or electron withdrawing. In electron donating substituents the negative end of the dipole points toward the acidic X–H group, whereas in electron withdrawing substituents the positive end of the dipole points toward the acidic X–H group.

imidazolium and pyridinium ions (Figure 5.17). Here again the acidic N–H bond involves an sp^2 hybrid orbital that lies in the plane of the ring. However, the *second nitrogen* atom in the imidazole ring does contribute its lone pair electrons into the π system, to satisfy Hückel's rule (Figure 5.18). This resonance donation makes imidazole more basic than pyridine. By the same token, pyridinium is a stronger acid because it cannot stabilize a positive charge in the way the imidazolium ion does—by sharing charge between its two nitrogen atoms. It might help to draw a resonance hybrid of the imidazolium ion to convince yourself of this!

5.9 Inductive Electronic Effects of Substituents on Acid/Base Strength

In the above sections we examined three factors that give rise to differences in relative acidities of X–H bonds within different functional groups. Most biological and drug molecules, however, have more than one functional group (substituents) and these may influence the electronic properties and acid/base properties of each other. The extent to which the properties are altered depends on the identity and placement of the substituents relative to one another, as well as on what types of bonds connect them. In this and the following two sections we examine the three main types of interactions between substituents: (1) inductive electronic effects, (2) combined resonance and inductive electronic effects, and (3) proximity effects.

As noted for resonance electronic effects, any structural feature that withdraws or pulls electron density away from a basic X atom decreases its basicity and increases the acidity of the corresponding X–H bond. Conversely, features that donate or push electron density toward a basic X atom increase its basicity and decrease the acidity of its corresponding X–H acid. While resonance effects result from direct delocalization of electron pairs into a conjugated π system, **inductive effects** result from *induced polarization* of σ *bonds* connecting the basic X atom of interest and a polarized substituent. The substituent is typically a functional group with a polarized bond, that is, a dipole moment. Inductive effects can be electron donating or electron withdrawing, depending on the direction of the dipole relative to the X–H bond (Figure 5.19).

Recall that the directionality and magnitude of the dipole in a polarized bond is determined by the relative electronegativities of the bonded atoms. Of the atoms found most often in organic molecules, only H is less electronegative than C, while all of the common heteroatoms (X = N, O, S, F, Cl, Br, I) are more electronegative than C (Table 5.3). Thus, H–C bonds are polarized with slight greater electron density on carbon and thus are *electron donating*. In contrast, the greater electronegativity of the X heteroatoms makes X–C bonds polarized in the opposite direction and *electron withdrawing*.

As an example of the effects of the donating versus withdrawing substituents, consider the relative acidities of the O–H bond in acetic acid as compared to formic acid or chloroacetic acid (Figure 5.20). Three electron

Figure 5.20 Structures and pK_a values for acetic acid as compared to either formic acid (left) or chloroacetic acid (right). Dipole moments are shown for specific substituents to illustrate inductive donating or withdrawing effects. In this figure and those that follow, the σ bonds connecting the basic O atom and the substituents being compared are shown as thick bonds.

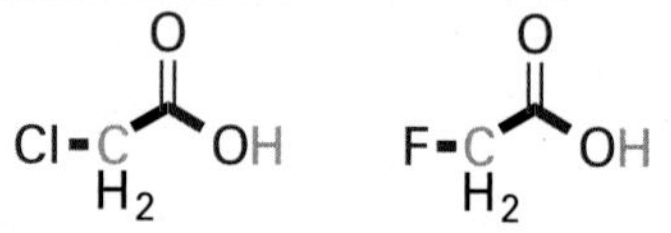

Figure 5.21 Structures and pK_a values for chloroacetic acid and fluoroacetic acid.

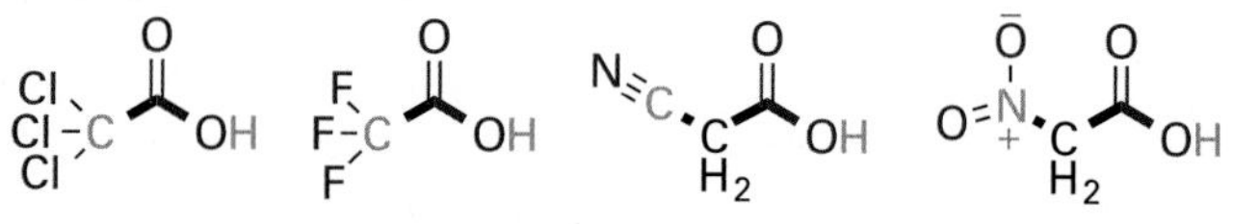

Figure 5.22 Examples of increased inductive electron withdrawing effect of substituents with multiple X–C bonds on the acidity of the O–H bond.

donating H–C bonds in the methyl group of acetic acid contribute electron density via σ bonds to the basic O, increasing its basicity and decreasing the acidity of the O–H bond in acetic acid (pK_a ~4.8) relative to that in formic acid (pK_a ~3.8). In contrast, replacement of methyl with chloromethyl reverses polarization of the substituent, which now pulls electron density away from the basic O, decreasing its basicity and increasing the acidity of the O–H bond in chloroacetic acid (pK_a ~2.8) relative to that in acetic acid (pK_a ~4.8).

Although alkyl groups are essentially the only electron donating substituents, there are a wide variety of electron withdrawing substituents of variable strength. To a first approximation, the polarization and consequent electron withdrawing effects will increase with increasing electronegativity of X in an X–C bond. Thus, the more electronegative atom fluorine is a stronger electron withdrawing substituent than chlorine, making fluoroacetic acid a stronger acid than chloroacetic acid (Figure 5.21).

Not surprisingly, the presence of multiple polarized X–C bonds, whether single (e.g., F_3C-, Cl_3C-), or double, or triple bonds (e.g., O=C–, N≡C–, O=N–), increases the polarization and consequent inductive withdrawing effect of a substituent (Figure 5.22). Note that the nitrile (N≡C–) and nitro groups (NO$_2$) in these examples exert their withdrawing effects via an inductive effect, since the basic O atom is not conjugated with the π bonds of these substituents.

Groups with double and triple bonds between C atoms (C=C or C≡C), although not polar themselves, are electron deficient and thus weakly pull electron density toward them through connecting σ bonds.

This effect is evident in the case of the phenyl substituent in benzoic acid, which reduces the pK_a slightly as compared to acetic acid. In contrast to the dramatic resonance effects observed in the cases of aniline and phenol, the effect in benzoic acid is more subtle and purely inductive since the aryl ring is connected to the basic O atom by two σ bonds rather than being conjugated with it (Figure 5.23).

In the remainder of this section we will examine how the *ionization state* (charge state) of functional groups can dramatically affect their inductive withdrawing or donating effects. This phenomenon is highly relevant for proteins, and especially enzyme active sites where a number of ionizable groups are usually found in close proximity. Here we will observe these effects in the context of small molecules with multiple ionizable groups.

First, we consider the carboxylic acid functional group (COOH) and its ionized (anionic) form, the carboxylate anion (COO⁻). To evaluate the inductive effect of COOH, we can compare the pK_a values of acetic acid with the dicarboxylic acids, succinic acid, and malonic acid (Figure 5.24). In the fully protonated diacids, the

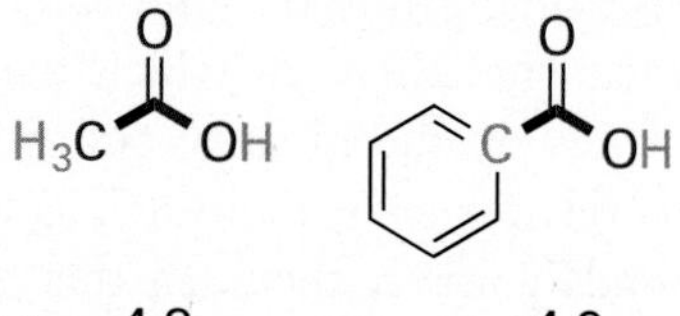

Figure 5.23 Structures and pK_a values for acetic acid and benzoic acid. The phenyl ring in the latter is weakly electron withdrawing by an inductive effect.

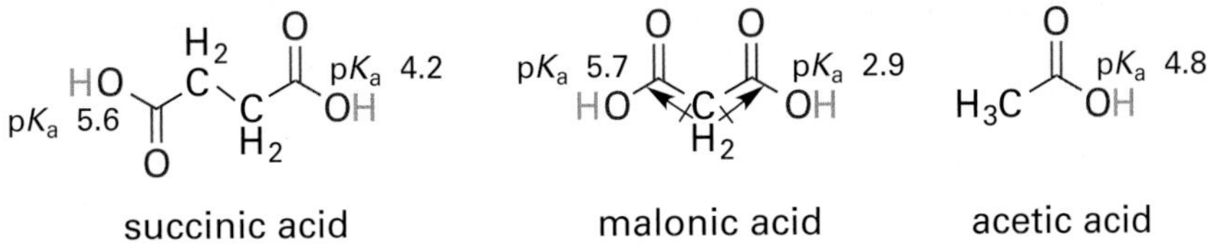

Figure 5.24 Comparison of the acidity of acetic acid with two related dicarboxylic acids. The uncharged COOH groups act as inductive electron withdrawing groups (dipole arrows shown on malonic acid), but the negatively charged COO⁻ group is inductively electron donating. The result of this is that the first pK_a of the diacids is lower than for acetic acid while the second pK_a is higher.

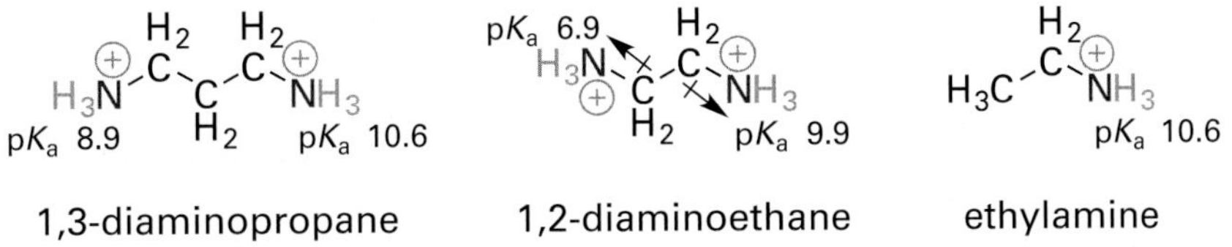

Figure 5.25 Comparison of acidities of diammonium ions relative to the mono-ammonium ion of ethylamine.

indistinguishable COOH groups are electron withdrawing, which we can see by noting that the *lowest* pK_a value for either of the diacids is lower (more acidic) than acetic acid. However, once a proton is lost from a diacid the negatively charged carboxylate anion COO⁻ exerts an *electron donating* effect on the remaining COOH group, decreasing its acidity substantially (higher second pK_a compared to acetic acid). Another thing to note is that the inductive withdrawing effect of COOH in the fully protonated diacids exhibits much stronger distance dependence than does the donating effect of the carboxylate anion COO⁻. This is in line with what we have learned about distance dependence in Chapter 2 for ion-dipole or ion-ion interactions (less distance dependence) as compared to directional dipole-dipole interactions (greater distance dependence). The inductive withdrawing effect of the COOH group is akin to a dipole-dipole interaction and thus stronger in malonic acid than in succinic acid. By contrast, the effect of the carboxylate anion in the second deprotonation step can be thought of as an unfavorable charge-charge interaction.

In contrast to the opposing effects of COOH and COO⁻, charged ammonium ions ($-NR_3^+$) and neutral amines ($-NR_2$) are both electron withdrawing, but the

charged forms are much more strongly withdrawing. These effects are apparent in comparing the acidities of two diammonium compounds with that of ethylammonium ion (Figure 5.25). The withdrawing effect of the ammonium group lowers the first pK_a for the diacids relative to ethylamine, an effect that can be viewed as a combination of a strong inductive withdrawing effect and a repulsive ionic interaction present only in the doubly charged forms (and which is relieved by deprotonation). After the first proton is lost, the resulting neutral amino group retains a weakly withdrawing effect as evidenced by the greater acidity of the second ammonium group in 1,2,-diaminoethane ($pK_a = 9.9$) as compared to ethylamine ($pK_a = 10.6$). In 1,3-diaminopropane, however, the inductive withdrawing effect is not significantly transmitted over the four σ bonds separating the amino groups, so the second pK_a value is only comparable to that of ethylamine.

The distance dependence of inductive electronic effects exemplified above with charged substituents can also be demonstrated by systematically moving a polarized bond further away from a basic atom X (Figure 5.26). In the mono-chlorobutanoic acids shown below, the inductive effect of the polarized C—Cl bond is strongest in chloroacetic acid ($pK_a = 2.8$) and

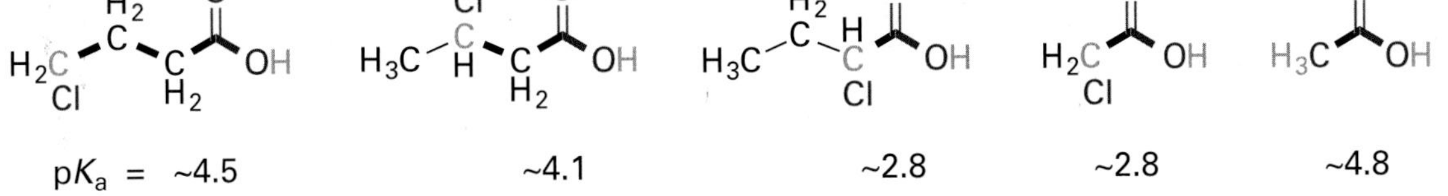

Figure 5.26 The distance dependence of inductive effects is illustrated with a series of carboxylic acids bearing a polarized C—Cl bond at various distances from the carboxylic acid. Acetic acid (far right) serves as a reference compound lacking the withdrawing substituent.

accordingly weaker as additional σ bonds are introduced between the withdrawing substituent and the basic O atom of the COOH function. Note that with just two σ bonds intervening, the withdrawing effect of the C–Cl bond is reduced significantly ($pK_a = 4.1$), and with three σ bonds intervening, the effect is nearly eliminated ($pK_a = 4.5$ vs. 4.8 for acetic acid).

5.10 Combined Inductive and Resonance Effects on Acid/Base Strength

When an acidic/basic functional group can interact with one or more substituents via a conjugated π system, a combination of inductive and resonance electron donating and withdrawing effects can occur. Resonance effects can arise from polarized substituents with π bonds such as C=O and S=O, which are resonance electron *withdrawing*, or from groups such as –NH₂, –OR, and halides with lone pairs of electrons, which are resonance electron *donating*. Thus, the inductive and resonance effects of substituents like C=O and S=O act in concert to withdraw electron density from the conjugated X–H group. For substituents with lone pairs of electrons, however, inductive and resonance effects will oppose one another so that the overall effect will depend on which individual effect (inductive withdrawing or resonance donating) is stronger. When a substituent of either type is not fully conjugated with the acidic X–H group or not conjugated with it at all, the resonance contribution is substantially diminished and the overall effect will be dominated by the inductive effect of the substituent. We will now examine several examples to help illustrate these contrasting behaviors.

The effect of the nitro (NO₂) group on the acidities of three different types of acidic functional groups is illustrated in Figure 5.27. The NO₂ group is a π-containing substituent that is electron withdrawing via both inductive and resonance effects. Compared to the unsubstituted acids in the figure, the molecules that bear a nitro group have pK_a values significantly lower. This indicates that the nitro-substituted analogs can better stabilize the deprotonated form of the acid (i.e., the conjugate base). Let us examine the source of this extra stabilization for the specific case of the *para-* and *meta*-substituted phenoxide anions.

If we draw resonance hybrids of these two phenoxide anions, we observe that the *para*-substituted phenoxide possesses a particularly attractive resonance form (Figure 5.28). This is one in which a positive charge is positioned immediately adjacent to the anionic oxygen. We might draw an additional resonance form in which a C=O bond is formed between the atoms in question. What the resonance hybrid tells us is that electrons from the anionic oxygen atom can be fully delocalized throughout the ring and into the π system of the *para*-NO₂ group as well, thus providing significant stabilization of the phenoxide anion. In contrast, the resonance hybrid for the *meta*-substituted analog does not allow for full delocalization of the negative charge on oxygen—one can "push electrons" from oxygen into the ring or from the ring onto the nitro group, but not both at the same time. The important thing to take away from this analysis is that the electron withdrawing effect of a *meta*-NO₂ group (and of *meta*-substituted π-type substituents in general) involves mainly inductive and not resonance effects. In contrast, substitution at the *para* (or *ortho*) position with such groups involves a stronger electron withdrawing effect resulting from a combination of inductive and resonance effects.

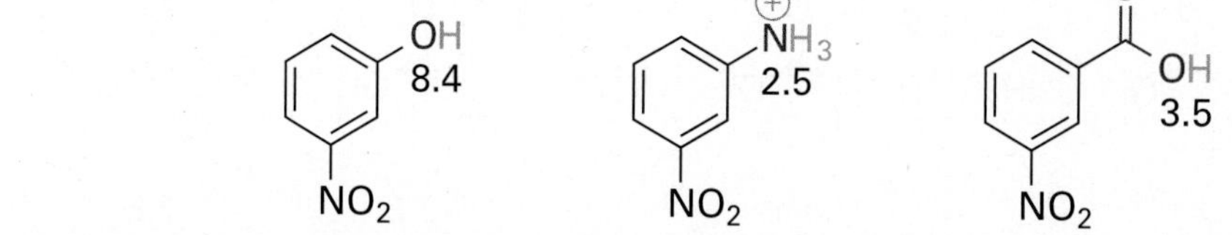

Figure 5.27 Illustration of the combined *inductive* and *resonance* effects of *para-* versus *meta*-nitro substitutions on the acidities of three different types of acidic groups—phenol, anilinium ion, and benzoic acids. The pK_as of the unsubstituted parent compounds (without a nitro group) are given at the top for reference.

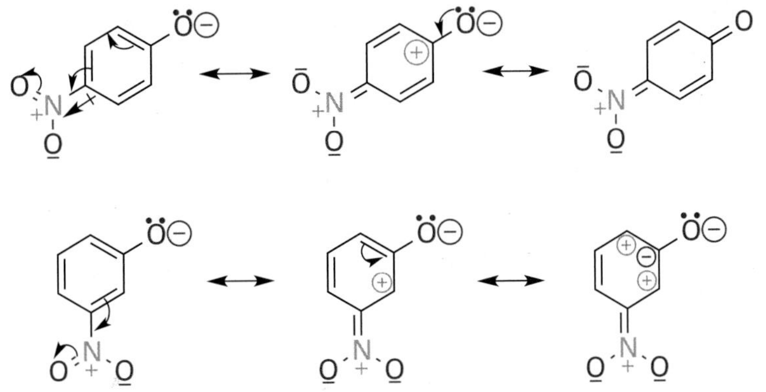

Figure 5.28 Comparison of key resonance structures for the *para*- and *meta*-nitro substituted phenoxide anions.

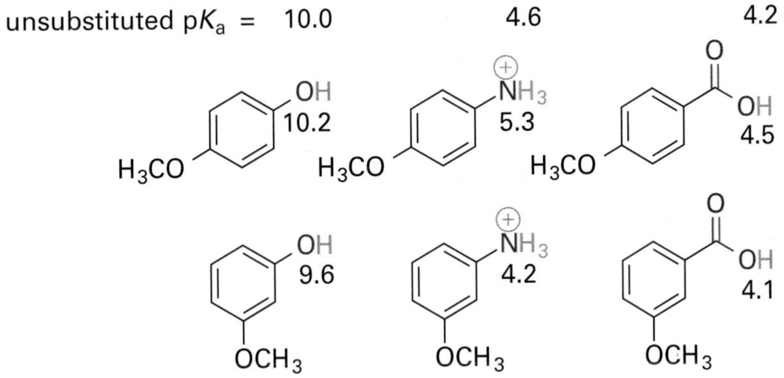

Figure 5.29 Comparison of the differences in the combined *inductive* and *resonance* effects of *para*- versus *meta*-methoxy substitutions on the acidities of three different types of acidic groups. The pK_as of the unsubstituted parent compounds are given at the top for reference.

Next, let us consider the case of *para*- or *meta*-substitution with a methoxy group (OCH$_3$) in an analogous series of acids (Figure 5.29). The methoxy group with its lone pair electrons is considered to exert a fairly strong resonance electron donating effect but also a fairly strong inductive electron withdrawing effect on account of the electronegativity of oxygen. In the examples at hand, the effect of *para*-methoxy substitution is electron donating (higher pK_a values compared to the unsubstituted systems), indicating that resonance electron donation overwhelms the inductive withdrawing effect for *para*-substitution. In contrast, the overall effects of methoxy in the *meta* position is electron withdrawing

(lower pK_a values compared to unsubstituted systems), indicating that resonance electron donation is either not effective at this position or is much smaller than the inductive electron withdrawing effect.

The above noted effect of the *para*-methoxy group on pK_a can be understood by examining key resonance structures for the corresponding conjugate bases (Figure 5.30). Resonance donation of a lone pair of electrons into the aromatic π system places a negative charge in proximity to other negatively charged or electron-rich atoms. The net contribution of these resonance forms then is to destabilize the conjugate bases slightly, leading to the observed increases in pK_a for the corresponding

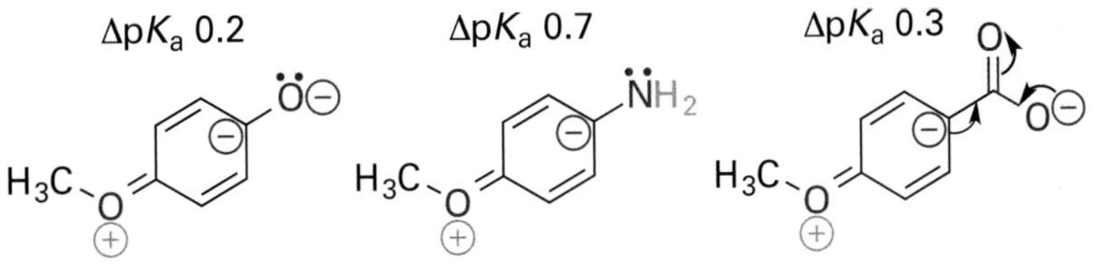

Figure 5.30 Comparison of key resonance structures for conjugate bases of three different *para*-OCH$_3$ acids. The ΔpK_a values refer to change in pK_a compared to unsubstituted parent compound ($\Delta pK_a = pK_{a\text{-subst}} - pK_{a\text{-parent}}$)

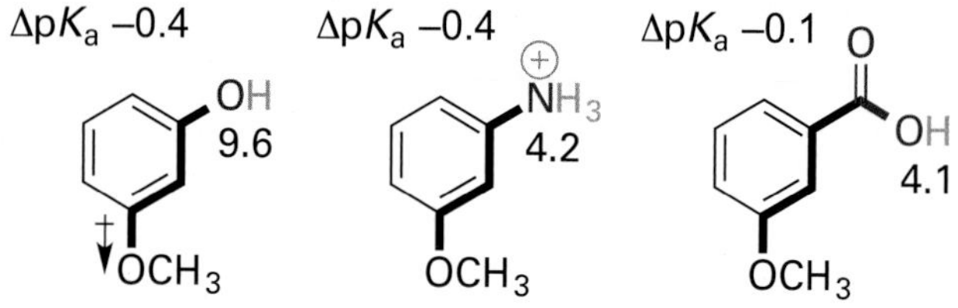

ΔpK_a −0.4 ΔpK_a −0.4 ΔpK_a −0.1

OH 9.6 NH_3^{+} 4.2   4.1

OCH₃   OCH₃   OCH₃

Figure 5.31 *Meta*-substituents primarily increase acidity through inductive electron withdrawal through σ bonds (bold bonds) and exhibit typical distance dependence.

acid forms. The effect of *meta*-methoxy substitution is primarily inductive withdrawal of electrons, and is distance dependent—thus larger for compounds with fewer σ bonds between the substituent and the acidic X–H bond (Figure 5.31).

The effects of other substituents bearing lone-pairs on electronegative atoms are demonstrated below in the context of phenolic and benzoic acids (Figure 5.32). The halogen atoms chlorine and fluorine are found to be slightly (for F) or moderately (for Cl) electron withdrawing at the *para* or *ortho* position, but most strongly withdrawing at the *meta* position. Why might this be so? The explanation is that these atoms exert a relatively modest resonance electron donating effect, less than the methoxy group but still significant. This resonance effect of the halogens is strongest at the *ortho* and *para* positions, for the same reason as it is in methoxy. Thus, the resonance effect partially offsets the dominant inductive withdrawing effect of the halogens when located at the *ortho* or *para* positions. At the *meta* position, resonance effects are minimal (as is generally the case) and so the strong inductive effect dominates.

Finally, comparison of the acidities for the *meta*- and *para*-aminobenzoic acids in Figure 5.32 shows that the intrinsically more basic N atom is overall electron

donating in both positions, but as expected, is much more strongly donating at the *para* position. This is due to the full conjugation of the amino group with the π system of the COO⁻ group, combined with a very weak inductive withdrawing effect. Amino groups are among the few substituents in which resonance electron donation dominates over inductive withdrawing effects, even at the *meta* position. Methyl groups are one of the few inductive electron *donating* groups, and since they have no resonance effect, a methyl (or other alkyl group) is electron donating at both the *para* and *meta* positions. This effect is similar to the amino group, albeit with a much smaller magnitude of electron donation.

To summarize, resonance electron withdrawal or donation is always strongest in the *para* and *ortho* positions because only in these positions can the substituent be fully conjugated with the acidic functional group. The four general categories of combined effects described in this section are as follows:

1. Substituents such as nitro with π bonds conjugated to aromatic rings, which are electron withdrawing by a combination of resonance and inductive effects. This effect is strongest at the *para* position.

2. Substituents such as the halides, which are strong inductive electron withdrawing groups at all positions, but are most withdrawing at the *meta* position. This is because of a weak and opposing electron donating resonance effect in the *para* or *ortho* position.

3. Other electronegative substituents such as OMe or OH are inductive electron withdrawing groups but have lone pairs of electrons that participate in resonance electron donation. These countering

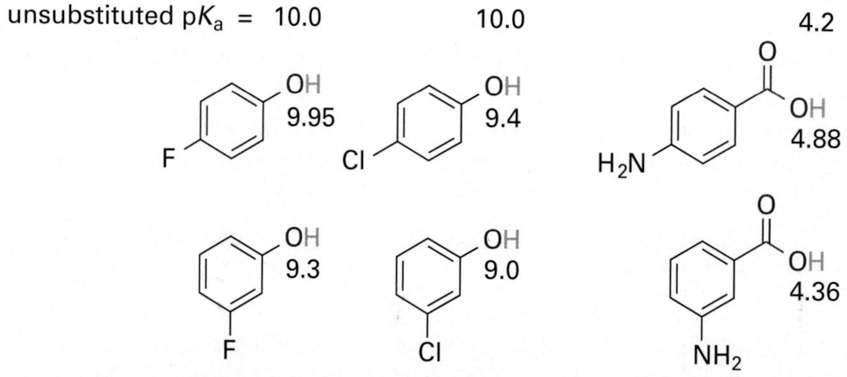

unsubstituted pK_a = 10.0   10.0   4.2

F — OH 9.95   Cl — OH 9.4 H_2N — COOH 4.88

F — OH 9.3   Cl — OH 9.0   COOH 4.36 / NH₂

Figure 5.32 Comparison of the combined *inductive* and *resonance* effects of *para*- and *meta*-halides and amino groups on the acidities of acidic groups. The pK_a values of the unsubstituted parent compounds are given at the top for reference and the pK_a values of the substituted analogs are given near each structure.

effects lead to an overall donating effect at the *para* and *ortho* positions, but an overall withdrawing effect at the *meta* position.

4. Less electronegative substituents like amino groups (:NR$_2$) have accordingly weaker inductive withdrawing properties and so act primarily as resonance electron donors. The effect is strongest at the *para* and *ortho* positions.

5.11 Proximity and Through-Space Effects on Acid/Base Strength

In addition to the through-bond electronic effects of substituents on acid/base strength discussed in Sections 5.8 through 5.10, substituents in close proximity to acidic groups can also alter the acid/base behavior via through-space hydrophobic effects or direct hydrogen bonding interactions.

This first example compares the effects of increasing the number of hydrophobic substituents in close proximity to neutral X–H versus charged BH$^+$ type acids (Figure 5.33).

In the first series, successive replacement of H atoms by –CH$_3$ groups leads to slight decreases in acidity of the uncharged alcohol O–H, as would be predicted for addition of more inductively electron donating methyl groups. In the second series, however, only the first replacement of H for ethyl (–C$_2$H$_5$) gives rise to a significant decrease in acidity for the positively charged +NH acid of the alkylammonium ion. The second replacement gives a further slight decrease in acidity, but the third replacement reverses the trend, indicating that another force is acting in opposition to the inductive donating effect of the alkyl groups.

If we imagine these molecules in aqueous solution we can better understand what is going on (Figure 5.34). As each hydrogen substituent is replaced by a hydrophobic ethyl group, stabilizing hydrogen bonds between water molecules and the charged BH$^+$ acid are lost. Thus, the change in the local environment of the +N–H acid from highly polar to more hydrophobic has the effect of destabilizing the charged acid form relative to the neutral N–H base. As a result of the opposing inductive and proximity effects, we find that primary, secondary and tertiary alkylammonium ions often have very similar pK$_a$ values in aqueous solution.

Similar effects are now recognized to operate with neutral O–H acids as well. As the microenvironment becomes more hydrophobic, the anionic conjugate base is disfavored relative to the neutral acid form. Thus, in the case of O–H acids, the local environment effect acts in concert with the inductive electron donation of

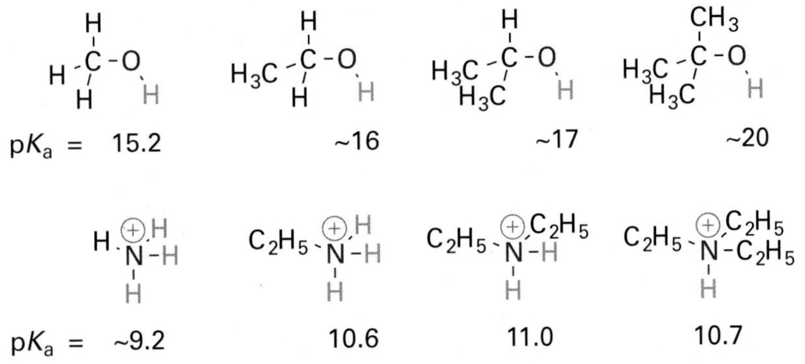

Figure 5.33 Comparison of the opposite effects of increasing numbers of hydrophobic substituents in close proximity to an uncharged X–H acid (top) versus a charged BH$^+$ acid (bottom).

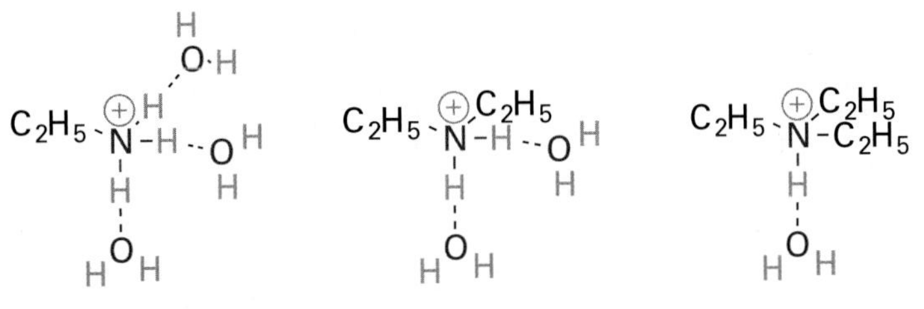

Figure 5.34 Increasing numbers of hydrophobic substituents decreases the number of stabilizing hydrogen bonds to water in the ionic BH$^+$ acid, which decreases the stability of the acid making it lose its proton more easily (increases its acidity).

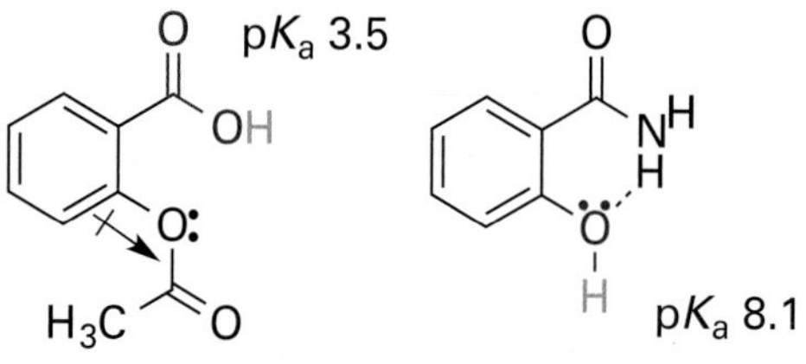

Figure 5.35 Arrow showing inductive electron withdrawing effect of the ester in acetylsalicylic acid (left) and combination of direct hydrogen bond and resonance electron withdrawing effects of the amide group in salicylamide (right).

the alkyl substituents, leading to significantly decreased acidity with each additional alkyl substituent.

Another common proximity effect occurs in molecules capable of forming intramolecular hydrogen bonds to an acidic functional group (Figure 5.35). In acetylsalicylic acid, the O-linked ester group provides a traditional inductive electron withdrawing effect that increases the acidity of the carboxylic acid function, lowering its pK_a to 3.5 (as compared to pK_a 4.2 for benzoic acid). In salicylamide, however, two factors are responsible for the significant reduction in pK_a to ~8.1 (from ~ 10 for phenol). First, the carbonyl (C=O) of the amide provides a modest resonance electron withdrawing effect. Second, the formation of a hydrogen bond (dashed line) between the amide N–H donor and the basic O: atom provides for stabilization of the conjugate base (phenoxide anion O$^-$).

Now consider the case of salicylic acid, where both an acidic phenol and carboxylic acid are present in close proximity (Figure 5.36). The overall effect is that the carboxylic acid O–H is a *stronger* acid than benzoic acid (pK_a = 3.0 vs. 4.2), while the phenolic O–H is a dramatically *weaker* acid as compared to phenol (pK_a 13.4 vs. 10). How can we understand these effects? Although the resonance donating effect of an *ortho* O–H would be expected to decrease the acidity of the COOH (contrary to what is observed), the O–H group is perfectly positioned to act as a hydrogen bond donor to the basic O of the carboxylic acid (Figure 5.36). This proximity effect is much more important than the resonance effect,

and reduces the basicity of the carboxylate anion (thus increasing COOH acidity). However, once the carboxylate anion has formed, the phenolic proton will be favorably hydrogen bonded to it. Moreover, to undergo a second deprotonation will involve the energetically unfavorable formation of two proximal negative charges. Overall, the combination of these forces raises the pK_a for the second deprotonation to pK_a = 13.4, making the phenolic O–H group in salicylic acid >1000-fold less acidic than the O–H group in phenol (pK_a = 10).

5.12 The Henderson–Hasselbalch Relationship and Acid/Base Equilibria as a Function of pH

As noted at the outset of this chapter, the charge states of acidic and basic groups can have important influences on the reactivities of drug molecules, on their aqueous versus lipid solubility, and on the specificity of the binding interactions with their target molecules. Thus, it is important to review the principles of acid/base equilibria that dictate how the charge state of the individual acidic and basic functional groups in a molecule, as well as of the whole molecule, change as a function of pH.

Starting with the definition of the equilibrium acid dissociation constants from Section 5.5:

$$H_2O: + HA \xrightleftharpoons{K_a} H_3O^+ + :A^- \qquad K_a = \frac{[H_3O^+][:A^-]}{[HA]}$$

Recall that when an acid or base is dissolved in a solution that is well buffered at a specific pH (i.e., $[H_3O^+]$ is constant), the relative concentrations of base $[A^-]$ and acid $[HA]$ (i.e., $[A^-]/[HA]$) is determined by the ratio of the equilibrium dissociation constant K_a to the constant $[H_3O^+]$.

Taking the negative log of the above equation for K_a gives the Henderson–Hasselbalch equation:

$$-\log K_a = -\log[H_3O^+] - \log \frac{[A^-]}{[HA]}$$

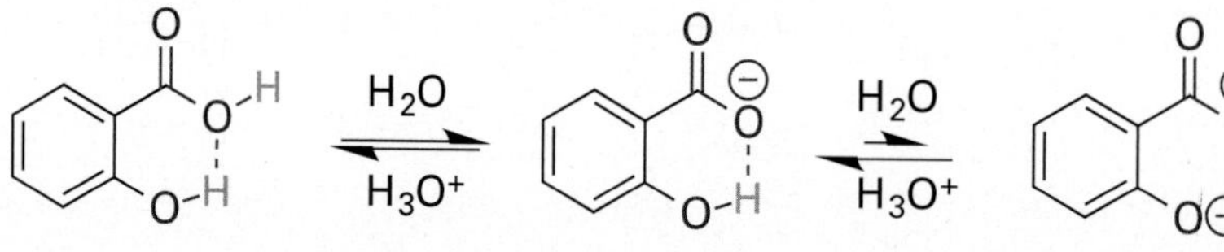

Figure 5.36 Successive loss of protons in salicyclic acid. Hydrogen bonding between phenolic O–H and O of COOH increases acidity of COOH, but decreases acidity of phenolic O–H in the monobasic anion (middle structure).

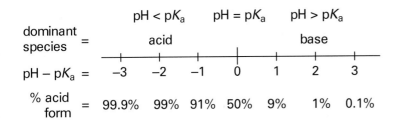

Figure 5.37 Relationship between fraction or percent of the acid (or base) forms of a functional group and the difference between the pH and pK_a.

Substituting $pK_a = -\log K_a$ and $pH = -\log [H_3O^+]$ gives the simpler relationship:

$$pK_a = pH - \log \frac{[A^-]}{[HA]}$$

Rearranging shows the amount of A^- relative to HA is simply determined by the difference between the pH and the pK_a:

$$pH - pK_a = \log \frac{[A^-]}{[HA]}$$

By definition, the pK_a for an acid is equal to the pH where $[HA] = [A^-]$, that is, the acid is 50% dissociated. At pH values below the pK_a, the acid is present at higher concentrations than its conjugate base ($[HA] > [A^-]$) and at pH values above the pK_a, the acid is present at lower concentrations than its conjugate base ($[HA] < [A^-]$). Figure 5.37 depicts this schematically.

From this relationship it is clear that for neutral H–A acidic groups, the uncharged HA state predominates at pH values below its pK_a while the charged anionic base A^- predominates at pH values above the pK_a.

The same equation can be derived from the equilibrium dissociation constant for BH^+ acids:

$$pH - pK_a = \log \frac{[B]}{[BH^+]}$$

where once again the acid form predominates at pH values below its pK_a while the base form predominates at pH values above the pK_a. Keep in mind that whereas H–A acids are charged (anionic) in the conjugate base form (A^-), BH^+ acids are charged (cationic) in the acid form and neutral in the conjugate base form (B:). The power of the Henderson–Hasselbalch equation is that it allows one to readily predict the charge state of drugs and specific functional groups at various pH values. The environment a drug might encounter ranges from quite acidic (e.g., the stomach, pH ~1–3) to mildly acidic (pH ~5 in the lysosome) to neutral (pH ~7.4 in the cytosol of a cell). Being able to predict the protonation/charge state of a drug in these various environments allows one to understand and make predictions about drug solubility, permeability, and interactions with their target molecules.

5.13 Summary

Section 5.1 Drug molecules often have one or more acidic and/or basic functional groups. The charge state of these groups varies with pH and affects a range of properties, including drug binding to its target, reactivity, and solubility.

Section 5.2 Three common theories have been used to describe the behavior of acids and bases. The Brønsted–Lowry theory defines an acid as a *proton donor* and a base as a *proton acceptor* in a *proton transfer reaction*. The Lewis theory defines an acid as an *electron pair acceptor* and a base as an *electron pair donor*.

Section 5.3 Water molecules are both weak Brønsted–Lowry acids and weak Brønsted–Lowry bases that react with each other with an equilibrium constant $K_w = [H_3O^+][OH^-] = 10^{-14}$. The relative acidity of aqueous solutions is measured using the pH scale where $pH = -\log [H_3O^+]$. In neutral water, $[H_3O^+] = [OH^-] = 10^{-7}$ M and pH = 7, in acidic solutions $[H_3O^+] > [OH^-]$ so pH < 7, and in basic solutions $[H_3O^+] < [OH^-]$ so pH > 7.

Section 5.4   Just as the terms "acid" and "base" can mean different things depending on which theory of acids and bases is being used, the terms "acidic" and "basic" and "acidity" and "basicity" can be used in different contexts. Acidic and basic are used to refer to the properties of solutions, properties of compounds, properties of functional groups, or properties of specific X–H bonds. Acidity and basicity typically refer either to how far the pH deviates from pH 7 or to the relative strength of an acid or base.

Section 5.5   Acid dissociation constants measured in water (K_a) for H–A acids and for the conjugate acids (BH$^+$) of bases are used to describe the relative strengths of acids and bases. As the range of values is very large (10^{-50}–10^{12}), acid dissociation constants are expressed as pK_a = –log K_a in analogy to the pH scale. Acids (X–H bonds) with pK_a < 0 are very strong and the acid strength decreases as pK_a increases above 0. Base strength changes in the opposite direction: strong acids have weak conjugate bases and weak acids have strong conjugate bases.

Section 5.6   The acidity of X–H bonds in the same molecular context is related to the intrinsic properties of the element X. For X atoms in the same row (period), the acidity increases as the electronegativity of X increases (C–H < N–H < O–H < F–H). For X atoms in the same column (group), the acidity increases with size (H–F < H–Cl < H–Br < H–I).

Section 5.7   The acidity of X–H bonds varies with the hybridization state of the X atom. As the "s" character increases, the acidity of X–H increases (sp^3 < sp^2 < sp).

Section 5.8   *Resonance electron withdrawal* or delocalization of electrons from a basic X atom into a conjugated π system *decreases the basicity* of X and *increases the acidity* of its corresponding X–H acid. Conversely, *resonance electron donation* of electrons from another basic X atom toward an sp^2 hybridized X atom of a +X–H acid *increases the basicity* of X and *decreases the acidity* of +X–H.

Section 5.9   *Inductive electronic effects* arise from induced dipoles in σ bonds connecting polarized substituents with acidic X–H bonds. Alkyl groups and negatively charged groups are *electron donating*, which *increases the basicity* of X and *decreases the acidity* of the corresponding X–H. Substituents with highly polar bonds to more electronegative atoms are *electron withdrawing*, which *decreases the basicity* of X and *increases the acidity* of its corresponding X–H acid. *Inductive effects* are highly distance dependent, that is, they become much weaker as the number of connecting σ bonds increases.

Section 5.10   Combined *inductive* and *resonance electronic effects* arise when substituents are conjugated with acidic functional groups via aromatic rings or other extended π systems. For substituents *meta* to the acidic group in aromatic rings, the *inductive* effects are dominant. For *para-* and *ortho*-substituents, the *resonance* effects are dominant. *Resonance electron donors* have lone pairs of electrons conjugated with the π system. *Resonance electron withdrawers* have polar π bonds (e.g., C=O or N=O) conjugated with the π system.

Section 5.11 The close proximity of hydrophobic substituents to acidic functional groups decreases the ability of water to solvate the ionic forms (anionic or cationic). Thus, hydrophobic substituents decrease the acidity of H–A acids and increase the acidity of BH⁺ acids. The close proximity of substituents that form hydrogen bonds with acidic groups can alter their acidity. Hydrogen bonds that stabilize the base increase the acidity, while hydrogen bonds that stabilize the acid decrease the acidity.

Section 5.12 The equilibrium between an acid and its conjugate base shifts as the pH of a solution changes by an amount defined by its acid dissociation constant (K_a). The concentrations of acid and base can be calculated using the Henderson–Hasselbalch equation: $pK_a = pH - \log([base]/[acid])$. In all cases, [acid] > [base] when pH < pK_a and [base] > [acid] when pH > pK_a. Thus, qualitatively the dominant form of an H–A acid is uncharged at pH < pK_a and becomes charged (anionic) at pH > pK_a. Conversely, the dominant form of a BH⁺ acid is charged (cationic) at pH < pK_a and becomes uncharged at pH > pK_a.

5.14 Case Study—Discovery of Tagamet

Gastric acid in the stomach (primarily hydrochloric acid) is essential to digest protein and emulsify fats. It breaks down food so it can go on to the small intestines where nutrients are absorbed. Insufficient levels of gastric acid can contribute to a myriad of discomforts and diseases. On the other hand, too much of a good thing can also be problematic. High levels of gastric acid can contribute to heartburn and ulcers. Nowadays, physicians have a fancy name for this condition: gastroesophageal reflux disease (GERD).

If GERD results from too much acid in the stomach, there would appear to be a simple solution—neutralize the acid with an orally administered base.

While this can work, it would require around 60 g of sodium bicarbonate ($NaHCO_3$) a day to treat patients with gastric ulceration! Meanwhile, calcium-based antacids like Tums or Rolaids can occasionally contribute to kidney stones while aluminum- or magnesium-based antacids like Mylanta and Maalox can sometimes be dangerous for people with kidney problems.

The emergence of histamine-2 receptor antagonists in the 1980s revolutionized the treatment of GERD. The first drug of this type, cimetidine (Tagamet), was so successful that it is now considered by many to be the first "blockbuster" drug. The

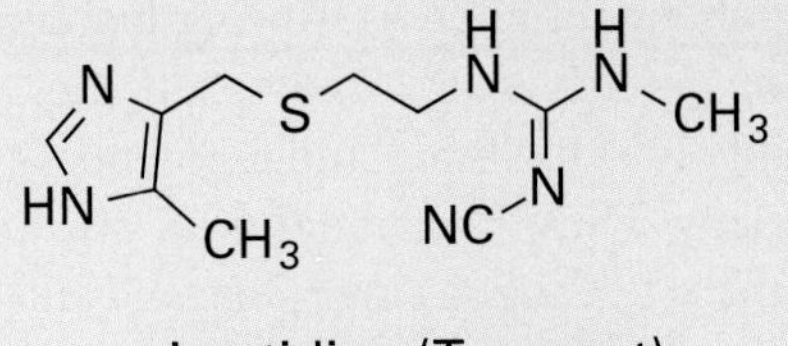

cimetidine (Tagamet)

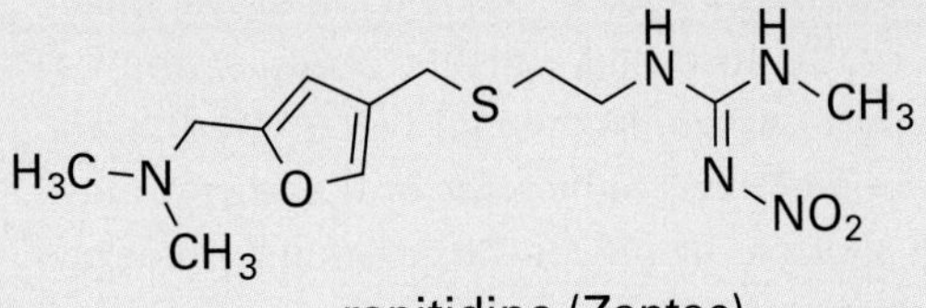

ranitidine (Zantac)

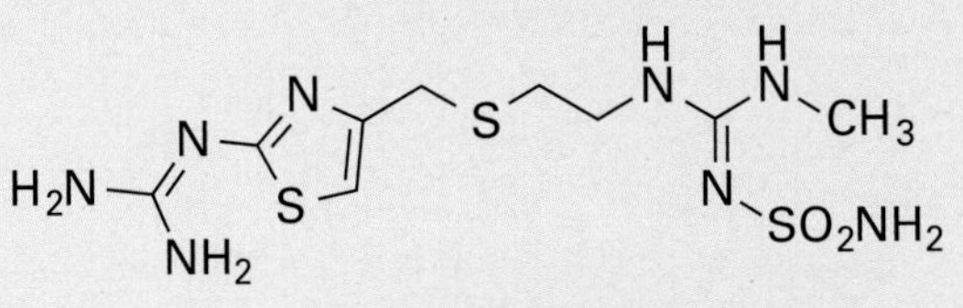

famotidine (Pepcid)

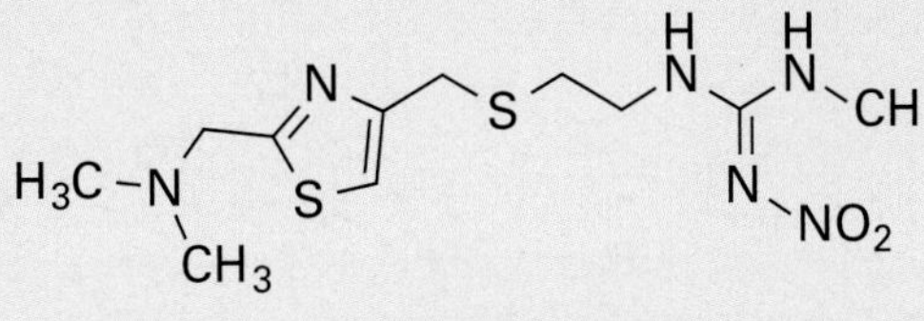

nizatidine (Axid)

4-methyl-histamine   guanylhistamine   burimamide

market success of cimetidine soon spawned additional drugs of the same type, such as ranitidine (Zantac), famotidine (Pepcid), and nizatidine (Axid). Interestingly, altering the pK_a of a key functional group was pivotal in the discovery of Tagamet and the later follow-on drugs.

In 1964, James Black, discoverer of the best-selling beta-blocker drug propranolol, led a group at SmithKline & French to pursue what he hoped would be a new class of drugs to treat stomach ulcers. These drugs would act directly to reduce stomach acid secretion by selectively antagonizing the histamine-2 (H_2) receptor. Starting from the natural ligand histamine, the group synthesized and tested a variety of new analogs. Among the early analogs was 4-methyl-histamine, a compound that turned out to be an *agonist* of the receptor and therefore *stimulated* acid secretion rather than suppressing it! Undeterred, the group pressed on and eventually found that by replacing the methylamine in 4-methyl-histamine with a guanidine function, they could produce compounds such as guanylhistamine that started to show antagonist-like behavior ("partial antagonists").

Unfortunately, guanylhistamine and related compounds were poorly absorbed from the stomach, most likely because they are strong bases and thus will be protonated (charged) in the acidic, gastric environment. Charged drug molecules can have trouble traversing the epithelial cells that line the small and large intestines, and across which drugs must pass to be orally absorbed. Further optimization of the H_2-receptor antagonists would be required, both to improve potency and to increase oral absorption—possibly by altering the pK_a of the guanidine function (reducing its basicity). Eventually, improved molecules like burimamide and metiamide were identified

in which a weakly basic thiourea function replaced the much more basic guanidine function. Burimamide was the group's first *bona fide* pure H_2-antagonist without agonist effects, and was also active in animals. Metiamide was an even more potent antagonist and also had improved oral bioavailability. Unfortunately, the story does not end here as the thiourea group turned out to have unforeseen liabilities of its own that included kidney toxicity and immune suppressive effects.

Abandoning the thiourea group would mean finding an alternative approach to reduce the basicity of the guanidine function. The solution that ultimately led to cimetidine (Tagamet) was to introduce a cyano (nitrile) group on the nitrogen atom of the guanidine group. The electron withdrawing effect of the cyano group lowered the pK_a (of the conjugate acid) into a range that allowed for good oral bioavailability while still retaining potency and also avoiding the toxicity observed with metiamide. The H_2-receptor antagonists that followed on the success of cimetidine also possess guanidine functions with reduced basicity. Instead of cyano, other electron withdrawing groups such as nitro or sulfonyl are employed to alter the pK_a of the guanidine function in drugs such as Zantac and Pepcid. Interestingly, a similar story is being played out in contemporary efforts to find Alzheimer's therapies that act on the aspartyl protease β-secretase. In these ongoing efforts, the basicity of cyclic guanidine and related inhibitors is being fine-tuned so as to balance potency with other properties such as permeability into the brain and a potentially serious cardiac toxicity. Thus, in seminal drug discovery efforts such as those leading to cimetidine and still today, attention to the acid-base properties of drug leads is central to the development of effective therapies.

cimetidine (Tagamet)   ranitidine (Zantac)

5.15 Exercises

Problem 5.1 What form of the amino acid shown below predominates at pH ~7?

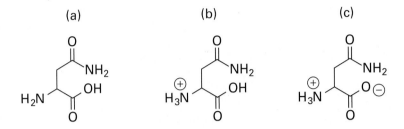

(a)   (b)   (c)

Problem 5.2 Order the compounds below from most acidic to least acidic. What factors influenced your analysis?

(a)   (b)   (c)   (d)

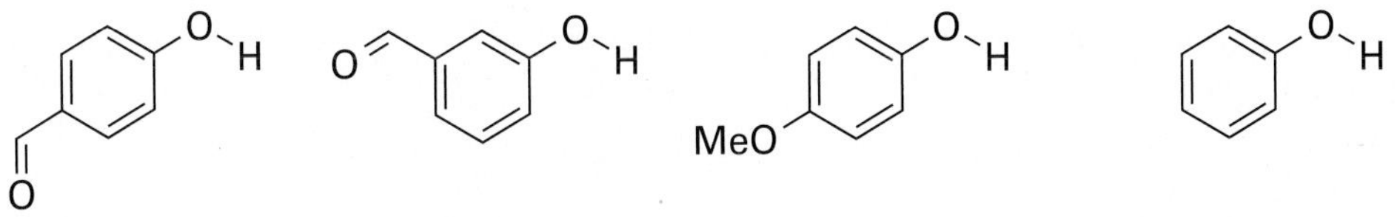

Problem 5.3 Order the compounds below from most basic to least basic. What factors influenced your analysis?

(a)   (b)   (c)   (d)

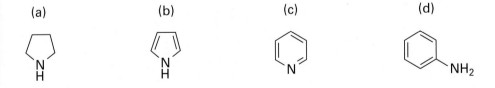

Problem 5.4 Each drug molecule below is shown in its neutral state along with its experimentally reported pK_a value. For each molecule, write the relevant acid/base equilibrium for the reported pK_a value.

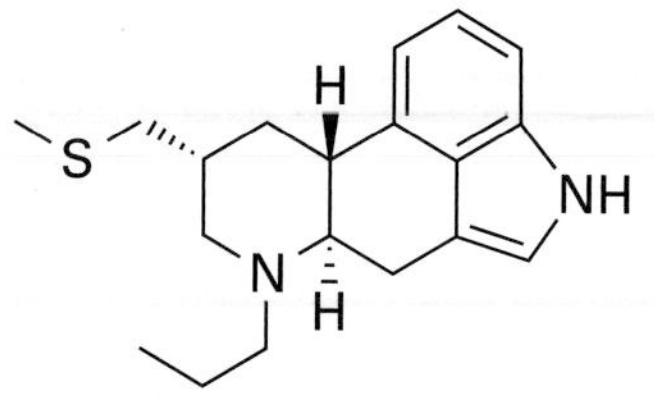

pergolide: pK_a ~8.0

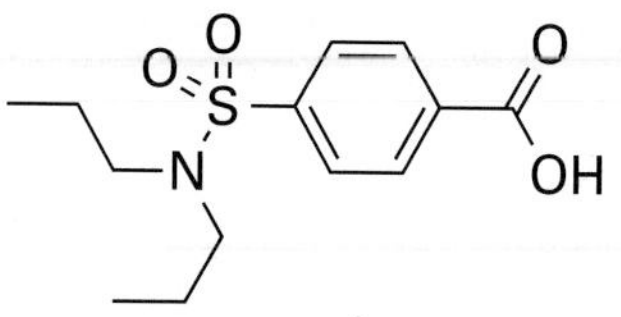

probenicid: pK_a ~3.4

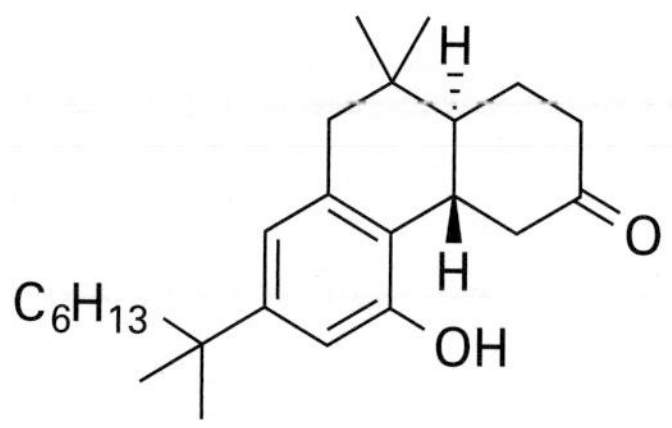

nabilone: pK_a ~9.7

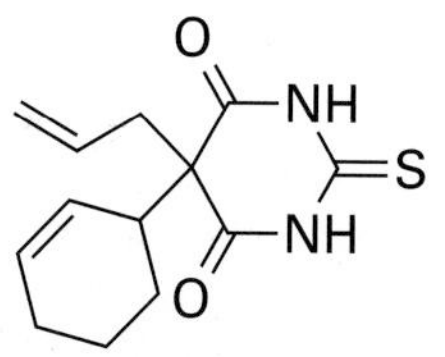

thialbarbitol: pK_a ~7.5

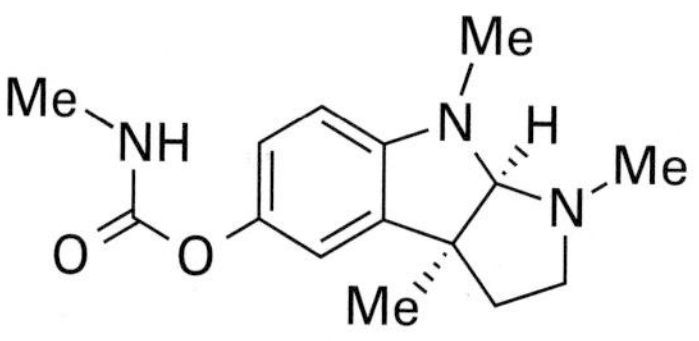

physostigmine: pK_a ~8.2

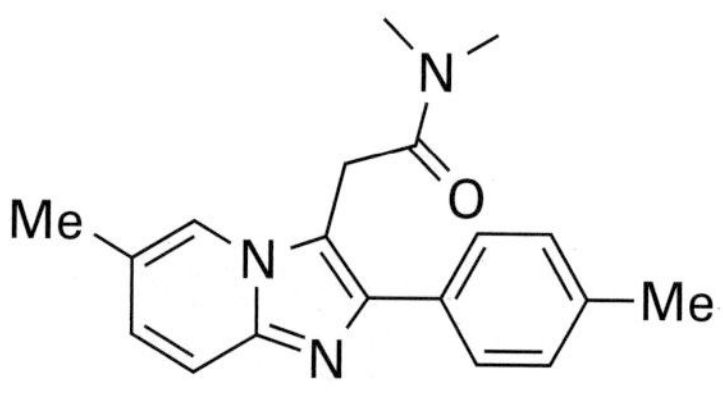

zolpidem: pK_a ~6.2

Problem 5.5 Shown below is a model of the drug paliperidone (Invega®) interacting with six amino acid side chains of a hypothetical target. The drug has a basic functional group with a BH^+ pK_a of ~8.1. Redraw paliperidone in its dominant protonation state at pH 7.4, labeling the basic group with its pK_a value. Finally, draw the side chains of the six amino acids making appropriate intermolecular interactions with the specific regions of the palperidone structure indicated below. Be sure to draw the interacting amino acid side chains in their appropriate protonation states.

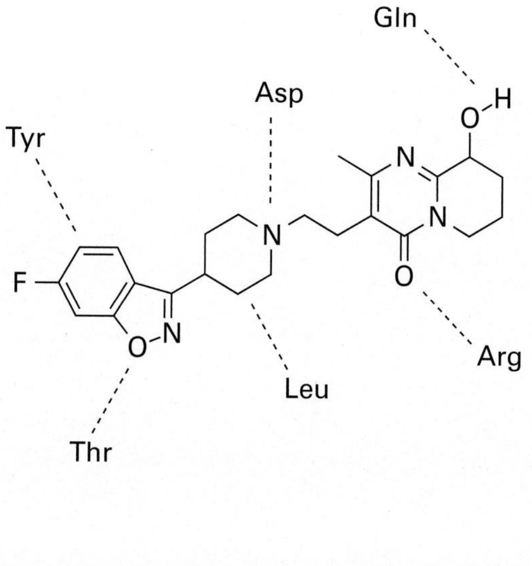

Problem 5.6 Shown below is a model of the drug lisinopril (Zestril®) interacting with six amino acid side chains of a hypothetical target. The drug has two acidic groups (HA pK_a of ~1.7 and ~3.3) and two basic groups (BH⁺ pK_a of ~7.0 and ~11). Redraw lisinopril in its correct protonation state at pH 7.4, labeling the acidic and basic groups with their correct pK_a values. Finally, draw the side chains of the six amino acids making appropriate intermolecular interactions with the specific regions of the lisinopril structure indicated below. Be sure to draw the interacting amino acid side chains in their appropriate protonation states.

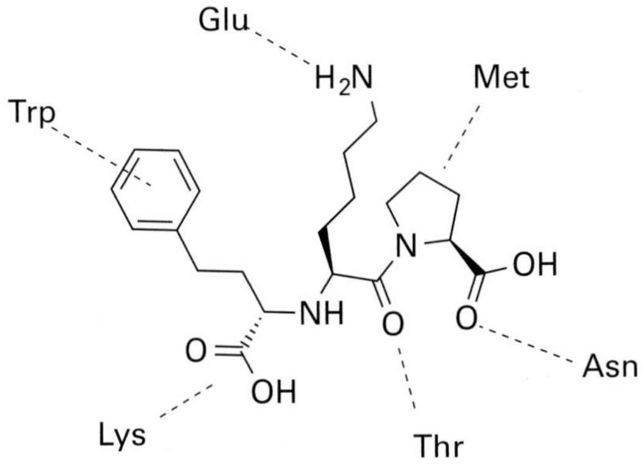

Problem 5.7 Shown below is a model of the drug moxifloxacin (Avelox®) interacting with five amino acid side chains of a hypothetical target. The drug has an acidic group (HA pK_a of 6.4) and a basic group (BH⁺ pK_a of 10.6). Redraw moxifloxacin in its correct protonation state at pH 7.4, labeling the acidic and basic groups with their correct pK_a values. Finally, draw the side chains of the five amino acids making appropriate intermolecular interactions with the specific regions of the moxifloxacin structure indicated below. Be sure to draw the interacting amino acid side chains in their appropriate protonation states.

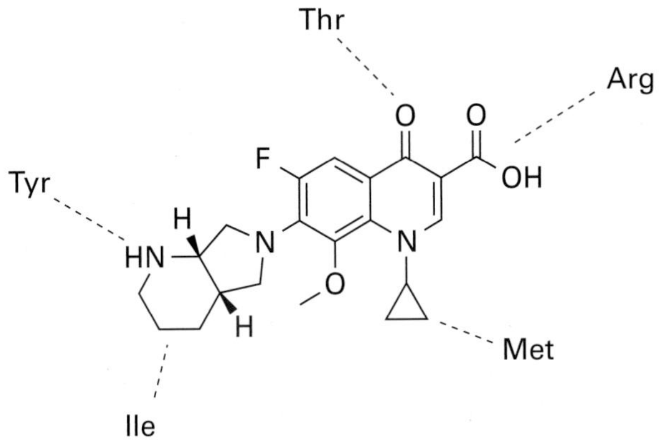

Problem 5.8 Shown below is a model of the drug arformoterol (Brovana®) interacting with six amino acid side chains of a hypothetical target. The drug has two pK_a values ~10 (one HA and one BH^+). Redraw arformoterol in its correct protonation state at pH 7.4, labeling the acidic and basic groups with their correct pK_a values. Finally, draw the side chains of the six amino acids making appropriate intermolecular interactions with the specific regions of the arformoterol structure indicated below. Be sure to draw the interacting amino acid side chains in their appropriate protonation states.

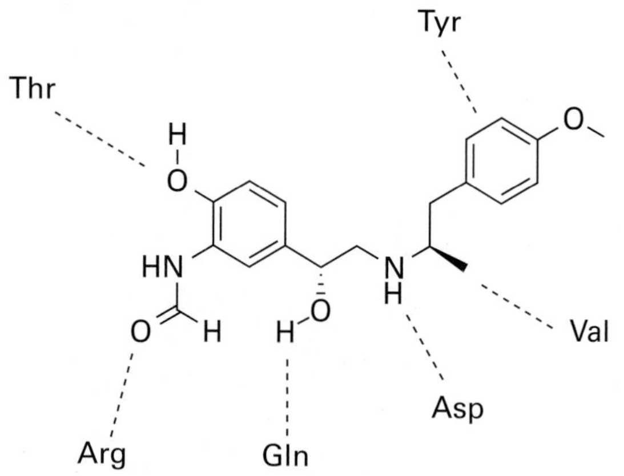
Tyr
Thr
H
O
HN
N
H
O
H
H
O
Val
Asp
Arg
Gln

Problem 5.9 One of the amino acids below has pK_a values of 10.2 and 3.6, while the pK_as of the other are 9.9 and 2.3. Assign the correct set of values to the functional groups in each structure and explain what factors influenced your analysis.

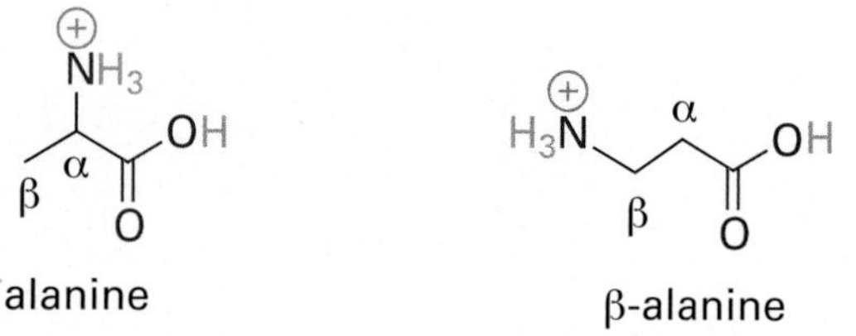
NH3
OH
α
β
O
alanine
H3N
α
OH
β
O
β-alanine

Problem 5.10 The pK_as for one of the following amino acids are 2.0, 3.9, and 10.0 and the pK_a values for the another are 2.1, 4.3, and 10.0. Assign the correct set of pK_as to the functional groups in each structure and explain what factors influenced your analysis.

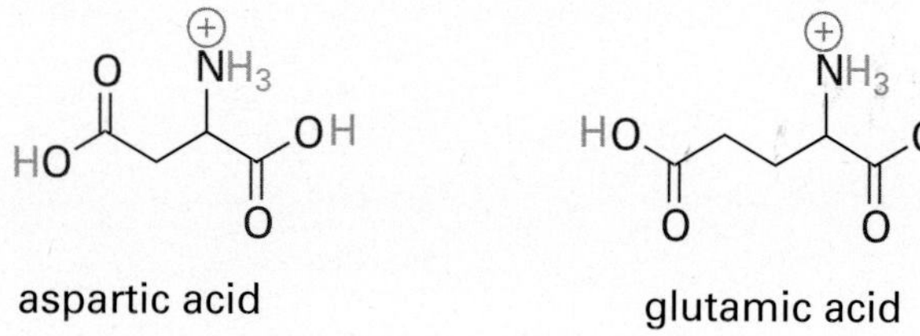
O
NH3
OH
HO
O
aspartic acid
NH3
HO
OH
O
O
glutamic acid

Chapter 6

Nucleophilic Substitution, Addition, and Elimination Reactions

Jie Jack Li & Adam Renslo

CHAPTER OUTLINE

6.1 Introduction
6.2 Nucleophiles
6.3 Electrophiles
    Box 6.1—Electrophiles in cancer drugs
6.4 Leaving Groups
6.5 Nucleophilic Aliphatic Substitution Reactions—S_N2
    Box 6.2—S_N2 reactions in biological chemistry
6.6 Nucleophilic Aliphatic Substitution Reactions—S_N1

6.7 Neighboring Group Assistance in S_N1 Reactions
6.8 Nucleophilic Aromatic Substitution Reactions—S_NAr
6.9 Addition reactions
6.10 Elimination Reactions—E1 and E2
6.11 Summary
6.12 *Case Study*—Drugs That Form a Covalent Bond to Their Target
6.13 Exercises

6.1 Introduction

The first few chapters of this text were focused on important properties of organic molecules and how these help determine the nature of a drug's interaction with its biological target. In this chapter and the ones that follow, we will discuss certain *reactions* of drug molecules and enzymes – biological macromolecules that break and form chemical bonds. In this chapter we discuss substitution, addition, and elimination reactions. The main focus is on substitution reactions, which are prevalent in physiological and metabolic processes, in the action

of some drugs, and in the chemical synthesis of nearly all drugs. The topic of addition reactions is introduced here and expanded upon in the following chapter on carbonyl chemistry.

Substitution reactions involve the reaction of **nucleophiles** with **electrophiles**. Nucleophiles are "nucleus seekers" that will donate a lone pair of electrons to the new bond that is formed with an electrophile. Electrophiles are "electron seekers" and thus accept a lone pair of electrons from a nucleophile. Some examples of nucleophiles and electrophiles are shown in Figure 6.1. Nucleophiles generally are anionic or neutral with

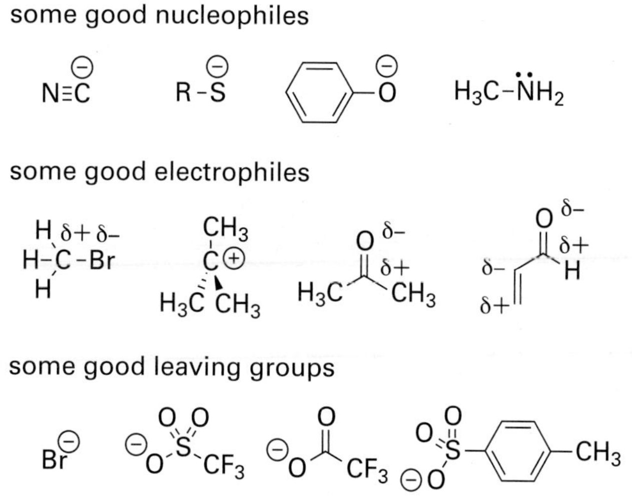

some good nucleophiles

some good electrophiles

some good leaving groups

Figure 6.1 Examples of some good nucleophiles, electrophiles, and leaving groups.

a lone pair of electrons to donate. Electrophiles are positively charged or have a polarized bond with partial positive character. Electrophiles capable of undergoing substitution reactions have a **leaving group**, a species that can accept and stabilize the pair of electrons that make up the bond being broken.

In the sections that follow, we will discuss in more detail the factors that make for a good nucleophile, electrophile, or leaving group. We will also review the various reaction mechanisms by which substitution, addition, and elimination reactions occur. By the end of the chapter you should have developed a sound understanding of the factors that govern these reactions and be able to predict reaction products when provided with the reactants and reaction conditions. You should also be able to write reasonable mechanisms for your reactions, making the proper use of curly arrows to show the movement of electrons as chemical bonds are formed and broken.

6.2 Nucleophiles

In the previous chapter, we used the Brønsted–Lowry definition of acids and bases—species that donate or accept a proton, respectively. A more general description of acids and bases is that first proposed by the chemist Gilbert N. Lewis, who described a covalent bond as the sharing of an electron pair between two atoms. Thus, a **Lewis acid** is a species that can accept an electron pair and a **Lewis base** is a species that can donate an electron pair in the formation of a covalent bond. A proton (H^+) qualifies as a species that can accept a lone pair of

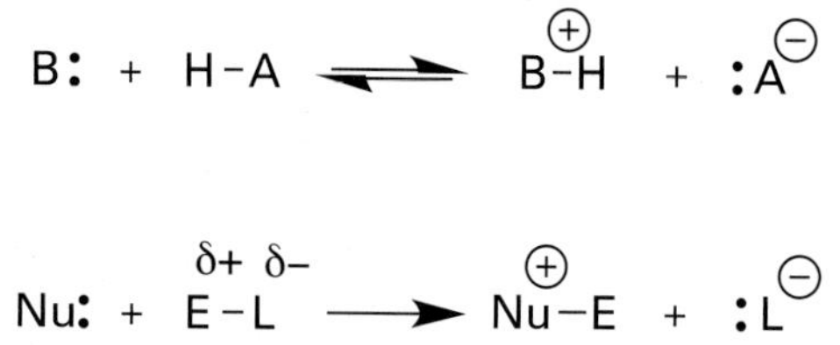

Figure 6.2 An acid-base equilibrium (top) shares many aspects of a nucleophilic substitution reaction (bottom). Both reactions involve species that donate an electron lone pair (Lewis bases, B: and Nu:) and species that accept an electron lone pair (Lewis acids, H–A and E–L).

electrons and thus the Lewis description of acids and bases encompasses the Brønsted–Lowry definition. However, Lewis' definition is more general and thus useful also to describe the reactions of nucleophiles and electrophiles (Figure 6.2). For example, we can say that a nucleophile acts as a Lewis base when it donates an electron pair in reaction with an electrophile (a Lewis acid) that accepts the electron pair. While acid-base reactions involve transfer of electrophilic protons, nucleophilic addition and substitution reactions involve a much broader range of electrophiles, as can be seen later in this chapter.

When describing nucleophilic substitution reactions, the term **nucleophilicity** is often used to describe the relative strength of a nucleophile—its ability to donate electrons. Table 6.1 compares the relative reactivity of a variety of common nucleophiles. What is apparent immediately is that most good nucleophiles in the table are anionic. This makes sense given that anionic species have an abundance of electrons. Now let us consider the four anionic species below derived from C, N, O, and F, which are immediately adjacent to one another in the second row of the periodic table. In this series of anions nucleophilicity decreases from left to right, with the methyl anion the strongest nucleophile, followed by the amide anion, hydroxide anion, and finally fluoride anion.

$$\overset{\ominus}{CH_3} > \overset{\ominus}{NH_2} > \overset{\ominus}{OH} > \overset{\ominus}{F}$$

This trend can be readily understood by considering the electronegativity of the atoms. Each anion possesses a full octet of valence electrons and a formal –1 charge, while the number of protons in the nucleus increases in the order C (6), N (7), O (8), F (9). Thus, proton-abundant and electronegative fluorine holds its electrons very tightly, making fluoride the least nucleophilic anion in the series. This trend in nucleophilicity is also correlated with the relative basicity of the anions, methyl anion being the strongest base and fluoride the weakest. Recall that weak bases have relatively little affinity for

Table 6.1 Nucleophilicity of Some Common Nucleophiles.

Reactivity class	Nucleophile	Relative reactivity
Very good nucleophiles	I^-, HS^-, RS^-	$>10^5$
Good nucleophiles	Br^-, HO^-, RO^-, CN^-, N_3^-	10^4
Fair nucleophiles	NH_3, Cl^-, F^-, RCO_2^-	10^3
Weak nucleophiles	H_2O, ROH	1
Very weak nucleophiles	RCO_2H	10^{-2}

Source: Reproduced, with permission, from Carey FA, Giuliano RM. *Organic Chemistry*. 9th ed. New York: McGraw-Hill Education; 2014.

protons, and we might expect them to have low affinity for other electrophiles as well. However, other factors can muddy the relationship between basicity and nucleophilicity, as in the case of the halides.

The halide anions iodide, bromide, chloride, and fluoride are nucleophilic anions from the same column or "group" of the periodic table. As in the previous case, nucleophilicity in this series is correlated with electronegativity and the order of relative nucleophilicity is that shown below.

$$\overset{\ominus}{I} \; > \; \overset{\ominus}{Br} \; > \; \overset{\ominus}{Cl} \; > \; \overset{\ominus}{F}$$

However, if we consider the relative acidity of the corresponding conjugate acids we find the order to be HI > HBr > HCl > HF. Thus, the trend with respect to basicity is opposite from what we might have predicted—the weakest base, iodide, is the best nucleophile. Why should the weakest base (the least proton-seeking) be the most nucleophilic (most nucleus-seeking)? The answer is related to the fact that basicity is a measure of affinity for *protons*, whereas nucleophilicity is more a measure of affinity for carbon-based electrophiles. In reactions with carbon electrophiles, the **polarizability** of the nucleophile is an important factor. Among the halide anions, iodide is the largest in size and its nucleus is least able to attract its outermost valence electrons. The highly polarizable iodide anion is most nucleophilic because it is most likely to react with the more diffuse positive charge that is characteristic of carbon electrophiles. At the other extreme in terms of polarizability is fluoride. Smallest in size and with its valence electrons held close to the nucleus, the electron cloud of fluoride is not at all polarizable and thus least reactive with carbon electrophiles.

The relationship between basicity and nucleophilicity may be further refined by a brief introduction to **hard-soft acid base** (HSAB) theory. In HSAB theory a

"hard" acid or base is a species with very little polarizability—think of a proton (a very hard acid) or fluoride anion (a very hard base). A "soft" acid or base then is a species with high polarizability and a more diffuse distribution of positive or negative charge. HSAB theory predicts that a hard base (or hard nucleophile) will prefer to react with a hard acid (or hard electrophile). Similarly, soft bases/nucleophiles will prefer to form bonds with soft acids/electrophiles. Using this concept we can understand how hydroiodic acid (HI) can be a strong acid while at the same time the iodide anion is a good nucleophile. In the molecule HI, the very hard proton is a poor match for the soft iodide anion. As a result, the covalent bond in HI is weak and prone to dissociate into ionic species in water (into H_3O^+ and $I^\ominus$ ions), thus making HI a strong acid. However, in substitution reactions with carbon-based (soft) electrophiles, HSAB theory predicts the soft iodide anion will be a good reaction partner and thus a good nucleophile.

Nucleophilicity is also affected by the presence of electron withdrawing or donating substituents that interact with the nucleophilic atom via inductive or resonance effects. This is illustrated below for substitutions on a pyridine ring (Figure 6.3). The ring nitrogen atom of pyridine is nucleophilic on account of this atom having a lone pair of electrons to donate. The presence of a *para*-dimethylamino group on the pyridine ring will be electron donating through resonance and this will produce a much more nucleophilic pyridine species. Conversely, an *ortho*-fluoro substituent will be electron withdrawing by an inductive effect, resulting in a much less nucleophilic pyridine species. For ionizable groups such as the −OH function in phenol, it is important to consider the concentrations of both the neutral and anionic forms. With a pK_a ~10, phenol exists primarily in its neutral form at physiological pH. The introduction of electron-withdrawing substituents may well *increase* nucleophilicity under physiological conditions, since the

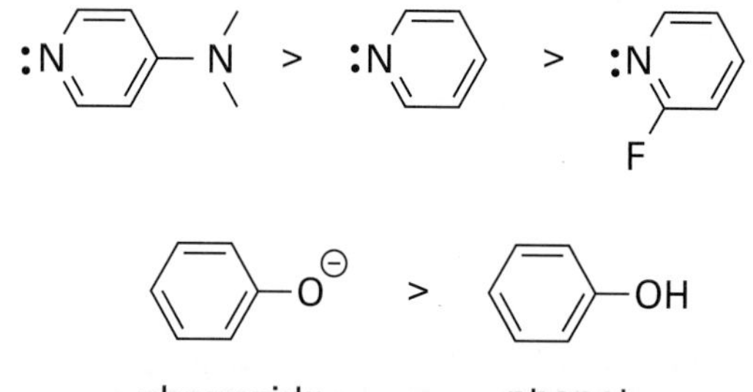

Figure 6.3 Relative nucleophilicity of substituted pyridines (top) and of phenol in its protonated and deprotonated forms.

effect will be to lower the pK_a and increase concentrations of the more nucleophilic phenoxide species.

Nucleophilic sulfur, nitrogen, and oxygen atoms in the side chains of amino acids play essential roles in various biological processes. Specific cysteine (R–SH) and serine (R–OH) residues in the active sites of cysteine and serine proteases serve as strong nucleophiles, reacting with the electrophilic amide (peptide) bonds of their protein substrates. Methylation and acetylation of specific lysine side-chain amines in histones is crucial for the regulation of gene expression. Phosphorylation of specific serine, threonine, or tyrosine hydroxyl (–OH) groups by kinases represents one of the most important mechanisms of controlling protein function and signaling in biology. The thiol containing tripeptide glutathione is sometimes referred to as the "guardian of the cell," on account of its various roles as an antioxidant and a nucleophilic scavenger of

potentially harmful electrophilic species. Glutathione is activated by the enzyme glutathione S-transferase, which functions to activate the thiol function (R–SH) for nucleophilic attack on electrophilic substrates (Figure 6.4). When the substrate is a xenobiotic small molecule, the effect of reaction with GSH is to produce a water-soluble product, thus promoting excretion and protecting the cell or organism from the potentially toxic effects of the xenobiotic agent. The role of GSH in drug metabolism will be discussed in more detail in Chapter 8.

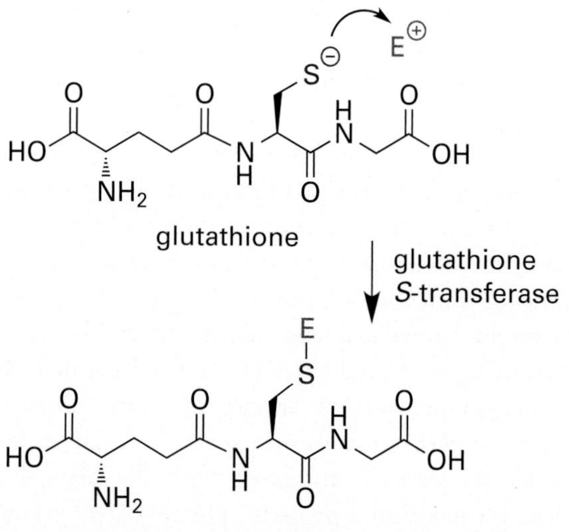

6.3 Electrophiles

Electrophiles are Lewis acids—species that accept an electron pair in the formation of a new covalent bond. Electrophiles can carry a formal positive charge or can be neutral overall but with partial positive charge at specific electrophilic sites. We will be most concerned with carbon-based electrophiles since these species are of greatest relevance in organic chemistry and in the chemistry of biological molecules and drugs. As illustrated in Figure 6.5, electrophilic sites in organic molecules can occur at both saturated and unsaturated carbon centers. The focus of this chapter is on saturated carbon electrophiles, electrophilic C–C double bonds, and aromatic systems. The reactions of electrophilic C=O double bonds (carbonyl species) are the topic of Chapter 7.

Let us now consider what makes the compounds in Figure 6.5 good electrophiles. Most obvious perhaps is the polarization of a C–X or C=X bond, producing a partial positive charge at one or more site(s) in the molecule. However, not all polarized C–X bonds are good electrophiles for substitution reactions. A perfect example of this is the C–F bond, which is highly polarized

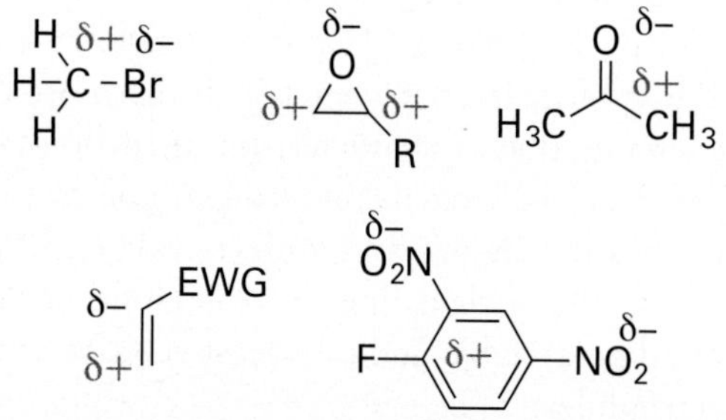

Figure 6.4 Reaction of the tripeptide glutathione with cellular electrophiles is promoted by the enzyme glutathione S-transferase.

Figure 6.5 Examples of both saturated and unsaturated carbon-based electrophiles. Electrophilic sites are those sites possessing partial positive character, shown in blue.

Box 6.1 Electrophiles in cancer drugs

Electrophilic centers on saturated carbon are found in various chemotherapeutics agents, including mechlor-ethamine and cyclophosphamide. Ironically, these life-extending drugs trace their chemical provenance back to the earliest chemical weapons, in particular mustard gas. Mechanistically, chemical mustards act by reacting in nucleophilic substitution reactions with DNA to form cross-links within and/or between DNA strands. The nucleophilic species in DNA are nitrogen atoms in the ring of nucleoside bases, particularly guanine. DNA cross-linking prevents cell division and ultimately leads to cell death. Unfortunately, these agents are not very selective and will also kill fast-growing non-cancerous cells in the bone marrow and in hair follicles, thus leading to some of the well-known side effects of cancer chemotherapy using such agents.

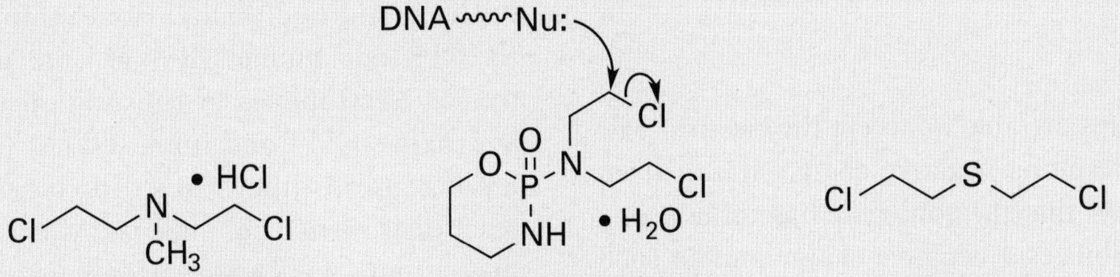

mechlorethamine
(nitrogen mustard)

cyclophosphamide
(Cytoxan)

mustard gas

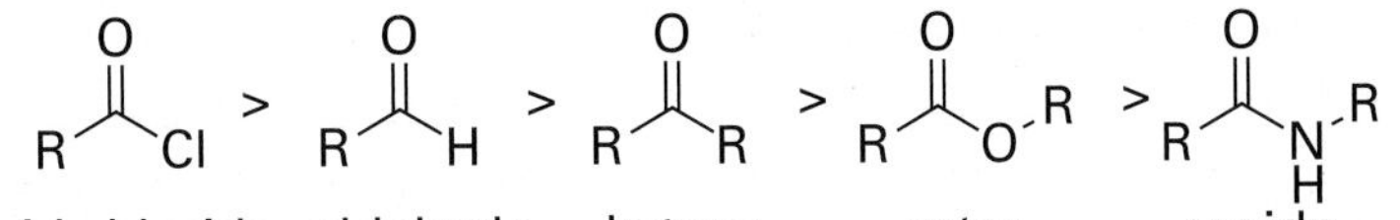

acid chloride   aldehyde   ketone   ester   amide

Figure 6.6 Relative reactivity of common carbonyl-containing electrophiles toward nucleophilic addition. The reactions of carbonyl species are more fully explored in Chapter 7.

(fluorine being most electronegative element) and yet not particularly reactive with nucleophiles. One reason for this poor reactivity is that the C–F bond, while highly polarized, is also a very strong bond. A second reason is that fluoride is a relatively poor leaving group (the topic of Section 6.4). This highlights the fact that in any nucleophilic addition or substitution reaction, certain bonds must be *broken* even as others are being formed. Hence, a good electrophile will possess a relatively weak bond to a good leaving group. An example of such a molecule is methyl bromide (CH$_3$–Br), with its relatively weak C–Br bond to a good leaving group (Br$^\ominus$). Epoxides are often good electrophiles because of their relatively weak and polarized C–O bonds, ring strain that is relieved upon breaking the C–O bond, and a reactive carbon atom that is sterically unhindered. Some examples of electrophilic chemotherapeutic agents are provided in Box 6.1.

Unsaturated sp^2 or sp-hybridized carbon atoms are generally poor electrophiles, except when directly bound to more electronegative atom, as is the case in the carbonyl (C=O) and nitrile (C≡N) functional groups. The reactivity of the carbonyl function is further impacted by the electronic and steric nature of the other substituent on the carbon atom (Figure 6.6 and Chapter 7). When a nucleophile reacts with a C=O bond, a tetrahedral intermediate is formed in which the negative charge is borne and stabilized by the electronegative oxygen atom. Similar reaction of a C=C double bond would place an unstabilized negative charge on carbon and thus simple C=C bonds are poor electrophiles. C=C double bonds can be rendered more electrophilic when they are substituted with one or more electron-withdrawing groups (EWG, Figure 6.5). Addition reactions of this type are covered in Section 6.9.

6.4 Leaving Groups

Substitution or elimination reactions involve breaking of a bond to a **leaving group**. If the breaking bond is C–Br, the leaving group is the bromide anion, which accepts the pair of electrons that formed the C–Br bond. The rates and mechanisms of substitution and elimination reactions are thus dependent on the ability of the leaving group to accept an electron pair from the breaking bond.

relative leaving group ability

$$F^{\ominus} \quad < \quad Cl^{\ominus} \quad < \quad Br^{\ominus} \quad < \quad I^{\ominus}$$

very poor   fair   good   excellent

relative acidity

$$HF \quad < \quad HCl \quad < \quad HBr \quad < \quad HI$$

weakest acid   strongest acid

Figure 6.7 Leaving group ability is correlated with the ability to stabilize a negative charge and thus is related to basicity. A good leaving group is a weak base—the conjugate base of a strong acid.

Good leaving groups are able to accept the electron pair and stabilize the resulting negative charge. Recall from the previous chapter that the conjugate base of a strong acid effectively stabilizes a negative charge and so such weak bases are generally good leaving groups. This relationship between basicity and leaving group ability is apparent with the halides, where iodide is both the weakest base and the best leaving group (Figure 6.7).

Basicity and the ability to stabilize a negative charge are determined by various factors, including inductive effects, resonance effects, and polarizability. The relative basicity of the halides is significantly impacted by the relative polarizability ("hardness") of the halide anion. Resonance and inductive effects are more dominant in the case of acetate and sulfonate anions, conjugate bases of acetic and sulfonic acids (Figure 6.8). Considering the acetate and trifluoroacetate anions, we might draw two resonance forms to show that the negative charge is shared equally by the two oxygen atoms, thus stabilizing the negative charge. What makes trifluoroacetate a much better leaving group (and a weaker base) is the strongly

electron-withdrawing inductive effect of the trifluoromethyl group. The methane sulfonate anion (mesylate) is a better leaving group than either of the acetate anions because the negative charge is shared between three electronegative oxygen atoms (rather than just two). Better still is the trifluoromethylsulfonate anion (triflate), which combines stabilizing inductive and resonance effects and is one of the best leaving groups known.

The reaction conditions employed in a substitution or elimination reaction can have a substantial effect on leaving group ability. For example, simple alcohols (R–OH) and amines (R–NH$_2$) are generally not reactive as electrophiles in substitution reactions since the hydroxide (OH$^{\ominus}$) and amide (NH$_2^{\ominus}$) anions are very poor leaving groups (they are strong bases). However, if the reaction is carried out under sufficiently acidic conditions these groups will become protonated to yield species like R–OH$_2^+$ and R–NH$_3^+$. Now the relevant leaving groups are the neutral species H$_2$O and NH$_3$, both weak bases and thus reasonably good leaving groups.

6.5 Nucleophilic Aliphatic Substitution Reactions—S$_N$2

The first type of substitution reaction we discuss in detail is the bimolecular nucleophilic substitution reaction, or S$_N$2 reaction for short. Two examples of S$_N$2 processes are shown in Figure 6.9. In the first reaction, hydroxide anion (HO$^{\ominus}$) is the nucleophile, methyl bromide is the electrophile and bromide anion is the leaving group. Experimentally, the rate of this reaction can be shown to obey a second-order rate law, Rate = k[HO$^-$][CH$_3$Br]. This rate law tells us that the nucleophile and electrophile

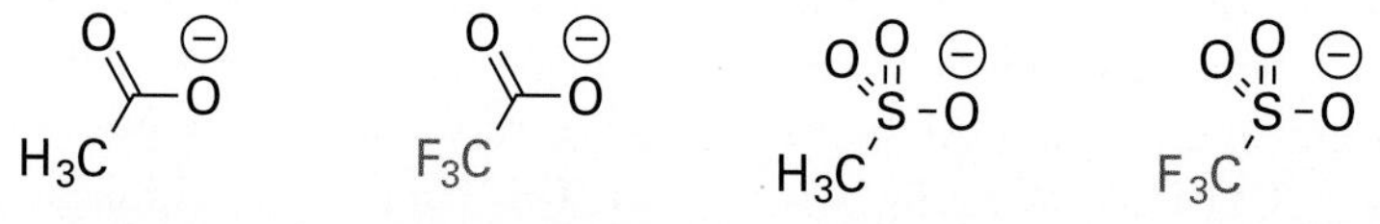

	acetate	trifluoroacetate	mesylate	triflate
k_{rel}	0.0000014	2.1	30,000	140,000,000

Figure 6.8 Relative rates of a solvolysis reaction involving acetate and sulfonate anions as leaving group. Resonance and inductive effects combine to make the triflate anion an exceptionally good leaving group.

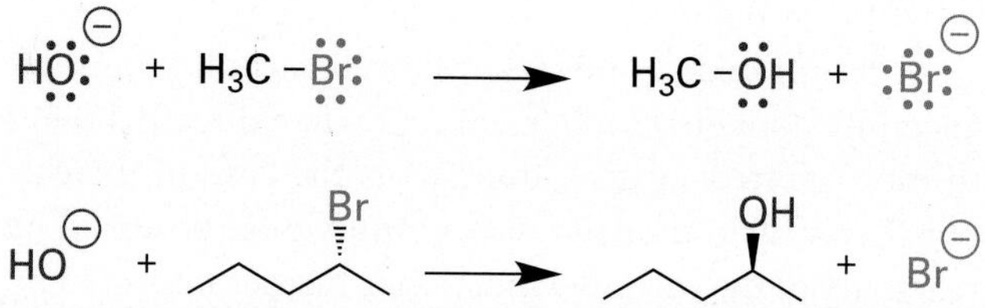

Figure 6.9 Examples of nucleophilic substitution reactions. Inversion of configuration as in the example at bottom is characteristic of the bimolecular nucleophilic substitution (S$_N$2) reaction.

The S$_N$2 Mechanism of Nucleophilic Substitution

THE OVERALL REACTION:

$$CH_3Br \quad + \quad HO^- \quad \longrightarrow \quad CH_3OH \quad + \quad Br^-$$

methyl bromide   hydroxide ion   methyl alcohol   bromide ion

THE MECHANISM: The reaction proceeds in a single step. Hydroxide ion acts as a nucleophile. While the C—Br bond is breaking, the C—O bond is forming.

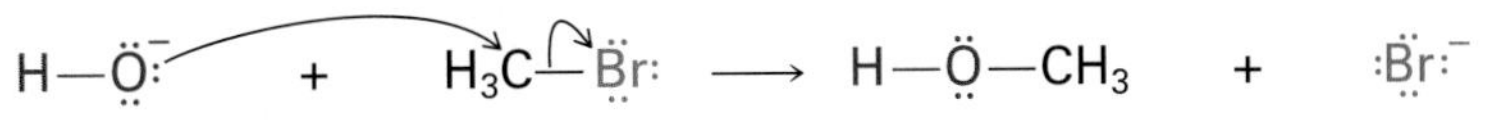

$$H—\ddot{O}{:}^- \quad + \quad H_3C—\ddot{B}r{:} \quad \longrightarrow \quad H—\ddot{O}—CH_3 \quad + \quad {:}\ddot{B}r{:}^-$$

hydroxide ion   methyl bromide   methyl alcohol   bromide ion

THE TRANSITION STATE: Hydroxide ion attacks carbon from the side opposite the C—Br bond.

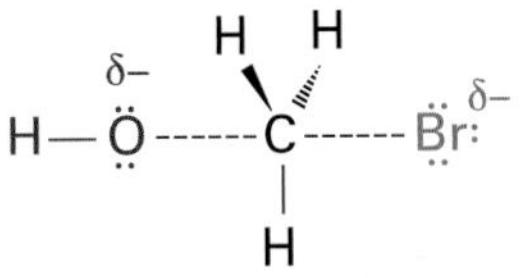

$$H—\overset{\delta-}{\ddot{O}}{-}{-}{-}{-}{-}{-}\underset{\underset{H}{|}}{\overset{\overset{H \quad H}{\diagup\diagdown}}{C}}{-}{-}{-}{-}{-}{-}\overset{\delta-}{\ddot{B}r{:}}$$

Carbon is partially bonded to both hydroxide and bromide. The arrangement of bonds undergroes

tetrahedral inversion from $\diagdown\!\!\!\overset{\diagdown}{C}\!\!-$ to $-\overset{\diagup}{C}\!\!\!\diagup$ as the reaction progresses.

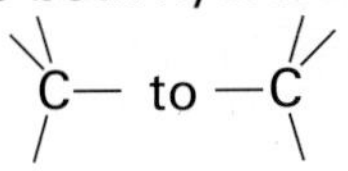

Figure 6.10 The S$_N$2 mechanism of nucleophilic substitution. (Reproduced, with permission, from Carey FA, Giuliano RM. *Organic Chemistry.* 9th ed. New York: McGraw-Hill Education; 2014.)

are involved in a bimolecular reaction that is rate determining. The reaction occurs in a single step with the new C–O bond forming at the same time the C–Br bond is breaking (Figure 6.10). We say that S$_N$2 reactions are **concerted** processes since bond formation and bond breaking occur simultaneously. Another characteristic of an S$_N$2 reaction is inversion of stereochemical configuration at the carbon atom undergoing reaction. This is illustrated in Figure 6.9 for the case of an S$_N$2 reaction involving one enantiomer of a chiral alkyl bromide.

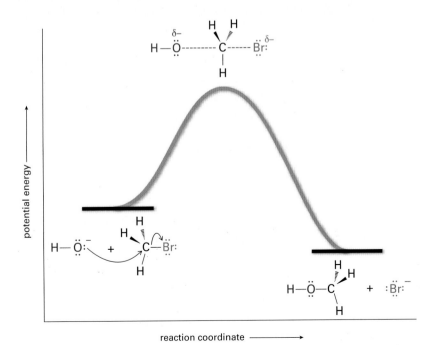

Figure 6.11 Potential energy diagram describing the one-step biomolecular S$_N$2 reaction of hydroxide anion with methyl bromide. (Reproduced, with permission, from Carey FA, Giuliano RM. *Organic Chemistry.* 9th ed. New York: McGraw-Hill Education; 2014.)

Et
N₃ ⊖ Et   ⊖
                                              Et
N₃ ──── Br   →   N₃   Br   →   N₃   + Br ⊖
H   H
Me   H Me   Me

chiral substrate   transition state   chiral product
S-configuration   (achiral)   R-configuration

Figure 6.12 The S$_N$2 reaction is concerted and stereospecific. An S$_N$2 reaction of a chiral substrate will produce a product with the opposite stereochemical configuration.

If we inspect a potential energy diagram of the S$_N$2 reaction we see that there are no intermediates formed along the reaction coordinate, only a single transition state whose energy corresponds to the activation energy of the reaction (Figure 6.11). The structure of the transition state also reveals why S$_N$2 reactions proceed with inversion of configuration. The hydroxide nucleophile attacks the carbon electrophile along the axis of the C–Br bond, a trajectory often refered to as backside attack. To accommodate a bond at this position, the other three substituents on carbon must invert, much as an umbrella turns inside out when hit by a strong gust of wind.

An example of a concerted S$_N$2 reaction involving backside attack and inversion of configuration is the reaction of S-2-bromobutane with nucleophilic azide (Figure 6.12). Note that while configuration will always invert upon S$_N$2 reaction at a chirality center, the actual CIP desination (R or S) at the reaction center may or may not change, depending on CIP priority rules and the nature of the nucleophile and leaving group. The necessary inversion of configuration for an S$_N$2 process makes this reaction a **stereospecific** one (i.e., it affords a single stereoisomeric product that can be predicted based on the reaction mechanism).

Another way to understand the backside trajectory of attack in S$_N$2 reactions is to inspect the molecular orbitals (MOs) involved. The relevant MOs will be the HOMO of the nucleophile (hydroxide) and the LUMO of the electrophile (methyl bromide), as illustrated below. It should be evident that the best overlap of MOs will occur along the axis of the C–Br bond. Since approach from the direction of the bromine atom cannot lead to a new C–O bond, the remaining possibility is overlap with the red lobe of the LUMO on the left, which is exactly opposite the C–Br bond. Thus, the molecular orbital description of the S$_N$2 reaction is consistent with the empirical observation of backside attack and inversion of configuration at the reacting center.

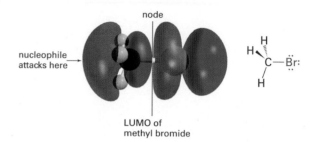

Another important characteristic of S$_N$2 reactions is sensitivity to the steric environment surrounding both the nucleophile and electrophile. This is a consequence of the need for the nucleophile to have unhindered access to the electrophilic carbon atom, opposite the breaking C–X bond. The best way to see this is to compare space-filling models of methyl bromide and the more hindered carbon atoms in ethyl-, isopropyl-, and finally *tert*-butyl bromide (Figure 6.13). As additional methyl groups are introduced, the electrophilic carbon atom becomes less and less accessible to nucleophiles. It is not surprising then that the order of relative reactivity for these species is CH₃–Br > CH₃CH₂–Br ≫ (CH₃)₂CH–Br ≫ (CH₃)₃C–Br.

While primary alkyl halides generally react readily in S$_N$2 reactions, there are cases where substitution farther out from the reactive center can still preclude reaction. This is illustrated for the alkyl halide electrophiles shown below. While all are primary alkyl halides, increasing steric bulk at the beta-carbon has a dramatic effect on reactivity. This is a consequence of the bulky isopropyl and *tert*-butyl substituents blocking approach of nucleophiles opposite the electrophilic C–Br bond. An example of an important S$_N$2 reaction in biology is provided in Box 6.2.

ethyl	propyl	isobutyl	neopentyl
1	0.8	0.036	0.00002

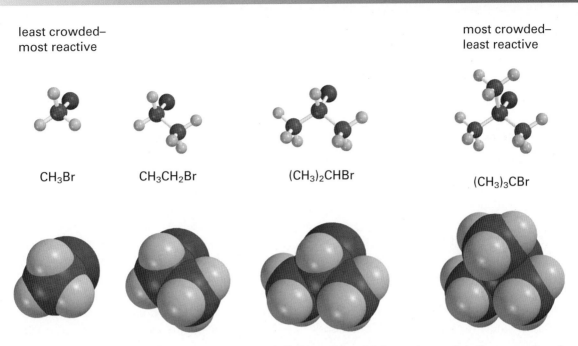

least crowded–
most reactive

most crowded–
least reactive

CH₃Br   CH₃CH₂Br   (CH₃)₂CHBr   (CH₃)₃CBr

Figure 6.13 Ball-and-stick and space-filling representations of alkyl bromides with increasing steric bulk surrounding the electrophilic carbon atom. Isopropyl and *tert*-butyl bromide are essentially unreactive in S$_N$2 reactions. (Reproduced, with permission, from Carey FA, Giuliano RM. *Organic Chemistry*. 9th ed. New York: McGraw-Hill Education; 2014.)

Box 6.2 S$_N$2 reactions in biological chemistry.

Mother Nature performs S$_N$2 reactions with ease and precision. An S$_N$2 reaction between the amino acid methionine and adenosine 5'-triphosphate (ATP) gives rise to *S*-adenosyl methionine (SAM). Neutral sulfur is the nucleophile in the reaction and the triphosphate of ATP is the leaving group. In the product SAM, a methyl group is attached to a charged sulfur atom, which makes for an excellent leaving group. SAM is therefore an excellent electrophile and its role in biology is to provide a methyl group to appropriate nucleophiles. When the nucleophile is norepinephrine, the S$_N$2 reaction between norepinephrine and SAM produces epinephrine (adrenaline).

methionine

adenosine 5'-triphosphate (ATP)   norepinephrine   *S*-adenosyl methionine (SAM)

epinephrine (adrenaline)   *S*-adenosyl homocysteine (SAH)

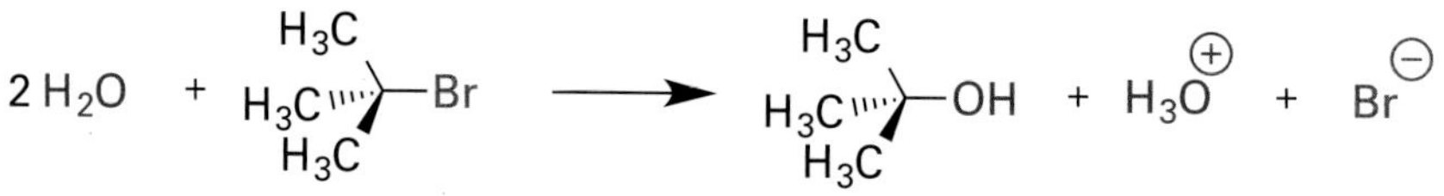

$$2\,H_2O \;+\; \underset{\substack{H_3C}}{\overset{\substack{H_3C}}{H_3C{\cdots}}}\!\!\!\!\!\!\!\!\text{—Br} \;\longrightarrow\; \underset{\substack{H_3C}}{\overset{\substack{H_3C}}{H_3C{\cdots}}}\!\!\!\!\!\!\!\!\text{—OH} \;+\; H_3\overset{\oplus}{O} \;+\; \overset{\ominus}{Br}$$

Figure 6.14 The hydrolysis reaction of *tert*-butyl bromide.

6.6 Nucleophilic Aliphatic Substitution Reactions—S_N1

Let us next consider a reaction that would appear unlikely to occur at all, the reaction of *tert*-butyl bromide with water (Figure 6.14). While the leaving group is a reasonably good one (bromide), the nucleophile is poor (water), and the electrophilic carbon of the C–Br bond is highly hindered and thus inaccessible for backside attack. However, not only does this hydrolysis reaction occur, it is actually much *faster* than the hydrolysis of ethyl or isopropyl bromide under the same reaction conditions!

In order to explain this surprising result, we must invoke a completely different reaction mechanism. A hint as to what is going on is provided by the empirically determined rate law of the reaction, Rate = $k[(CH_3)_3 C\text{–}Br]$. The rate law tells us that the reaction rate is determined solely by the nature and concentration of the electrophile. We call this type of reaction a unimolecular nucleophilic substitution reaction, or S_N1 **reaction** for short. The first, rate-determining step in the hydrolysis of *tert*-butyl bromide is dissociation of the C–Br bond to form a carbocation intermediate (Figure 6.15). Once formed, this highly electrophilic species will react very

The S_N1 Mechanism of Nucleophilic Substitution

THE OVERALL REACTION:

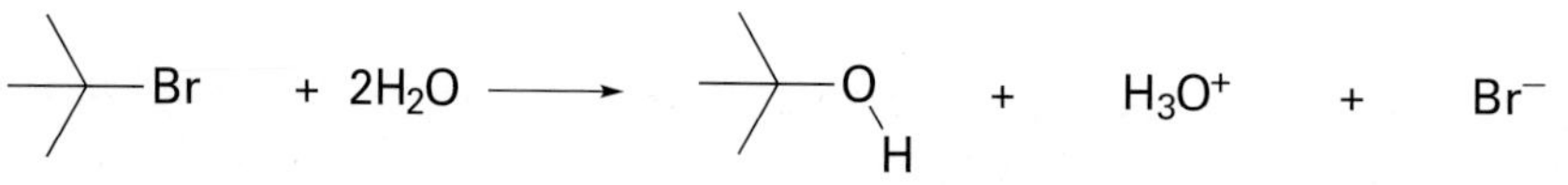

tert-butyl bromide   water   *tert*-butyl alcohol   hydronium ion   bromide ion

THE MECHANISM:

Step 1: The alkyl halide dissociates to a carbocation and a halide ion.

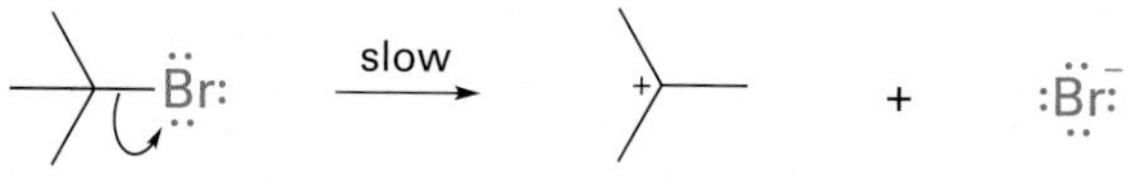

tert-butyl bromide   *tert*-butyl cation   bromide ion

Step 2: The carbocation fromed in step 1 reacts rapidly with water, which acts as a nucleophile. This step completes the nucleophilic substitution stage of the mechanism and yields an alkyloxonium ion.

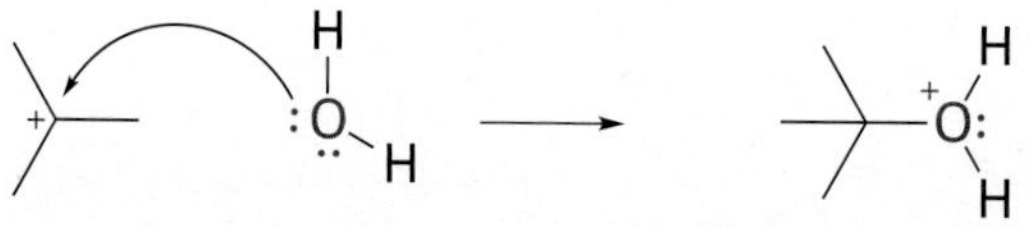

tert-butyl cation   water   *tert*-butyloxonium ion

Step 3: This step is a fast acid—base reaction that follows the nucleophilic substitution. Water acts as a base to remove a proton from the alkyloxonium ion to give the observed product of the reaction, *tert*-butyl alcohol.

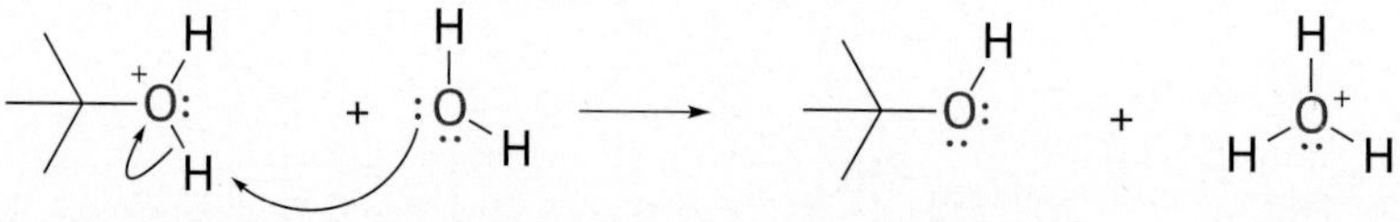

tert-butyloxonium ion   water   *tert*-butyl alcohol   hydronium ion

Figure 6.15 The mechanism of the S_N1 reaction between water and *tert*-butyl bromide. (Reproduced, with permission, from Carey FA, Giuliano RM. *Organic Chemistry*. 9th ed. New York: McGraw-Hill Education; 2014.)

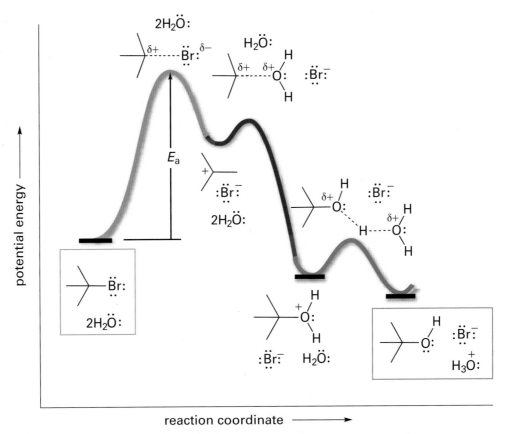

Figure 6.16 Potential energy diagram for the S_N1 reaction of tert-butyl bromide with water. (Reproduced, with permission, from Carey FA, Giuliano RM. *Organic Chemistry.* 9th ed. New York: McGraw-Hill Education; 2014.)

Figure 6.17 Relative rate for the hydrolysis reaction of alkyl bromides within aqueous formic acid. These reaction conditions favor S_N1 reaction via initial ionization of the C–Br bond. (Reproduced, with permission, from Carey FA, Giuliano RM. *Organic Chemistry.* 9th ed. New York: McGraw-Hill Education; 2014.)

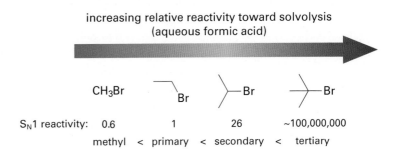

rapidly with nucleophile (water in this case) to give the product. Note that the nucleophile in this reaction need not be an especially strong one since the carbocation is such a powerful electrophile.

Inspection of a potential energy diagram for this S_N1 reaction reveals several reaction intermediates and transition states along the reaction coordinate (Figure 6.16). The energetic barrier to reaction (the activation energy) is that required to form the initial carbocation intermediate. The height of this barrier will then depend on both the stability of the carbocation and the nature of the leaving group. Although an S_N1 reaction requires a reasonably good leaving group, even more important

is the stability of the carbocation intermediate. What determines this stability? To answer this question, consider the rate of the hydrolysis reaction for various alkyl bromides, carried out under acidic conditions (Figure 6.17). Acidic conditions minimize competing S_N2 reactions (no nucleophilic hydroxide anion is present) and thus the measured rates should reflect reaction via the S_N1 mechanism.

What we find is a reactivity trend quite the opposite of that we saw for S_N2 reactions. The reaction is fastest with the tertiary bromide because this substrate can most readily form a carbocation intermediate (the tertiary carbocation is much more stable than a

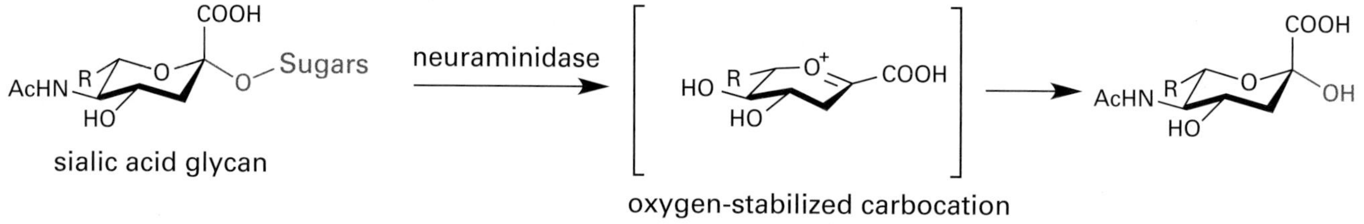

Figure 6.18 Formation of an oxygen-stabilized carbocation in the hydrolysis of a glycosidic bond by the enzyme neuraminidase. In this reaction neuraminidase accelerates an S_N1-like substitution reaction by forming favorable non-covalent interactions with the carbocation intermediate.

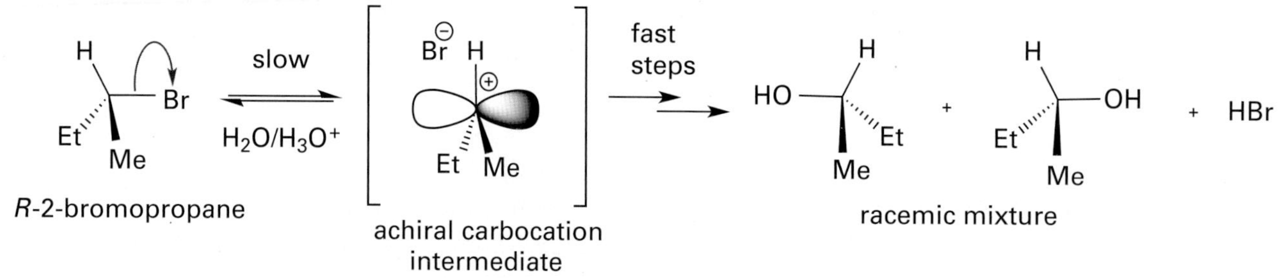

Figure 6.19 Mechanism of S_N1 reaction of R-2-bromopropane. The reaction proceeds via the planar, achiral carbocation intermediate shown and affords a racemic mixture of the 2-propanol product.

secondary or primary carbocation). Thus, we find that tertiary alkyl halides react by S_N1 mechanisms, whereas primary halides react via the S_N2 mechanism. The formation and breaking of glycosidic bonds in carbohydrates is one important example of an S_N1-like process in biological systems. Recall, for example, the case study from Chapter 4 where we have seen how the influenza drug oseltamivir has been designed to mimic an oxygen-stabilized carbocation formed during the removal of sialic acid groups by the enzyme neuraminidase (Figure 6.18).

In Section 6.5 we have seen that S_N2 reactions are concerted processes that occur with inversion of configuration at the carbon center undergoing reaction. By contrast, S_N1 reactions are neither concerted nor stereospecific—they typically proceed to afford mixtures of products resulting

from retention and inversion of configuration. This is a consequence of the fact that the carbocation intermediate in S_N1 reactions is planar and therefore achiral (Figure 6.19). The nucleophile can add to either side of this intermediate and so a mixture of products results. In the specific example shown in Figure 6.19, R-2-bromopropane is hydrolyzed to afford a racemic mixture of R- and S-2-propanol.

6.7 Neighboring Group Assistance in S_N1 Reactions

Next, consider two nucleophilic substitution reactions performed on very similar substrates that nonetheless produce two very different outcomes (Figure 6.20).

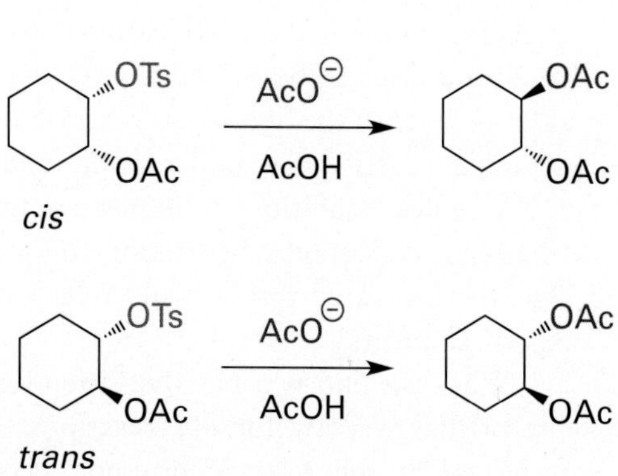

	stereochemical outcome	rate dependent on [AcO$^{\ominus}$]	k_{rel}
cis	inversion	yes	1
trans	retention	no	670

Figure 6.20 Nucleophilic substitution reactions involving two similar substrates that proceed at very different rates and with different stereochemical outcomes.

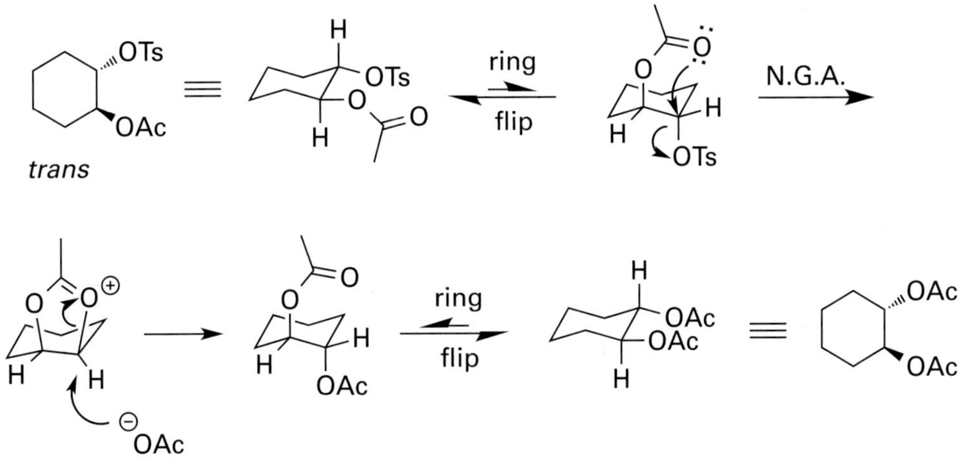

Figure 6.21 Mechanism of an S_N1-type reaction with neighboring group assistance. The acetate substituent both promotes dissociation of the C–OTs bonds and shields one side of the resulting oxygen-stabilized carbocation from reaction with acetate nucleophile, thus affording a single stereoisomeric product with retention of configuration.

The reaction of the *cis* diastereomer appears to be a normal S_N2 reaction. The acetate nucleophile reacts at the carbon bearing the better leaving group (tosylate) to afford a product with inversion of configuration at the reacting carbon center. The rate of the reaction is dependent on the concentration of the nucleophile and electrophile. When the same conditions are applied to the *trans* diastereomer, the result is unexpected and puzzling. The stereochemical outcome is that of retention of configuration and the reaction rate is independent of the concentration of nucleophile. Finally, the reaction rate is 670-fold faster for the *trans* diastereomer than for the *cis* diastereomer.

Neither the S_N1 nor S_N2 reaction mechanism seems to be fully consistent with the observed result, although the rate law suggests an S_N1-type mechanism. The reaction of the *trans* diastereomer is an example of **neighboring group assistance** in an S_N1-type reaction. Ionization of the C–OTs bond is rate-determining and is accelerated by the neighboring acetate group, which acts as a kind of "internal" nucleophile (Figure 6.21). Note that neighboring group assistance is only possible when the molecule adopts

the less-favored diaxial conformation. The acetate group is simply too far away from the reacting carbon center while in the more favored diequitorial conformation. The final step in the reaction mechanism is the addition of the "external" nucleophile (acetate) to the oxygen-stabilized carbocation intermediate. Note here that this addition is possible only from the side of the ring opposite the breaking C–O bond. This then explains why only the product with retention of configuration is formed.

We consider this reaction to be an S_N1-type process since the rate is dependent only on the substrate. Formation of the oxygen-stabilized carbocation via neighboring group participation is rate determining. The overall rate of reaction is faster with the *trans* diastereomer because the **intramolecular** addition of the internal acetate group is a much faster process than the **intermolecular** S_N2 addition of acetate to the *cis* diastereomer. Intramolecular processes are almost always much faster than equivalent intermolecular ones. Finally, note that neighboring group assistance is not possible in the *cis* diastereomer because the acetate substituent is never

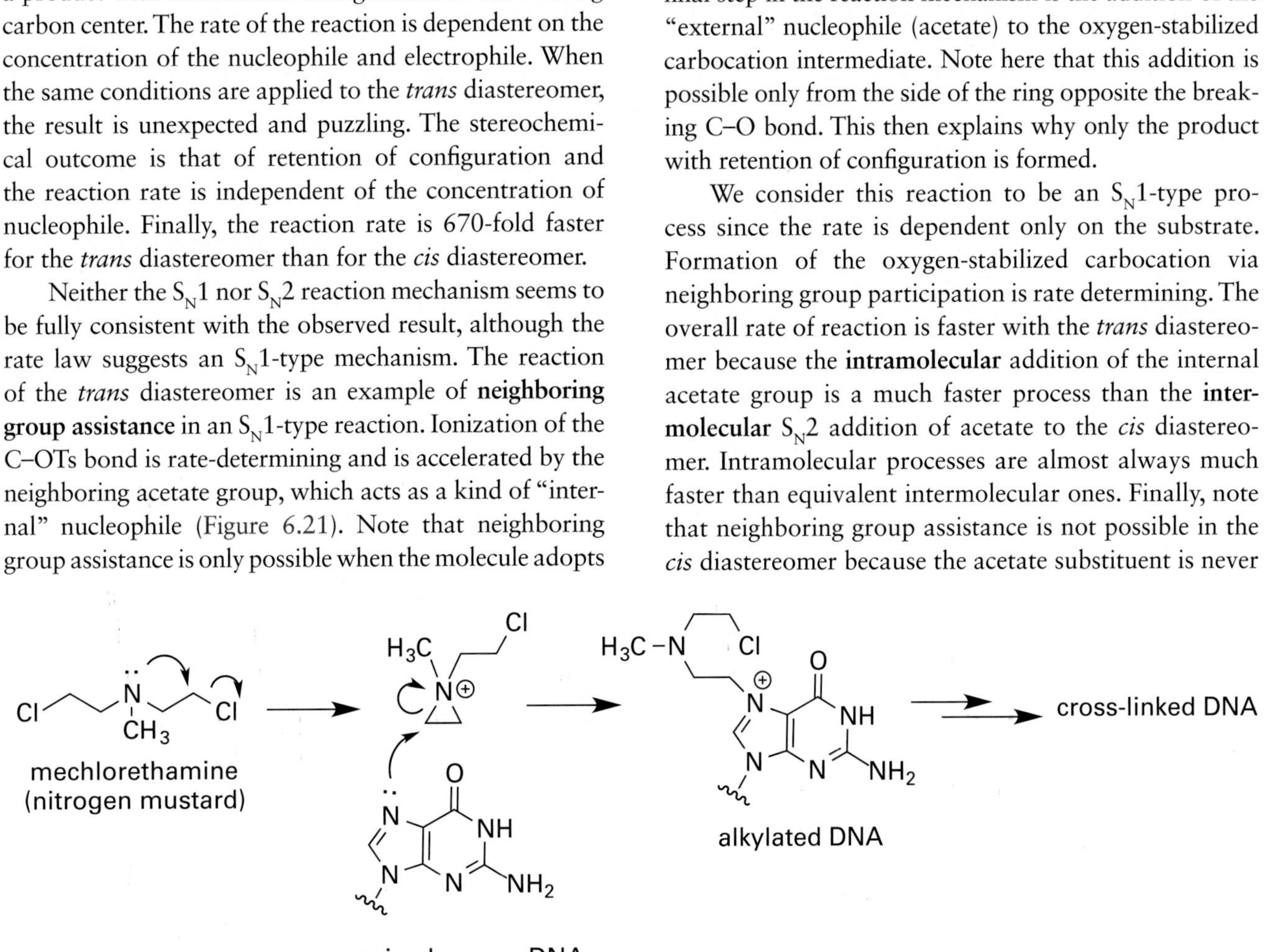

Figure 6.22 Mechanism of DNA alkylation by the nitrogen mustard mechlorethamine, a prototypical chemotherapeutic agent.

situated close enough to assist in breaking of the C–OTs bond (draw the two chair conformers of the *cis* substrate to convince yourself that this is true).

Another example of neighboring group assistance is found in the S_N1 reaction between mechlorethamine and DNA (Figure 6.22). As shown in this figure, ionization of the C–Cl bond is promoted by the neighboring nitrogen atom, leading to a cyclic nitrogen-stabilized carbocation (an aziridinium ion). This reactive intermediate reacts rapidly with a nucleophilic nitrogen atom in a nucleotide base of DNA. The remaining N–Cl bond can become activated similarly and the resulting aziridinium ion can react with a second DNA base on the same or a different strand of DNA. Thus, two S_N1 reactions with neighboring group assistance lead to cross-linking of DNA strands and eventually to cell death.

6.8 Nucleophilic Aromatic Substitution—S$_N$Ar

Nucleophilic substitution reactions of aromatic systems occur via a completely different mechanism since the sp^2 bonds involved can neither react via backside attack nor easily ionize to afford stable cationic species. For a

nucleophilic substitution reaction to occur on an aromatic substrate, it has to be activated by one or more strong electron-withdrawing groups. While such highly activated aryl rings are uncommon in drugs, they are sometimes employed as intermediates in the synthesis and manufacture of drugs. Thus, a nucleophilic aromatic substitution reaction (S_NAr for short) is the first step in the synthesis of the highly successful drug quetiapine (Seroquel®), an atypical antipsychotic used for the treatment of schizophrenia. In this S_NAr reaction, 1-chloro-2-nitrobenzene reacts with benzenethiol to produce a diaryl thioether that is then converted through additional steps to quetiapine (Figure 6.23).

For an S_NAr reaction to proceed requires both a good leaving group and at least one (often two) strongly electron-withdrawing groups such as nitro or cyano. The mechanism of the reaction involves attack of the nucleophile on the activated aryl ring to form an anionic species known as a Meisenheimer complex. This initial addition step is slow and rate-determining for S_NAr reactions since it requires breaking the aromatic character of the ring. The position of the activating group is important since only addition at the *ortho* and/or *para* position (relative to the withdrawing group) can stabilize the Meisenheimer complex (Figure 6.24). The second step in

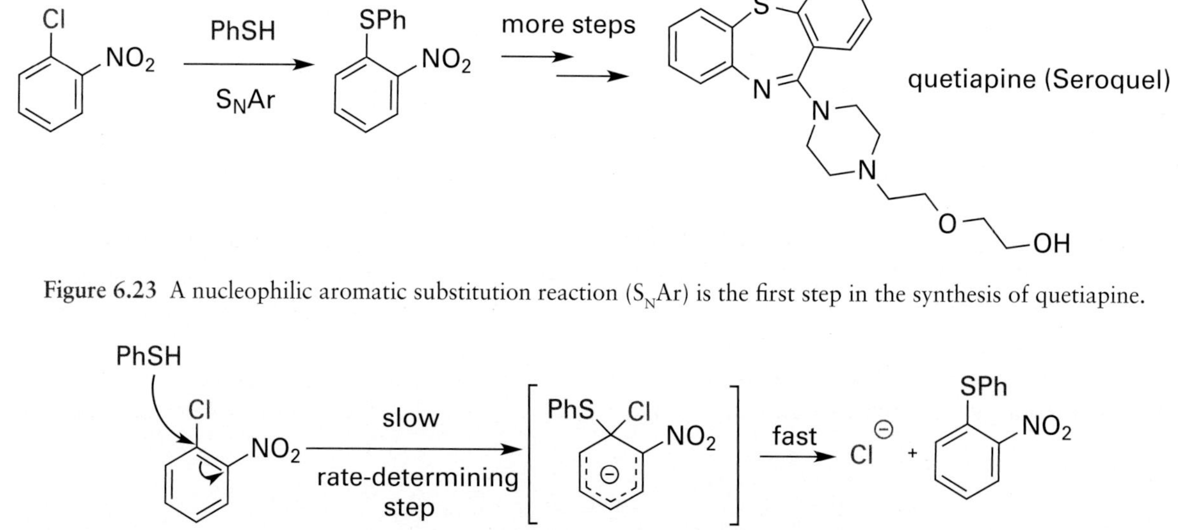

Figure 6.23 A nucleophilic aromatic substitution reaction (S_NAr) is the first step in the synthesis of quetiapine.

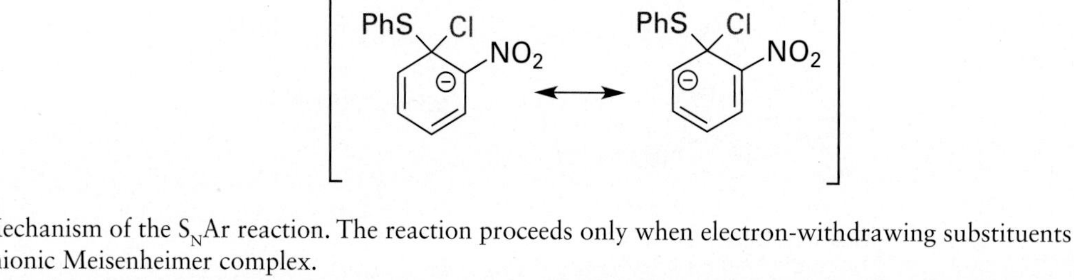

Figure 6.24 Mechanism of the S_NAr reaction. The reaction proceeds only when electron-withdrawing substituents are present to stabilize the anionic Meisenheimer complex.

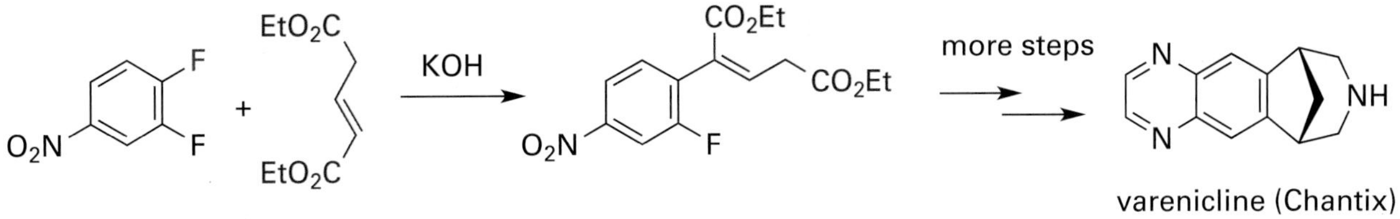

Figure 6.25 Example of an S_NAr reaction used in a synthesis of varenicline.

an S_NAr reaction is rapid and involves the loss of the leaving group and formation of the product, with aromaticity restored. The S_NAr reaction has a bimolecular rate law since the slow, rate-determining step involves both the nucleophile and electrophile. Unlike an S_N2 reaction, however, the S_NAr reaction is not a concerted process since it involves substitution via two separate steps—addition and elimination. In this sense the reaction is conceptually related to substitution reactions at the sp^2 hybridized carbon atom of a carbonyl, a topic we will explore in detail in Chapter 7.

Another example of the S_NAr reaction in the context of drug synthesis is found in a synthesis of the smoking cessation drug varenicline (Chantix®). The aromatic electrophile in this case bears a fluorine atom as the leaving group and a nitro group to activate the ring toward S_NAr reaction (Figure 6.25). Only the *para*-fluoro group reacts via S_NAr reaction. Can you explain why this might be? (Hint: Draw resonance forms of the two possible Meisenheimer complexes.)

6.9 Addition Reactions

When the reddish brown colored liquid bromine is added to a solution of 1-methylcyclohex-1-ene, the color disappears to form a colorless solution. What has happened is that the bromine molecule has undergone addition to the double bond of the cyclohexene to afford a dibromide product. This is an example of an addition reaction. Unlike a substitution reaction, all the atoms present in the two reactants are also present in the single reaction product.

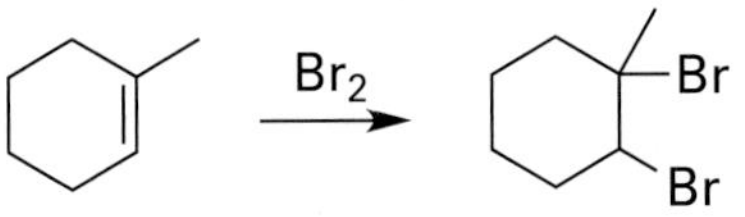

The mechanism of this reaction is quite interesting; in the first step Br–Br reacts with the π electrons of the alkene to produce a three-membered bromonium ion intermediate and a bromide anion (Figure 6.26). In the second step, the bromide anion acts as nucleophile

to open the three-membered bromonium ion ring and produce the dibromide product. Because bromide addition must occur opposite the breaking C–Br bond in the bromonium ion, the dibromide product will have *trans* stereochemistry. It was in fact the stereospecificity of this addition reaction that first suggested the possible intermediacy of a bromonium ion in the reaction.

Next, let us consider the similar addition reaction of hydrogen bromide (H–Br) to the same alkene substrate, 1-methylcyclohex-1-ene (Figure 6.27). Since the two atoms involved in the addition are now different, we might expect to observe a mixture of two reaction products. In fact, however, such reactions are usually **regioselective**, meaning that they produce primarily one product. In the 1870s, Markovnikov observed that in additions of H–X acids to unsymmetrical alkenes, the H atom usually ends up bonded to the less substituted carbon atom. This is now known as Markovnikov's rule, and may be explained by considering the reaction mechanism, as it is understood today. The molecule H–Br will be polarized according to atom electronegativity, with a significant partial positive character on hydrogen. Thus, the H atom will serve as the more electrophilic atom in reaction with the alkene π electons serving as nucleophile. If addition of H^+ occurs at the less substituted carbon atom, the resulting carbocation intermediate will be tertiary and thus relatively stable (Figure 6.27). If on the other hand addition occurs at the more substituted carbon, the resulting intermediate will be a secondary carbocation and thus less stabilized. Accordingly, the reaction proceeds primarily through the more favored tertiary carbocation intermediate and addition of bromide anion to the tertiary carbocation produces the observed product.

Another important type of addition reaction is that involving nucleophilic addition to a suitably polarized, and thus electrophilic, double bond. This is the case when a C=C bond is substituted with an electron-withdrawing group such as a carbonyl, sulfonyl, nitro, or cyano function. Addition reactions at such double bonds are known as **Michael addition** reactions and the alkene electrophiles are often referred to as Michael acceptors. The effect of the

Bromine Addition to Cyclopentene

THE OVERALL REACTION:

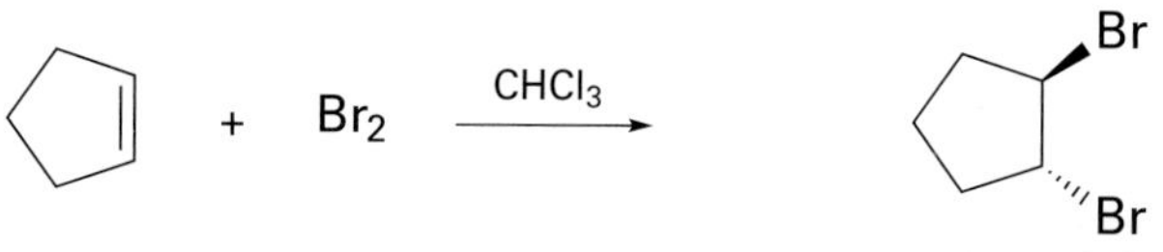

cyclopentene   bromine   trans-1,2-dibromocyclopentane (80%)

THE MECHANISM:

Step 1: Bromine acts as an electrophile and reacts with cyclopentene to form a cyclic bromonium ion. This is the rate-determining step.

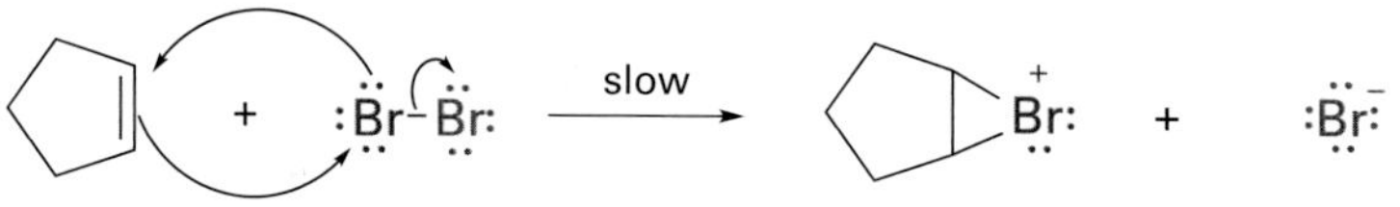

cyclopentene   bromine   bromonium ion   bromide ion
                                          intermediate

Step 2: Bromide ion acts as a nucleophile, forming a bond to one of the carbons of the bromonium ion and displacing the positively charged bromine from that carbon. Because substitutions of this type normally occur with the nucleophile approaching carbon from the side opposite the bond that is broken, the two bromine atoms end up in a *trans* relationship in the product.

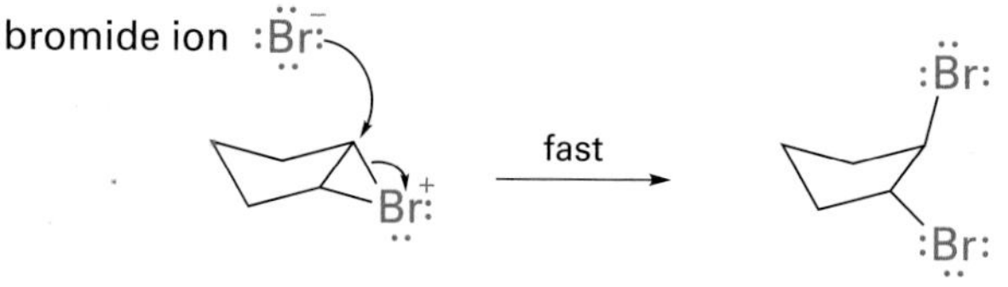

bromonium ion   trans-1,2-
intermediate   dibromocyclopentane

Figure 6.26 Bromide addition to cyclopentene. (Reproduced, with permission, from Carey FA, Giuliano RM. *Organic Chemistry.* 9th ed. New York: McGraw-Hill Education; 2014.)

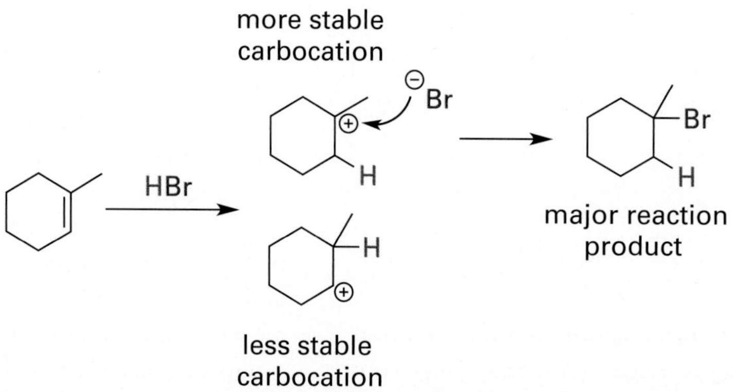

more stable
carbocation

less stable
carbocation

major reaction
product

Figure 6.27 Addition of hydrogen bromide across the double bond of an alkene substrate. The reaction is regioselective, with the major product resulting from the more stable tertiary carbocation intermediate.

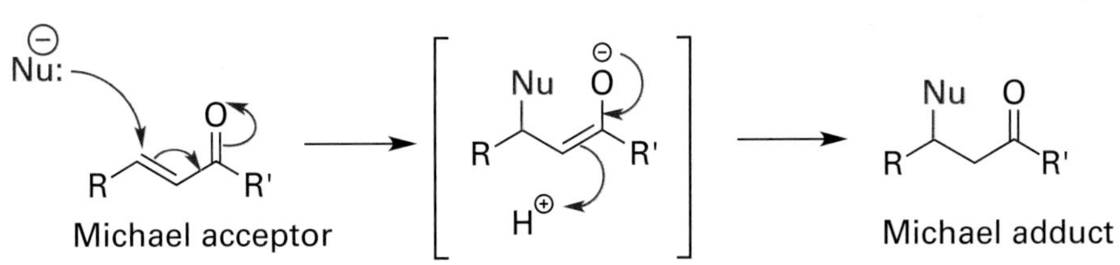

Figure 6.28 Reaction mechanism of the Michael addition reaction between a nucleophile and a polarized double bond.

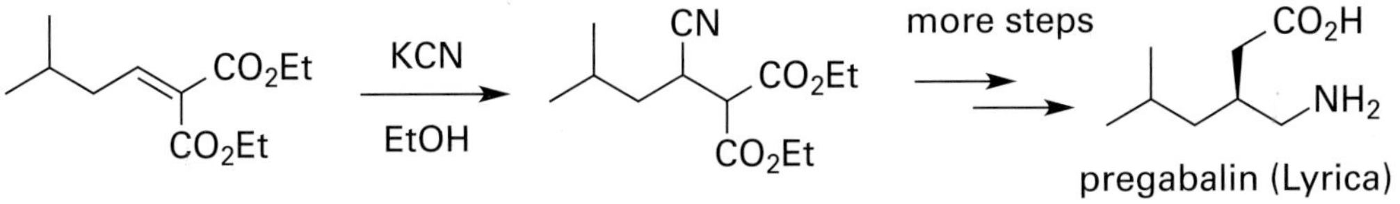

Figure 6.29 Example of a Michael addition reaction used in a synthesis of the drug pregabalin.

electron-withdrawing group in a Michael acceptor is to polarize the double bond such that the β-carbon has partial positive character and is thus electrophilic. The reaction mechanism is illustrated for a generic nucleophile in Figure 6.28. The carbonyl function (the EWG) serves both to polarize the double bond for reaction and then, after nucleophilic addition, to stabilize the resulting negative charge on an electronegative (oxygen) atom. The second step of the reaction is usually protonation of the anionic intermediate to afford the final addition product.

Michael addition reaction is a useful reaction in the synthesis of some drugs. The synthesis of pregabalin (Lyrica®), for example, involves the Michael addition of cyanide anion to an α,β-unsaturated diester (Figure 6.29). Michael reaction between a drug molecule and nucleophilic residues (usually cysteine thiols) on its target can be an effective mechanism of drug action. Of course, such an approach carries with it the risk of undesired Michael addition to other non-targeted biomolecules. This might lead to undesired side effects and can provoke an immune response to the resulting drug-protein conjugate.

Nevertheless, the targeting of nucleophilic residues on kinases and proteases is an area of growing interest in drug discovery, with some recent examples described in the case study at the end of this chapter.

6.10 Elimination Reactions— E1 and E2

Whereas addition reactions see the addition of H–Br or Nu–H across a double bond, elimination reactions are effectively the reverse of these same processes. The two most common mechanisms of the reaction, denoted **E1** and **E2**, share aspects of the S_N1 and S_N2 mechanisms discussed in previous sections. Thus, whereas an addition reaction adds H–Br across a double bond to form a saturated product, the corresponding elimination reaction extrudes H–Br from a saturated substrate to form a double bond in the product (Figure 6.30). Similarly, the product of Michael addition can undergo elimination to reform a double bond, in what is sometimes called a

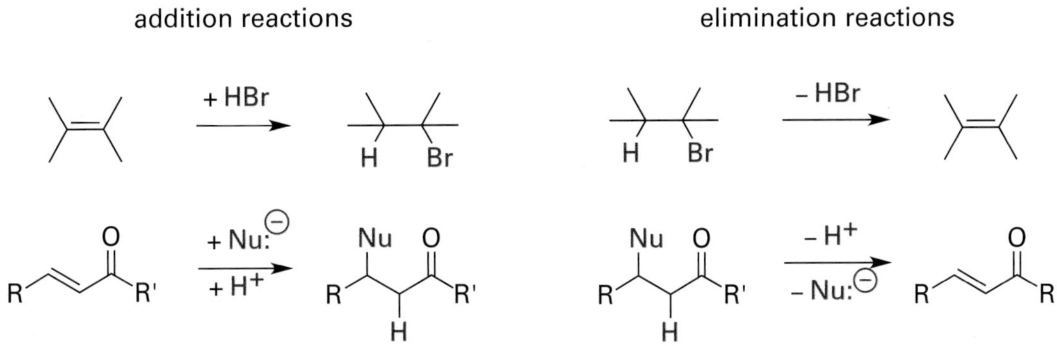

addition reactions   elimination reactions

Figure 6.30 Elimination reactions are conceptually the reverse of addition reactions.

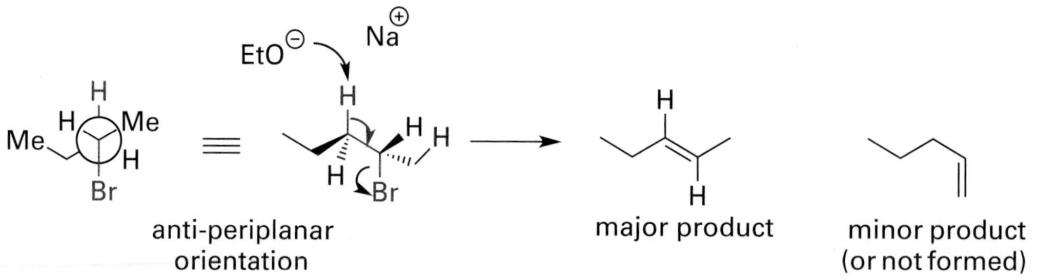

Figure 6.31 Newman projection and wedge-and-dash drawings illustrating the anti-periplanar orientation of bonds required for an E2 elimination reaction. Note also that the proton (shown in blue) on the more highly substituted carbon atom reacts preferentially to afford the product with the more highly substituted double bond.

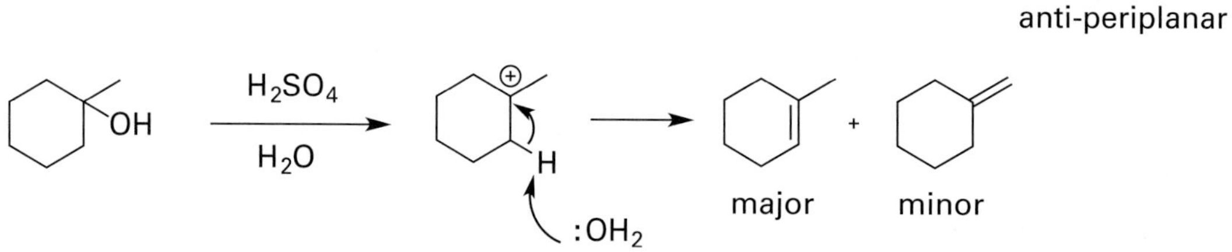

Figure 6.32 Mechanism of the E1 elimination reaction. The initial rate-determining step involves formation of the tertiary carbocation intermediate.

retro-Michael reaction. Elimination reactions require the presence of a base, ideally a relatively strong base that is also not very nucleophilic. In fact, elimination reactions are often an undesired side-reaction in nucleophilic substitution reactions; the degree of elimination versus substitution will depend on the nature of the nucleophile/base. Generally speaking, strong nucleophiles prefer to undergo nucleophilic substitution reactions and strong bases tend to promote elimination reactions.

The first mechanism of elimination we discuss is the bimolecular elimination, or E2 for short. The rate of an E2 elimination reaction depends on the concentrations of both the base and the substrate. This rate law implies that bond breaking and bond making occur simultaneously and thus the E2 reaction, like the S_N2 reaction, is a concerted process. In a typical E2 reaction, the base (e.g., sodium ethoxide in the example in Figure 6.31) extracts a proton from the substrate, which leads to the simultaneous loss of a leaving group (e.g., bromide anion) and the formation of a double bond (Figure 6.31). If we view this elimination reaction in Newman projection we see that the C–H and C–Br bonds are positioned opposite one another (i.e., in an anti-conformation). This **anti-periplanar** orientation of breaking bonds is in fact a requirement for E2 elimination reactions. In molecular orbital terms, the σ orbitals of the breaking bonds must be anti-periplanar because these bonds will become the

p orbitals of the new π-bond that is formed in the E2 reaction. When a proton might be abstracted from more than one different carbon atoms, **Zaitsev's rule** predicts that the major product is the one with the more highly substituted double bond. Thus in the example in Figure 6.31, the proton in blue is abstracted in preference to that in red and the resulting product is that with carbon substitution on both sides of the double bond.

Elimination reactions can also occur by a mechanism that is closely related to the S_N1 substitution reaction. Thus, the rate law for a unimolecular elimination reaction (E1 for short) depends only on the concentration of the substrate. As in an S_N1 reaction, the rate-determining step involves breaking of a bond in the substrate to form a carbocation intermediate. Thus, E1 reactions will be favored when the substrate can easily stabilize a carbocation, as in the case of 1-hydroxy-1-methylcyclohexane, which upon heating in aqueous sulfuric acid produces a tertiary carbocation by ionization of the C–OH bond (Figure 6.32). The second, fast step of an E1 reaction is the breaking of a neighboring C–H bond to liberate a proton (H⁺) and produce the alkene product. Once the carbocation is formed, the neighboring C–H bonds will become quite acidic, so that even a weak base such as water is sufficiently basic to accept the proton that is liberated in the elimination. Note that Zaitsev's rule also applies to E1 elimination reactions and predicts formation of the more highly substituted alkene product.

6.11 Summary

Section 6.1   **Substitution** reactions involve bond making between a **nucleophile** and **electrophile** with the loss of a **leaving group**. These processes are prevalent in physiological and metabolic processes and in the manufacture of drugs.

Section 6.2   A **nucleophile** is a Lewis base that can donate an electron pair in the formation of a new bond. Nucleophilicity refers to the relative reactivity of a nucleophile in reaction with electrophiles. It is determined by several factors including electronegativity, basicity, and polarizability.

Section 6.3   **Electrophiles** are Lewis acids that can accept an electron pair in the formation of a new bond. The polarization of bonds produces electrophilic sites in molecules. A strong electrophile possesses a weak bond to a good leaving group, such as in the molecule methyl iodide (CH_3–I).

Section 6.4   Leaving groups are species that can readily accept and stabilize an electron pair upon the breaking of a bond to the leaving group. Weak bases (the conjugate bases of strong acids) generally make good leaving groups.

Section 6.5   The bimolecular nucleophilic substitution reaction (S_N2) is a **concerted** process in which bond making occurs concurrently with bond breaking. These reactions occur with backside attack of the nucleophile on the breaking bond, resulting in inversion of configuration at the reacting center. The rate of the S_N2 reaction is also affected by the steric environment around the reacting carbon center.

Section 6.6   The S_N1 reaction occurs via discreet steps and involves a carbocation intermediate. The rate-determining step in an S_N1 reaction is the formation of a carbocation intermediate. The reaction rate is highly impacted by the nature of the electrophilic carbon center and leaving group but less so by the nature of the nucleophile.

Section 6.7   Substitution reactions can be significantly accelerated when an internal nucleophile is positioned to promote loss of a leaving group and/or stabilization of a carbocation intermediate. This effect is known as **neighboring group assistance** and can affect both the rate and stereochemical outcome of the reaction.

Section 6.8   Nucleophilic aromatic substitution (S_NAr) involves a slow, rate-determining addition step to form an anionic Meisenheimer complex, followed by a rapid elimination step. The aromatic electrophile must be activated by one or more electron-withdrawing substituents such as nitro or cyano positioned *ortho* or *para* to the leaving group.

Section 6.9   The **addition reaction** of HBr across an unsymmetrical alkene occurs according to Markovnikov's rule to produce the more highly substituted bromide product. This results from preferential formation of the more stabilized carbocation intermediate. The addition of nucleophiles to highly polarized double bonds is known as the **Michael reaction**.

Section 6.10   **E1** and **E2** elimination reactions are conceptually the reverse of addition reactions. Both reactions follow Zaitsev's rule, which states that the more highly substituted alkene product will predominate when multiple regioisomeric alkene products are possible.

6.12 Case Study—Drugs That Form a Covalent Bond to Their Target

We have seen in this chapter that some cancer drugs exert their cytotoxic effects by forming covalent bonds with their target (e.g., the reaction of mechlorethamine with DNA bases). A number of well-known drugs including aspirin and omeprazole work by covalent modification of their targets. In most such cases, however, the reactive nature of the drug was not appreciated at the time of its discovery or approval. In modern drug discovery, the idea of *intentionally* designing drugs to react with their target is controversial. Avoiding covalent modification of the target is probably advisable in the case of chronic conditions (e.g., pain, autoimmune disease) where a drug must be administered over years or even a lifetime. In the case of more acute conditions such as cancer or infection, however, the potential benefits of covalent drugs may outweigh the risks.

One area where the idea of covalent drugs has garnered attention is the treatment of cancer, and specifically in the development of kinase inhibitors. Kinases mediate a wide variety of cellular signaling events by transferring a phosphate group to specific oxygen atom(s) on their substrate(s). When a kinase is aberrantly activated or inactivated, the resulting effects on signaling pathways can result in the unrestrained cell growth that is characteristic of cancer. The first kinase inhibitor approved to treat cancer was imatinib (Gleevec®). The success of this drug in treating certain kinase-driven cancers demonstrated the potential of kinase inhibition as a new therapeutic

approach in oncology. However, producing selective kinase inhibitors can be challenging because most kinase inhibitors target the ATP-binding site, which is quite similar across the roughly 500 known human kinases. One approach to improve selectivity has been to design kinase inhibitors to react with the thiol (–SH) group of specific cysteine residues present only in a subset of kinases. Two recently approved kinase inhibitor drugs that were intentionally designed to react with their kinase targets are ibrutinib (Imbruvica®) and afatinib (Gilotrif®). Both drugs possess a side chain with an electrophilic Michael acceptor (Figure 6.33).

Afatinib is an irreversible inhibitor of a family of membrane-bound receptor tyrosine kinases that includes EGFR and HER2. Mutations in EGFR are implicated in some head and neck tumors while overproduction of HER2 is associated with some breast cancers. Afatinib binds in the ATP-binding site of EGFR with its electrophilic side chain positioned in close proximity to cysteine-797. Afatinib targets an analogous cysteine residue (Cys805) on HER2. With the electrophilic drug and nucleophilic cysteine thiol in close proximity, a nucleophilic addition (Michael reaction) can occur (Figure 6.34). Note that non-covalent binding of afatinib to EGFR (or HER2) must occur prior to the subsequent covalent reaction; the initial non-covalent binding is what brings the reacting groups into proximity. This proximity effect may explain why such drugs react selectively with specific

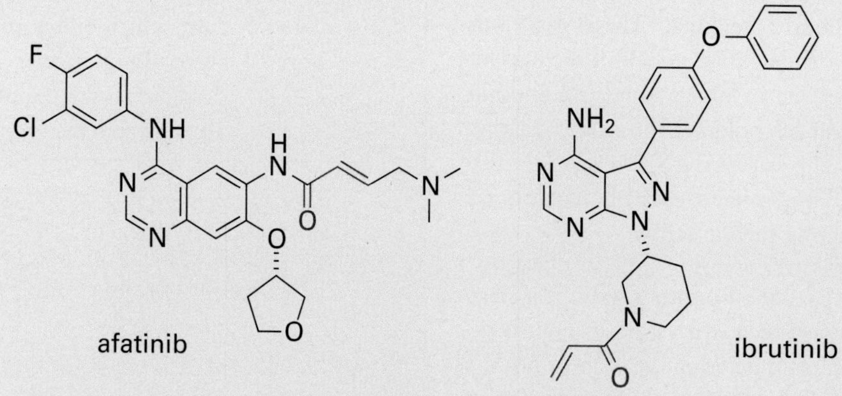

Figure 6.33 Structures of irreversible kinase inhibitors afatinib and ibrutinib. Each compound bears an electrophilic side chain (shown in red) intended to react with a nucleophilic cysteine residue on the kinase target.

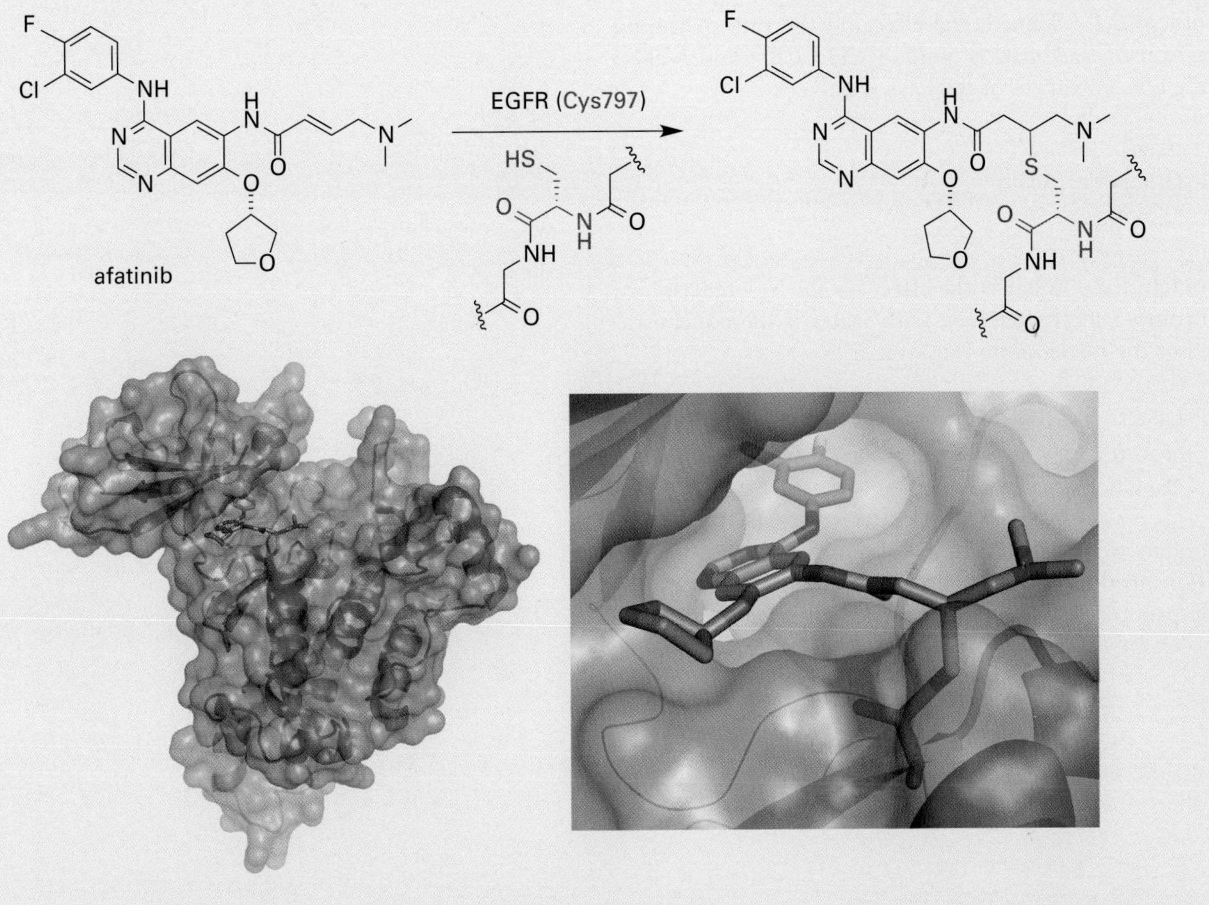

Figure 6.34 Top: Michael addition reaction between the electrophilic side chain of afatinib and the nucleophilic thiol of Cys797 on the receptor tyrosine kinase EGFR. Bottom: Two images created from the X-ray crystal structure of EGFR with afatinib bound. The covalent bond between afatinib and Cys797 is apparent in the close-up image of the ATP-binding site (bottom, right).

cysteine residues on their target and do not react randomly with any exposed cysteine thiol.

Ibrutinib is an irreversible inhibitor of a different kinase, Bruton's tyrosine kinase (BTK), and is currently approved to treat mantel cell lymphoma and chronic lymphocytic leukemia. The drug binds covalently to Cys-481 in the ATP-binding site of BTK, resulting in potent inhibition of kinase activity.

Initial indications are that ibrutinib is well tolerated and effective in CLL patients that have typically had a poor prognosis, such as those with relapsing disease. Time will tell if the success of new drugs like ibrutinib and afatinib leads to greater interest in drugs designed to form covalent bonds with their biological targets.

6.13 Exercises

Problem 6.1 What is the effect on the rate of the E2 reaction of *tert*-butyl bromide [$(CH_3)_3CBr$] and NaOH if the concentration of the base is halved?

> Faster
> Slower
> No Change

Problem 6.2 What is the effect on the S_N1 reaction of 3-bromo-3-methylpentane with water if the concentration of the nucleophile is doubled?

> Faster
> Slower
> No Change

Problem 6.3 Predict and draw the structures of the *major* product in the following reactions. If a minor side-product is also expected, suggest what it might be.

(a)

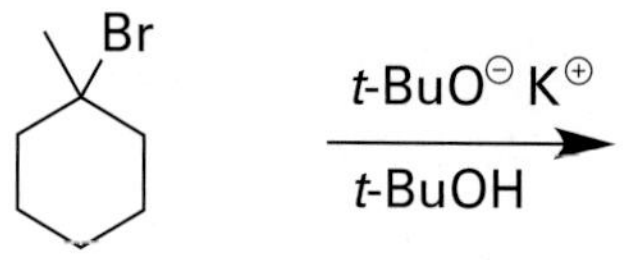

$$\xrightarrow[\text{t-BuOH}]{\text{t-BuO}^\ominus\text{K}^\oplus}$$

(b)

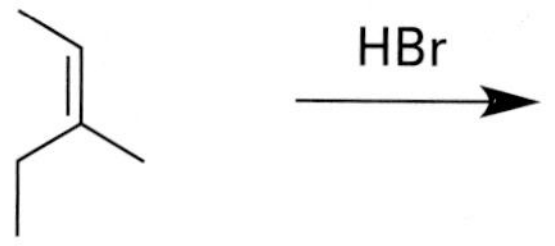

$$\xrightarrow{\text{HBr}}$$

(c)

$$\xrightarrow{\text{MeO}^\ominus\text{Na}^\oplus}$$

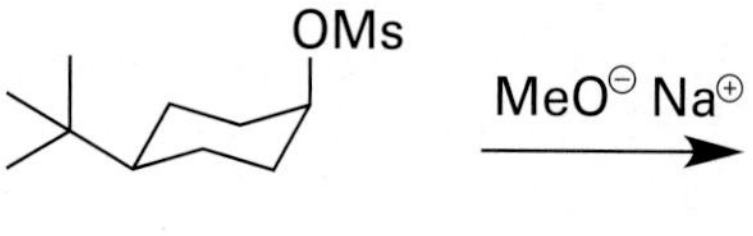

Problem 6.4   Predict the major product for reaction (i) and (ii) shown below. What is the reaction mechanism (S_N1, S_N2, E1, E2, etc.) leading to the major product you predicted? Explain your reasoning in each case.

(i)

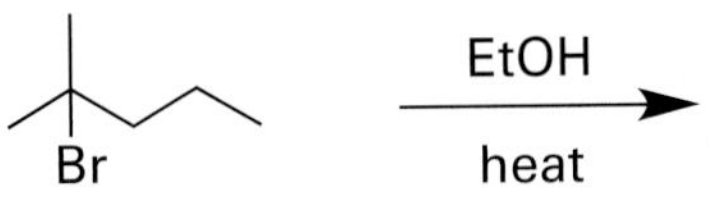

EtOH
heat

(ii)

$t\text{-BuO}^{\ominus}\,\text{Na}^{\oplus}$
$t\text{-BuOH}$

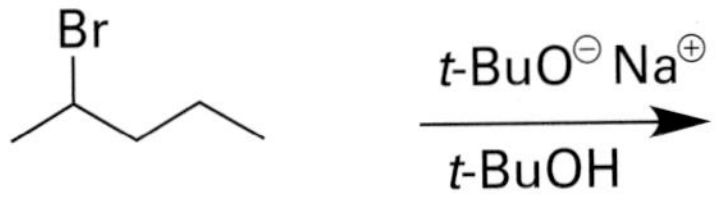

Problem 6.5   Predict the product(s) of the following reactions. Explain your predictions based on the likely reaction mechanism.

(a)

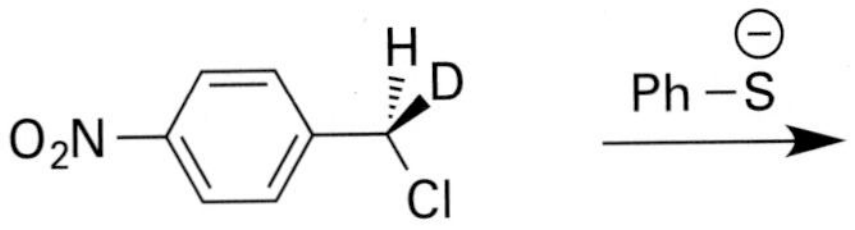

$Ph-\overset{\ominus}{S}$

(b)

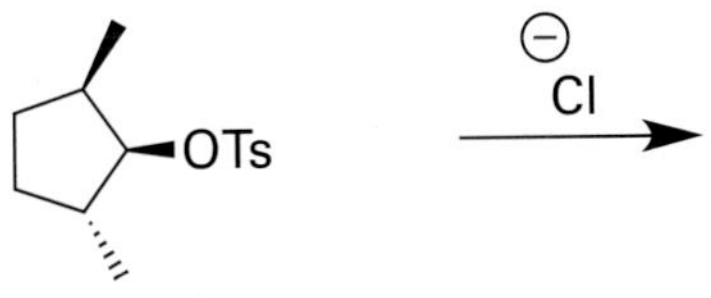

$\overset{\ominus}{Cl}$

(c)

$\overset{\ominus}{C}\equiv N$

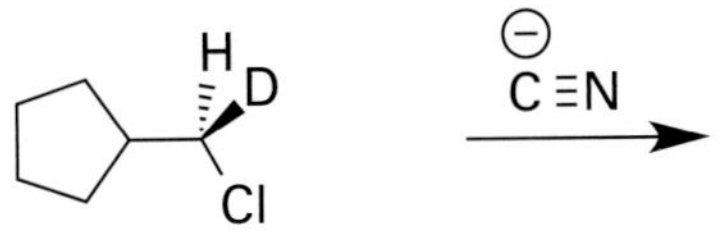

Problem 6.6 For the following reactions two different starting materials are shown. In each case, predict which compound will react faster and draw the product(s) of that reaction. Explain your prediction, considering factors such as the likely reaction mechanism, the strength of nucleophile or electrophile, and, where relevant, steric or conformational effects.

(a)

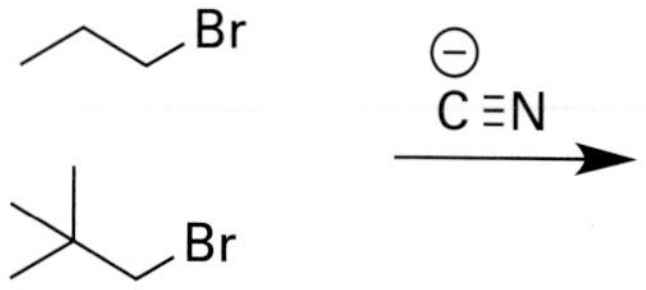

(b)

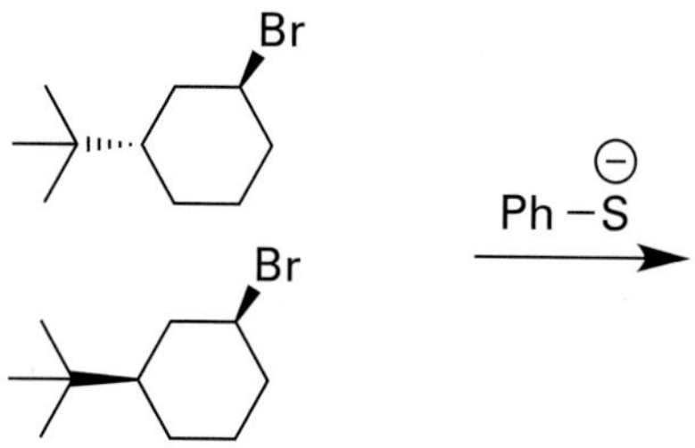

(c)

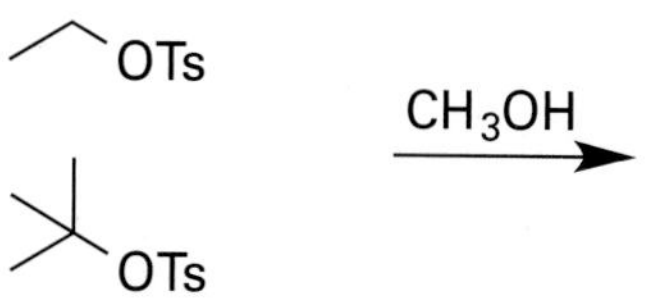

(d)

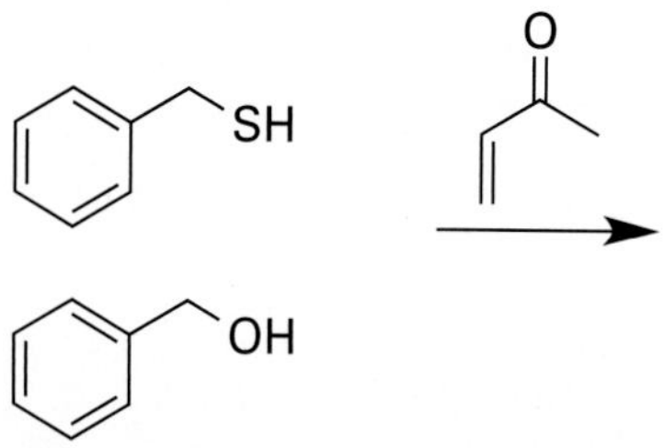

(e)

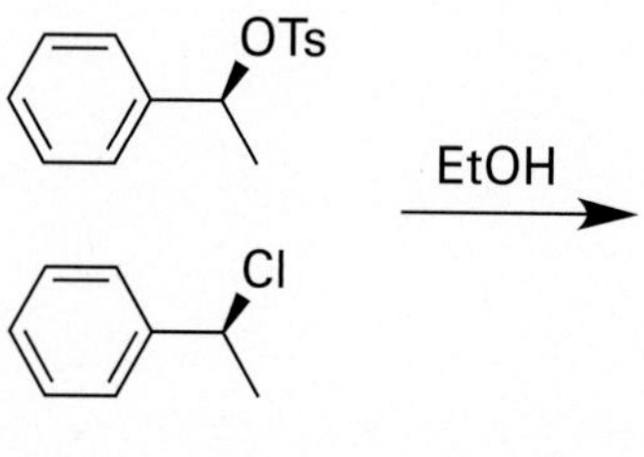

Problem 6.7 Consider the two reactions shown below and then answer questions (a) through (d).

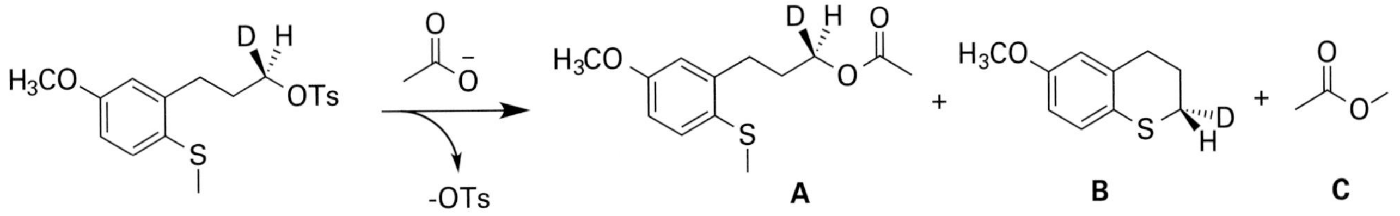

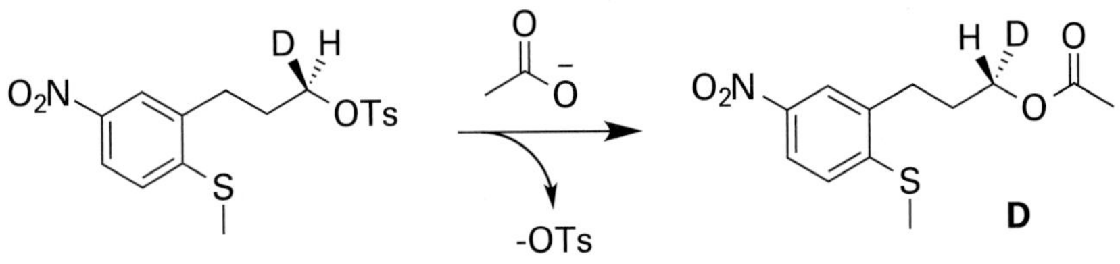

(a) For each of the products **A**, **B**, and **D**, indicate whether stereochemical configuration is retained or inverted?

(b) Write a mechanism that accounts for the formation of products **A–C**.

(c) Write a mechanism that accounts for the formation of product **D**.

(d) Explain in words why these two reactions proceed via different mechanisms.

Chapter 7

Reactions of Carbonyl Species

Adam Renslo

CHAPTER OUTLINE

7.1 Introduction

7.2 Nature of the Carbonyl Group

7.3 Relative Reactivity of Carbonyl-Containing Functional Groups

7.4 Hydration of Aldehydes and Ketones

7.5 Reactions of Aldehydes and Ketones with Alcohols

　　Box 7.1—Glucuronidation in the metabolism of drugs

7.6 Imines and Enamines

　　Box 7.2—Imines in drug-protein conjugates

7.7 Oximes and Hydrazones

7.8 Chemical Hydrolysis of Ester and Amide Bonds

7.9 Enzymatic Hydrolysis of Peptide Bonds by Proteases

　　Box 7.3—Drugs designed to inhibit proteases

7.10 Summary

7.11 *Case Study*—Odanacatib

7.12 Exercises

7.1 Introduction

In this chapter we explore the structure and reactivity of the **carbonyl** (C=O) bond and related carbon–heteroatom (C=X) double bonds. These functional groups are ubiquitous in both biological molecules and in the structures of drugs. A prominent example in biological molecules is the amide bond (peptide bond), which serves as the structural backbone of proteins and also helps determine how proteins fold into the specific three-dimensional shapes that lead to function. Other biological molecules containing ketone or thioester functions are involved in cellular metabolism and in sterol biosynthesis in animals and terpene biosynthesis in plants.

Carbonyl-containing functional groups are also found in the structures of many drugs. Often these groups play a structural role, linking and helping to properly orient other functionality for interaction with the drug's target. These groups can also make direct contact with the target, forming hydrogen bonds and other intermolecular interactions as we have seen in Chapter 2. The chemical reactivity of carbonyl functional groups can also be important in drug action, as is the case for the cyclic amide (β-lactam) present in penicillins and related β-lactam antibiotics. This chapter examines many important classes of carbonyl-containing functional groups and reviews the biologically relevant chemistry of the carbonyl.

7.2 Nature of the Carbonyl Group

Carbonyl-containing functional groups are those possessing a double bond between a carbon and oxygen atom (C=O). The molecular orbital description of a carbonyl involves a σ bond between sp^2 hybrid orbitals on carbon and oxygen atoms and a π bond involving the $2p$ orbitals on the bonded atoms. It is the interacting p orbitals of the π bond that prevents rotation about the

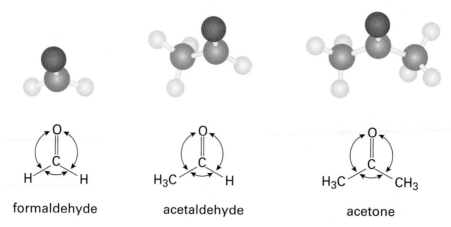

| formaldehyde | acetaldehyde | acetone |

Figure 7.1 Structures and stick models of carbonyl groups in formaldehyde, acetaldehyde, and acetone. (Reproduced, with permission, from Carey FA, Giuliano RM. *Organic Chemistry*. 9th ed. New York: McGraw-Hill Education; 2014.)

C=O bond. The two remaining sp^2 hybrid orbitals on carbon form σ bonds with additional substituents that lie in the plane of the carbonyl bond, and separated by ~120° (Figure 7.1). Two electron lone pairs on oxygen project out at a ~120° angle and can accept hydrogen bonds or be protonated under acidic conditions.

The bonding between carbon and oxygen in a carbonyl is analogous to that between the carbon atoms of ethylene. The greater electronegativity of oxygen as compared to carbon, however, means that electron density in the carbonyl function is polarized. This polarization can also be understood in resonance terms, the resonance forms shown below implying partial positive character at carbon and partial negative character at oxygen. These partial charges can be indicated as a dipole or using the δ+ and δ− nomenclature we have used previously (Figure 7.2).

This polarization is an important contributor to the reactivity of the carbonyl group as it makes the carbon atom electrophilic and thus reactive with nucleophiles. Substituents that reduce polarization of the C=O bond make the carbonyl less reactive while substituents that increase polarization make the carbonyl more reactive. Hydrogen bonding to (or protonation of) the lone pair electrons of a carbonyl increases its polarization and thus enhances its reactivity with nucleophiles.

Steric effects between carbon substituents represent another important contributor to carbonyl reactivity. Reaction of a carbonyl with a nucleophile results in a change from planar sp^2 hybridization to tetrahedral sp^3 hybridization. The introduction of a new substituent (from the nucleophile) combined with the smaller 109.5° bond angle associated with sp^3 hybridization

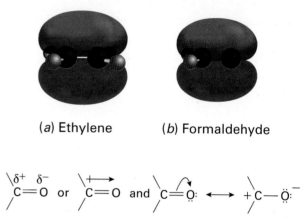

(a) Ethylene   *(b)* Formaldehyde

Figure 7.2 Shown at top is a molecular orbital view of formaldehyde showing the π bond formed by overlap of *p* orbitals on carbon and oxygen. Polarization of the carbonyl bond can be illustrated using resonance structures, as partial charges, or as a dipole. (Reproduced, with permission, from Carey FA, Giuliano RM. *Organic Chemistry*. 9th ed. New York: McGraw-Hill Education; 2014.)

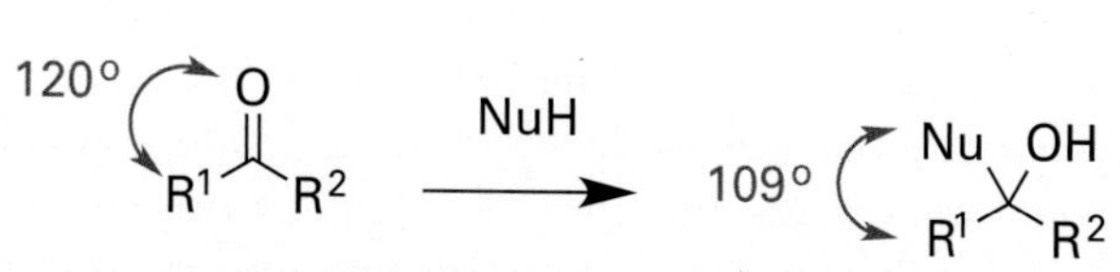

Figure 7.3 Nucleophilic addition to a carbonyl results in a change from sp^2 to sp^3 hybridization and a reduction in bond angle from ~120° to ~109.5° at carbon. The smaller bond angle results in greater steric strain in the product of the reaction.

leads to greater steric strain in the tetrahedral product (Figure 7.3). This steric effect will be greatest when the transition state for the addition reaction is "late" (i.e., when it resembles the tetrahedral product). As we discuss the reactivity of various functional groups in the sections that follow it will be helpful to keep in mind the two main contributors to carbonyl reactivity—polarization of the carbonyl bond and the size of the carbonyl substituents.

7.3 Relative Reactivity of Carbonyl-Containing Functional Groups

The simplest carbonyl-containing functional group is the **aldehyde** and the simplest aldehyde is formaldehyde. The hydrogen atoms in formaldehyde can do little to stabilize the positive character of the carbonyl carbon and hence this carbonyl is quite polarized. Add to this the very small size of the carbonyl substituents (hydrogen atoms) and we might expect that formaldehyde should be quite reactive with nucleophiles. Indeed, the reaction of formaldehyde with even a weak nucleophile

such as water is very favorable, and in aqueous solution >99.9% of formaldehyde exists in the "hydrated" form (Table 7.1). Acetaldehyde, with methyl and hydrogen substituents, is less reactive than formaldehyde for both electronic and steric reasons and only about 50% hydrated in aqueous solution. Addition of a second methyl group on carbon leads to a **ketone** (acetone) that is only ~0.14% hydrated in aqueous solution.

Electronic effects on carbonyl reactivity can be mediated through both inductive and resonance effects. A striking example of carbonyl activaton by an inductive effect is evident in comparing the hydration equilibrium constants for acetaldehyde and trifluoroacetaldehyde. The trifluoromethyl group is significantly bulkier than methyl, yet the highly electron-withdrawing nature of this substituent results in a hydration equilibrium constant even greater than that of formaldehyde (Table 7.1).

Table 7.1 Hydration Reaction for Selected Aldehydes and Ketones.

Reaction	K_{hydr}	Percent hydrate
Formaldehyde + water 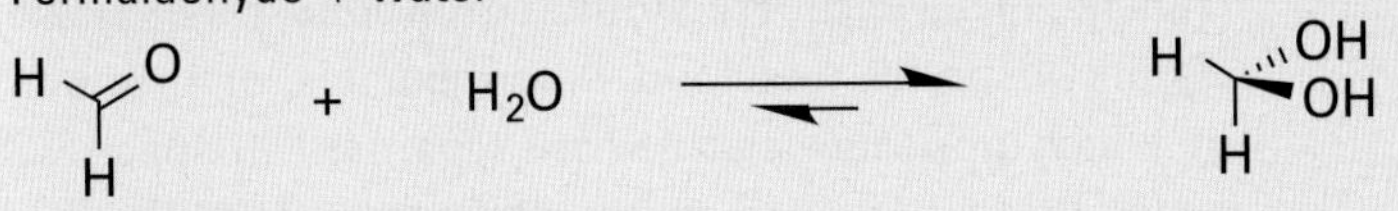	2300	>99.9
Acetaldehyde + water 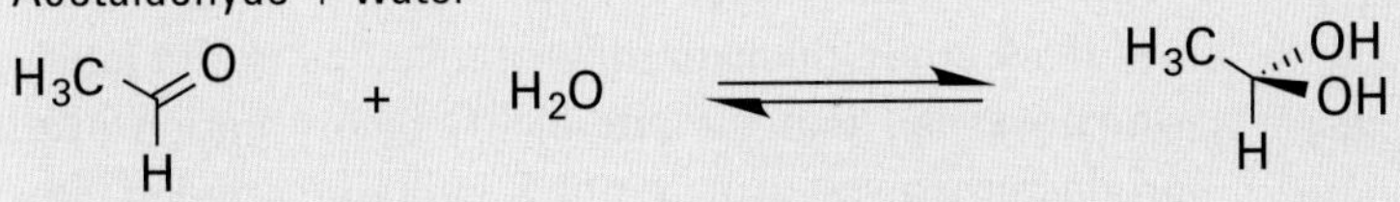	1.0	50
Pivaldehyde + water 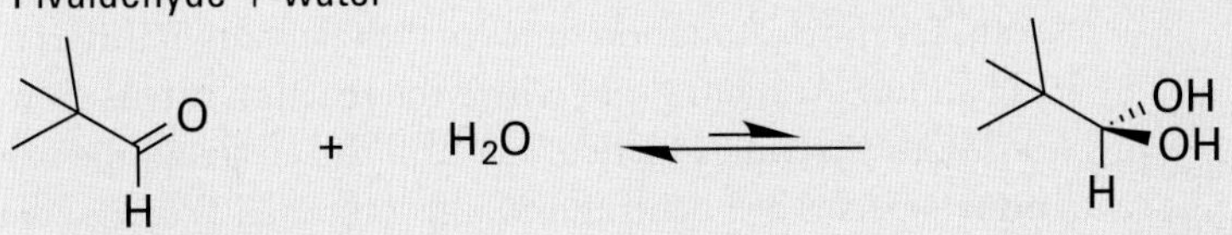	0.2	17
Acetone + water 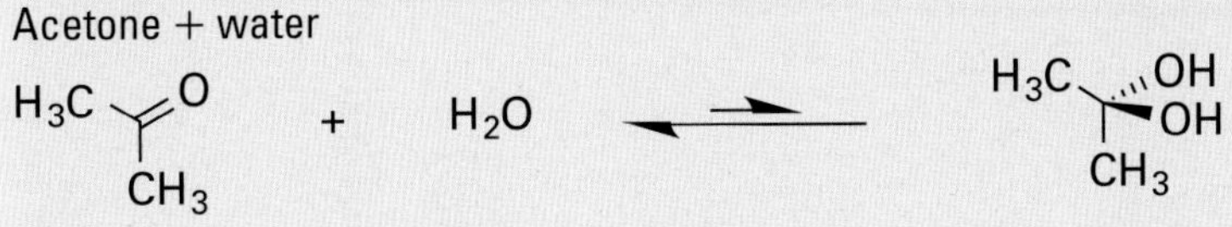	0.0014	0.14
Fluoroacetaldehyde + water 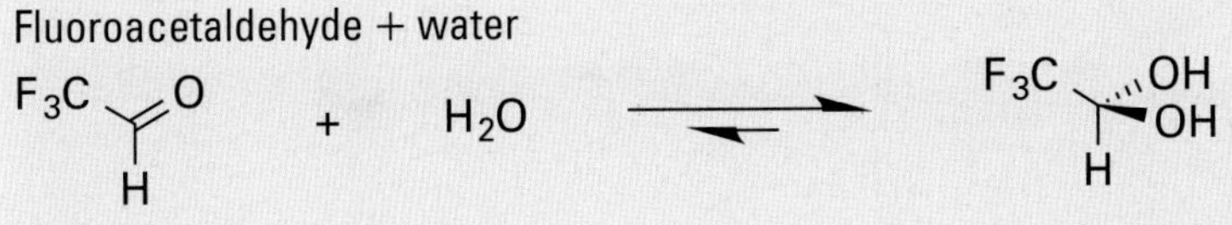	29,000	>99.9
Benzaldehyde + water 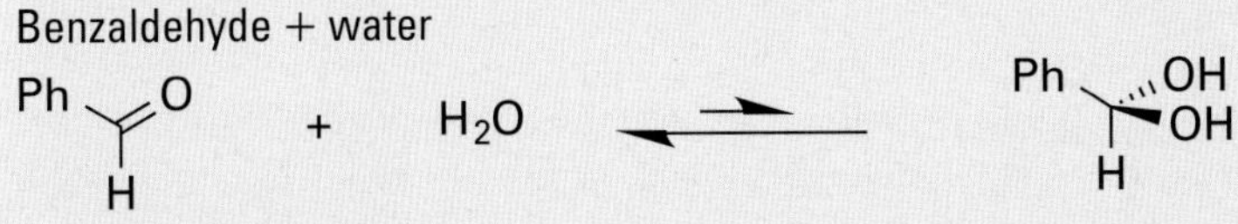	0.008	0.8

K_{hydr}, Equilibrium constant.

Resonance effects can also have a dramatic effect on the reactivity of aldehydes and ketones. In the case of benzaldehyde, for example, the carbonyl π bond is delocalized into the π system of the aromatic ring, thereby reducing the degree of carbonyl polarization. As a result, benzaldehyde is much less electrophilic than acetaldehyde or even pivaldehyde with its very bulky *tert*-butyl group. When a C=O bond is immediately adjacent to a C=C bond, the effect is to reduce polarization of the C=O bond while increasing polarization of the C=C. These effects in the molecule acrolein are illustrated using resonance structures and partial charge nomenclature (Figure 7.4).

Inductive and resonance effects also help determine the reactivity of C=O bonds substituted with non-carbon atoms like oxygen, sulfur, nitrogen, or chlorine (Figure 7.5). Acid chlorides have highly reactive carbonyls because of the strong inductive electron-with-drawing effect of the chlorine atom and also because chloride (Cl⁻) is a good leaving group (it is the conjugate base of hydrochloric acid, a strong acid). Acid anhydrides are nearly as reactive as acid chlorides, having a leaving group (acetate) in which negative charge is shared between two electronegative oxygen atoms. Next in order of reactivity are aldehydes and ketones, followed by esters, which are generally less reactive than ketones or aldehydes because the −OR substituent donates significant electron density by a resonance effect. Thioesters are *more* reactive than esters since the lone pair electrons on sulfur are in *d* orbitals that have poor overlap with the carbonyl π bond and thus provide less resonance stabilization than in an ester. Amides are significantly less electrophilic than esters because of the reduced electronegativity of nitrogen compared to oxygen combined with a stronger electron-donating resonance effect. We generally consider carboxylic acids to be non-electrophilic since under physiological conditions these groups exist in the carboxylate form with

the negative charge fully delocalized into the carbonyl bond. This leaves no significant electrophilic character at carbon in a carboxylate.

7.4 Hydration of Aldehydes and Ketones

Water serves as solvent for the chemistry of life and so the reactions of water, whether acting as a nucleophile or serving as an acid or base, are of significant interest. In this section, we explore in depth the mechanism of the hydration of aldehydes and ketones under different reaction conditions. In the previous section we have seen how the types of substituents on a carbonyl function can greatly impact the equilibrium constant (K_{hydr}) of the hydration reaction (Table 7.1). While equilibrium constants can tell us about the *thermodynamics* of a hydration reaction, studying the *kinetics* of these reactions can shed light on the reaction mechanism. In the mechanistic discussions that follow, it will be helpful to remember two general points. The first is that C–O bond forming reactions, such as in the addition of water to a carbonyl, are usually much slower processes than proton transfer (acid-base) reactions. The second point is that chemical species (reactants, intermediates, or products) in which opposing charges are separated in space will generally be higher in energy than neutral species with more evenly distributed charge.

If we study the hydration of a ketone in ¹⁸O-labeled water, we find that the rate of ¹⁸O incorporation in the product is slowest around pH 7 and more rapid at either acidic or basic pH. To understand why this is so, we must consider the protonation states of the reactants at different pH values. At neutral pH where the reaction rate is slowest, both the water nucleophile and the electrophilic carbonyl species are neutral and unprotonated (Figure 7.6).

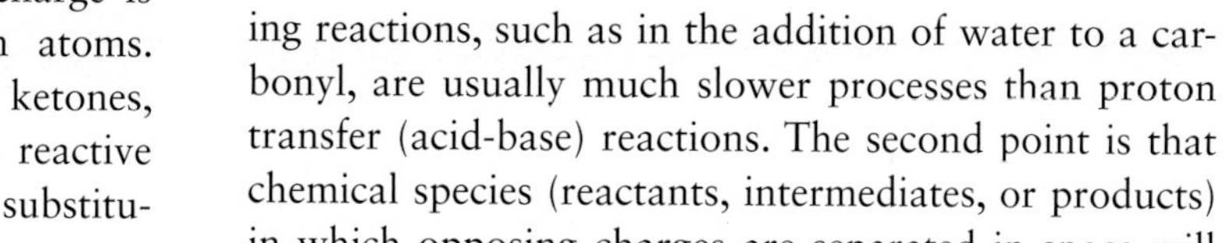

Figure 7.4 The carbonyl in acrolein is depolarized by delocalization of the carbonyl and alkene π systems. The alkene bond, however, is more polarized than in a simple unsubstituted alkene.

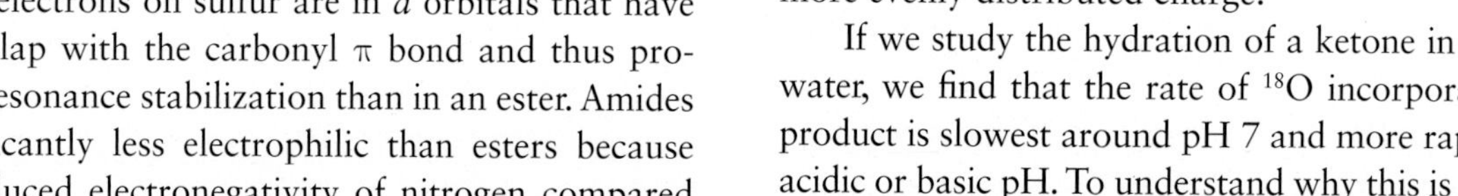

acid chloride   acid anhydride   aldehyde   ketone   thioester   ester   amide

Figure 7.5 Carbonyl-containing functional groups in order of decreasing reactivity from left to right.

THE OVERALL REACTION:

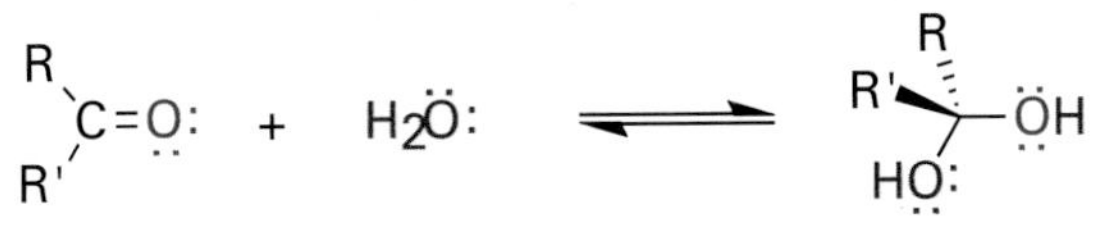

THE MECHANISM:

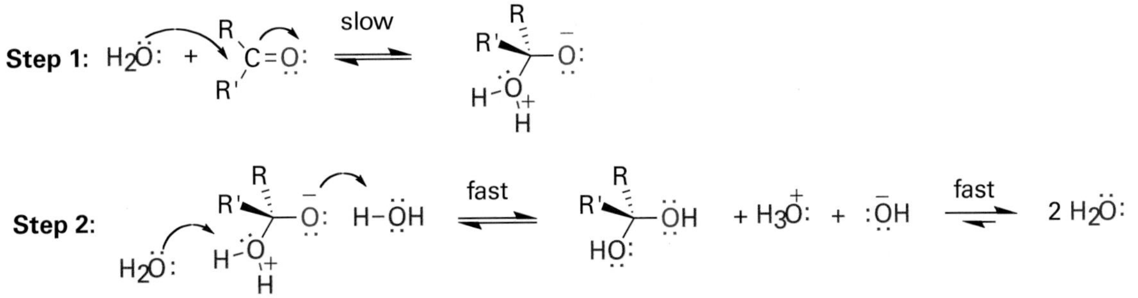

Step 1:

Step 2:

Figure 7.6 Hydration of an aldehyde or ketone under neutral conditions (pH ~7).

Hydration of an Aldehyde or Ketone in Acid Solution

THE OVERALL REACTION:

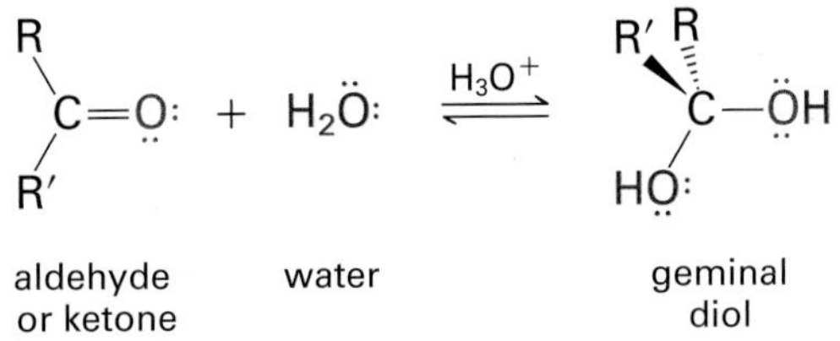

aldehyde   water   geminal
or ketone   diol

THE MECHANISM:

Step 1: Protonation of the carbonyl oxygen

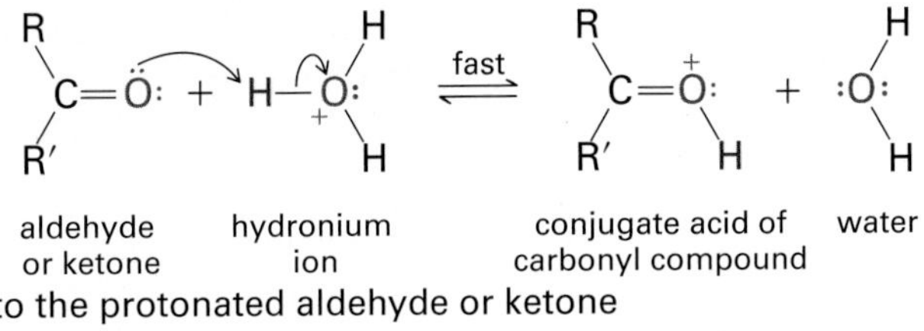

aldehyde   hydronium   conjugate acid of   water
or ketone   ion   carbonyl compound

Step 2: Nucleophilic addition to the protonated aldehyde or ketone

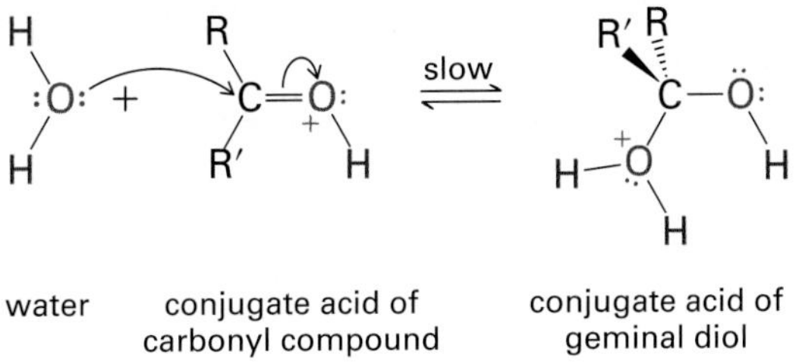

water   conjugate acid of   conjugate acid of
       carbonyl compound   geminal diol

Step 3: Proton transfer from the conjugate acid of the geminal diol to a water molecule

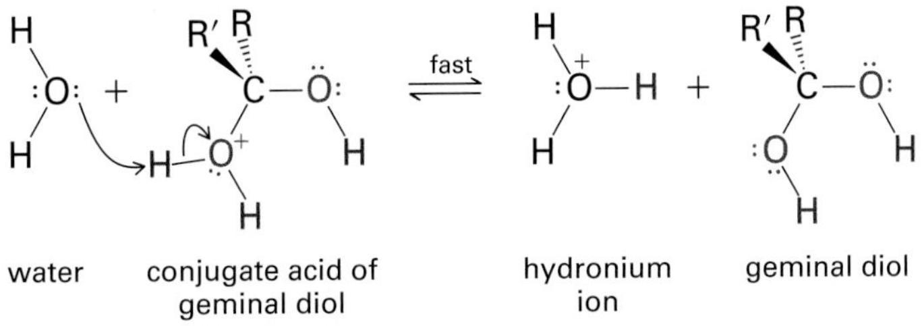

water   conjugate acid of   hydronium   geminal diol
       geminal diol   ion

Figure 7.7 Hydration of an aldehyde or ketone under acidic conditions. (Reproduced, with permission, from Carey FA, Giuliano RM. *Organic Chemistry.* 9th ed. New York: McGraw-Hill Education; 2014.)

The rate-determining step of the reaction is the C–O bond forming reaction—the addition of water to the carbonyl (step 1, Figure 7.6). This addition reaction involves neutral reactants and produces an intermediate in which positive and negative charges are separated in space. The significant energy difference between the neutral reactants and the charged intermediate corresponds to a high **activation energy** and this is what accounts for the slow reaction rate. Once formed, the charged intermediate will either revert back to the neutral reactants or undergo a rapid proton transfer reaction (step 2, Figure 7.6) to afford the product.

Next, let us consider the mechanism of the same reaction when carried out under acidic conditions (Figure 7.7). Under acidic conditions where hydronium ion (H_3O^+) concentrations are significant, the carbonyl species can become protonated on oxygen. This has the effect of further polarizing the carbonyl bond and increasing its reactivity as an electrophile. The reactivity of the water nucleophile, by contrast, has not changed

significantly when compared to the reaction under neutral conditions. Following the nucleophilic addition step, a single proton transfer to water produces the neutral product and regenerates the hydronium ion catalyst. Since hydronium ion is present on both sides of the reaction equation, the equilibrium constant is not affected—acid catalysis simply accelerates the rate of the reaction.

Finally, consider the hydration reaction under basic conditions (Figure 7.8). At higher pH values, hydroxide ion ($OH-$) is present at significant concentrations. Hydroxide is a much stronger nucleophile than neutral water and thus reacts more rapidly with the carbonyl electrophile (which is no more reactive than at neutral pH). A proton transfer with water then produces the diol product and regenerates hydroxide ion catalyst. As with acid catalysis, basic catalysis affects the rate of the reaction but does not impact the equilibrium constant. To summarize, the hydration of aldehydes and ketones is accelerated under acidic conditions due to activation of the carbonyl electrophile and is accelerated under basic conditions due to a more reactive nucleophile.

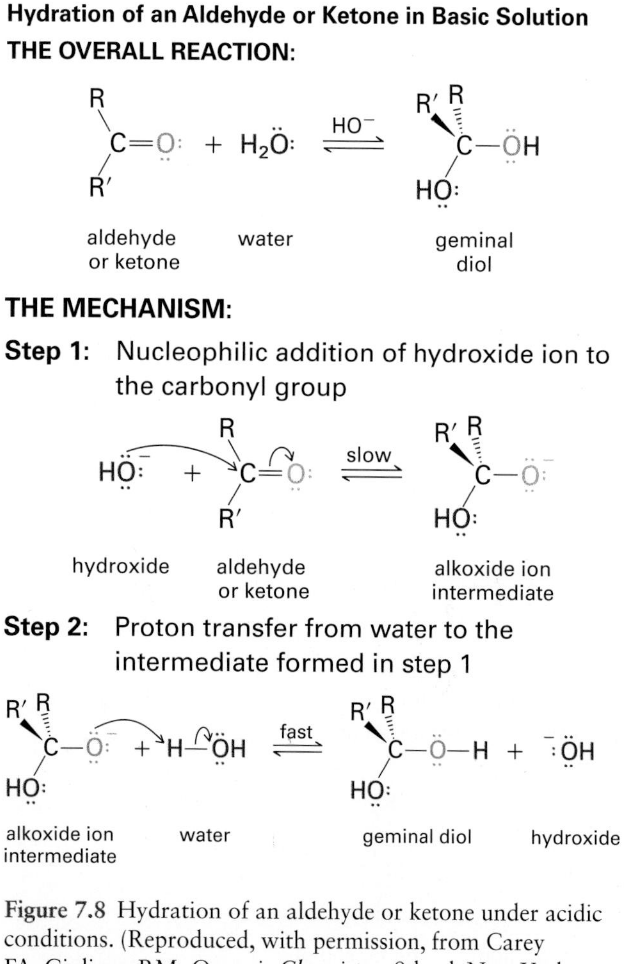

7.5 Reactions of Aldehydes and Ketones with Alcohols

The reaction of a carbonyl species with an alcohol as nucleophile is similar in many ways to the hydration reaction, but with some interesting additional features. Addition of an alcohol to an aldehyde or ketone results in the formation of a **hemi-acetal** or **hemi-ketal**, tetrahedral species that are analogous to the diol product of the hydration reaction. These reactions are slow and reversible at neutral pH, with the equilibrium generally favoring the carbonyl starting material over the hemi-acetal or hemi-ketal. If, however, the reaction is carried out under acidic conditions, a second equivalent of the alcohol nucleophile can be incorporated, producing stable **acetal** or **ketal** products. The mechanism of this reaction reveals two important roles for the acid catalyst and also reveals why acetal formation does not occur under basic conditions (Figure 7.9).

The initial role of the acid catalyst is to protonate and thereby activate the carbonyl electrophile (benzaldehyde in the example shown in Figure 7.9). Reaction with nucleophile (Et–OH in this example) then leads ultimately to a hemi-acetal intermediate (steps 1–3). Next, the hemi-acetal can be protonated on the hydroxyl function and the C–O bond cleaved with loss of water, a good leaving group (steps 4 and 5). The loss of water

Hydration of an Aldehyde or Ketone in Basic Solution
THE OVERALL REACTION:

| aldehyde or ketone | water | geminal diol |

THE MECHANISM:

Step 1: Nucleophilic addition of hydroxide ion to the carbonyl group

| hydroxide | aldehyde or ketone | alkoxide ion intermediate |

Step 2: Proton transfer from water to the intermediate formed in step 1

| alkoxide ion intermediate | water | geminal diol | hydroxide |

Figure 7.8 Hydration of an aldehyde or ketone under acidic conditions. (Reproduced, with permission, from Carey FA, Giuliano RM. *Organic Chemistry*. 9th ed. New York: McGraw-Hill Education; 2014.)

Acetal Formation from Benzaldehyde and Ethanol
THE OVERALL REACTION:

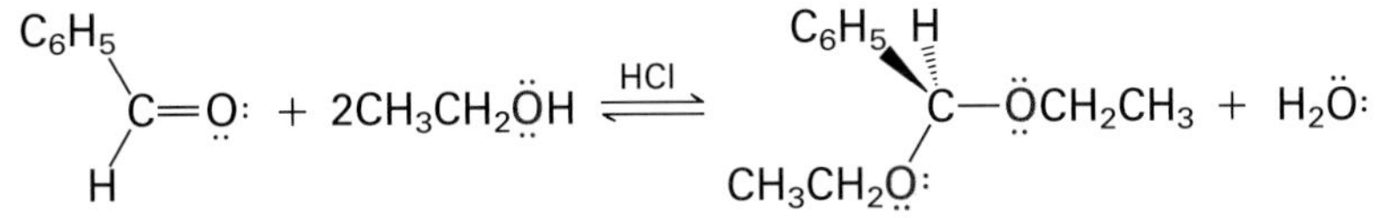

benzaldehyde   ethanol   benzaldehyde   water
                                   diethyl acetal

THE MECHANISM:

Steps 1–3: Acid-catalyzed nucleophilic addition of 1 mole of ehtanol to the carbonyl group. The details of these three steps are analogous to the three steps of acid-catalyzed hydration in Figure 7.7. The product of these three steps is a hemi-acetal.

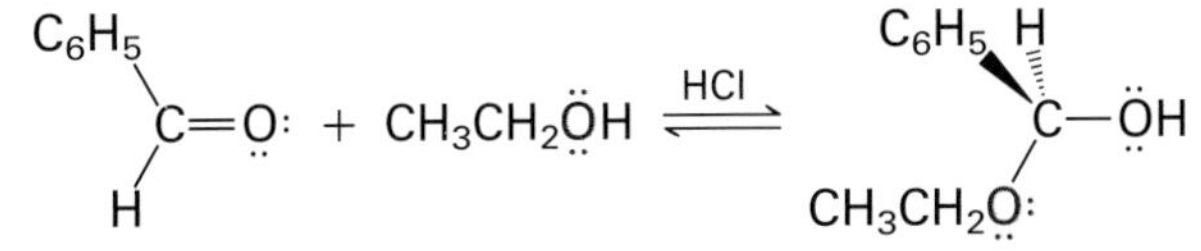

benzaldehyde   ethanol   benzaldehyde
                                   ethyl hemi-acetal

Step 4: Steps 4 and 5 are analogous to the two steps in the formation of carbocations in acid-catalyzed reactions of alcohols. Step 4 is proton transfer from hydronium ion to the hydroxyl oxygen of the hemi-acetal.

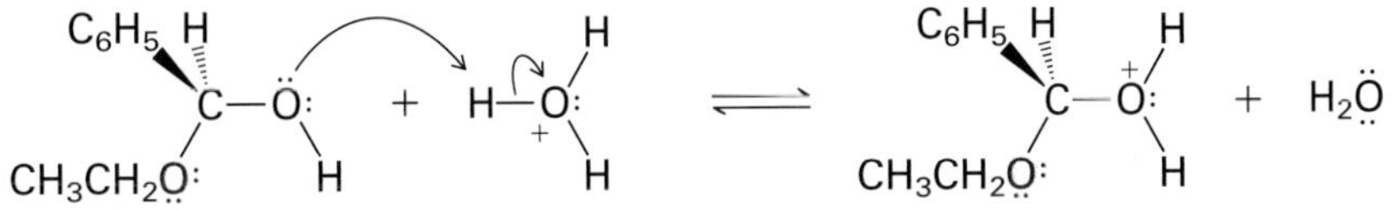

benzaldehyde   hydronium   conjugate acid of   water
ethyl hemi-acetal   ion   benzaldehyde ethyl hemi-acetal

Step 5: Loss of water from the protonated hemi-acetal gives an oxygen-stabilized carbocation. Of the resonance structures shown, the more stable contributor satisfies the octet rule for both carbon and oxygen.

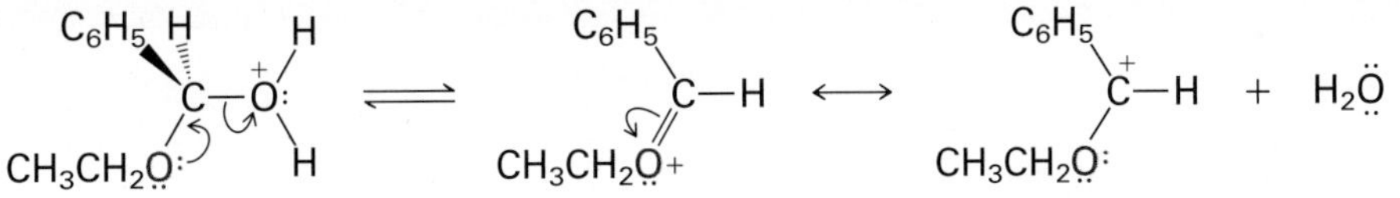

conjugate acid of   more stable   less stable   water
benzaldehyde ethyl hemi-acetal   contributor   contributor

Step 6: Nucleophilic addition of ethanol to the oxygen-stabilized carbocation

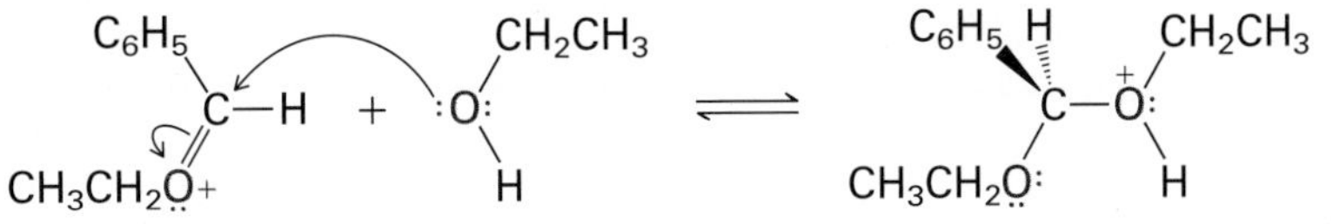

oxygen-stabilized   ethanol   conjugate acid
carbocation   of acetal

Step 7: Proton transfer from the conjugate acid of the product to ethanol

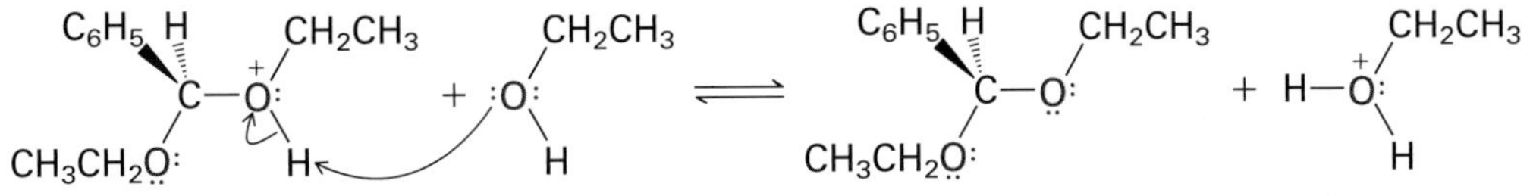

conjugate acid   ethanol   benzaldehyde   conjugate acid
of acetal   diethyl acetal   of ethanol

Figure 7.9 Acetal formation in the reaction of benzaldehyde with ethanol. (Reproduced, with permission, from Carey FA, Giuliano RM. *Organic Chemistry*. 9th ed. New York: McGraw-Hill Education; 2014.)

results in formation of an oxygen-stabilized carbocation, which can be drawn in different resonance forms but is most often shown with a C=O double bond. This cationic species is of course an excellent electrophile and will react readily with an available nucleophile (water or Et–OH). Reaction with water leads back to the hemi-acetal, while reaction with alcohol generates the acetal product (had the carbonyl reactant been a ketone, the product would be a ketal). Because each step in this process is reversible, the reaction can be driven in either direction depending on the reaction conditions. For example, acetal formation is favored if the alcohol nucleophile is used as solvent and so is in large excess. Conversely, acetals can be converted back to

aldehydes by reaction with aqueous acid. Acetals do not form under basic conditions because there is no means to produce the requisite oxygen-stabilized carbocation intermediate.

Earlier in this section we have noted that hemi-acetals and hemi-ketals are generally not stable and prefer to decompose to their component carbonyl and alcohol species. An exception to this rule is the case of *cyclic* hemi-acetals, which are often more stable than the corresponding acyclic hydroxy-aldehyde form. For example, the common sugars D-glucose and D-fructose exist chiefly in the form of a cyclic hemi-acetal and cyclic hemi-ketal, respectively (Figure 7.10). Whereas glucose exists primarily as a six-membered "pyranose" ring,

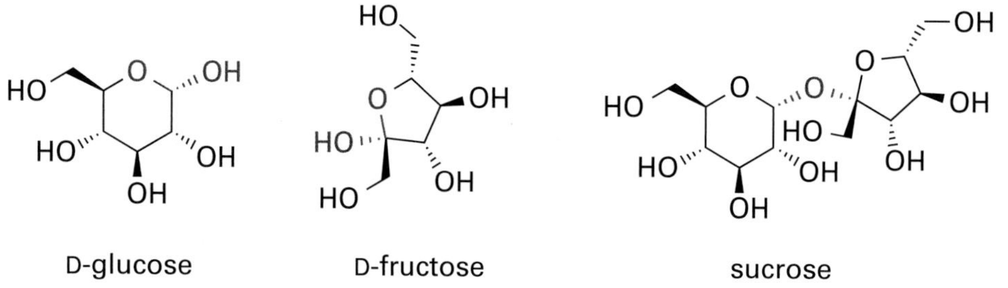

Figure 7.10 Structures of D-glucose in D-fructose it their cyclic forms. The hemi-acetal and hemi-ketal bonds are highlighted in blue. Sucrose (table sugar) is a disaccharide formed by joining D-glucose and D-fructose via a glycosidic bond (also shown in blue).

Box 7.1 Glucuronidation in the metabolism of drugs.

A particularly important type of glycosidic bond with respect to drug action is that formed between some drug species and glucuronic acid. Glucuronic acid is an oxidized form of glucose and is highly water-soluble. The enzyme UDP-glucuronosyltransferase (UGT) catalyzes the formation of a glycosidic bond between glucuronic acid and alcohol- or acid-bearing drugs, drug metabolites, or other xenobiotic molecules. The resulting conjugate, called a **glucuronide**, is usually highly water-soluble and this allows it to be more rapidly eliminated from the body. This process of glucuronidation is one of the mechanisms by which the body clears drugs and other xenobiotic small molecules. In fact, phase 1 metabolism of drugs in the liver often involves oxidation of drug molecules to produce a new alcohol function. Such metabolites are then subject to phase 2 metabolism to form glucuronides. Shown below is the glucuronidation reaction of the NSAID anti-inflammatory drug zomepirac. Note that in this case glucuronidation occurs at the carboxylate function of the drug itself—no initial oxidation is required. As described later in Box 7.2, further reactions of the zomepirac glucuronide are believed to be responsible for rare but serious side effects that led the drug to be pulled from the market only a few years after its introduction.

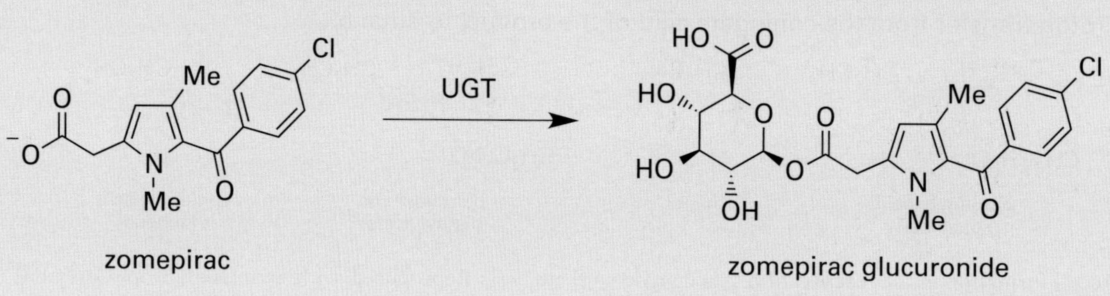

zomepirac   zomepirac glucuronide

fructose exists as a mixture of pyranose and five-membered "furanose" forms (the furanose form is shown in Figure 7.10). The hemi-acetal function of a sugar molecule (or monosaccharide) can react with an alcohol function of a second sugar to produce a disaccharide in which the two sugars are linked by an oxygen atom. In the context of carbohydrate chemistry, these acetal linkages are known as **glycosidic** bonds. Glycosidic bonds can be found in a wide variety of biologically important macromolecules, including in polysaccharides, that play important structural and energy-storage roles in biology. An example of a glycosidic bond relevant to drug metabolism is that formed between glucuronic acid and nucleophilic drugs or drug metabolites (Box 7.1).

7.6 Imines and Enamines

The addition of amines to aldehydes and ketones is similar in many respects to the addition of alcohols but with some important differences. While amines are generally better nucleophiles than alcohols, they are also more basic and this fact has interesting ramifications in terms of the products that are ultimately formed. The reaction of aldehydes or ketones with primary amines (R–NH$_2$) leads to **imines** while similar reactions of secondary amines (R$_2$NH) result in **enamines**. Imines are sometimes further categorized as aldimines if formed from aldehydes and ketimines if formed from ketones (Figure 7.11). Imines are sometimes called **Schiff bases** and can be formed under physiological conditions from amines present in amino acids and other biological and drug molecules.

The mechanism of imine formation is shown below and begins with the addition of a primary amine

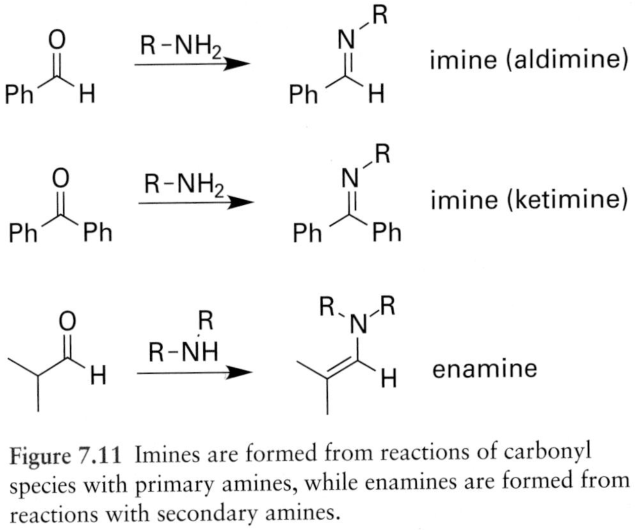

Figure 7.11 Imines are formed from reactions of carbonyl species with primary amines, while enamines are formed from reactions with secondary amines.

nucleophile to the carbonyl electrophile (Figure 7.12). The resulting tetrahedral intermediate is called a **hemi-aminal** and is analogous to a hemi-acetal. Protonation of the hemi-aminal on oxygen leads to elimination of water and the formation of a nitrogen-stabilized carbocation or **iminium ion**. While the iminium ion is potentially reactive as an electrophile, the more rapid reaction is to simply lose a proton from nitrogen to afford the neutral imine. Another way of seeing this is to recognize that the iminium ion is just the conjugate acid of the imine. Iminium ions formed from secondary amines do not have a proton on nitrogen to lose and so these species will either react with a nucleophile (if present) or will be deprotonated at the neighboring carbon atom to afford an enamine (Figure 7.13).

Recall that the rate of water or alcohol addition to a carbonyl is accelerated under acidic or basic conditions and is slowest at neutral pH (Section 7.4). In contrast, amine addition reactions are fastest under mildly acidic conditions (pH ~5) and are slower at either lower or higher pH values. Considering the mechanism of the reaction we can readily understand the pH dependence of reaction rate. Under highly acidic conditions (pH < 4) the amine nucleophile will be mostly or entirely protonated, making it unreactive as a nucleophile (no free lone pair electrons). At the optimal pH for reaction (pH ~5) there will be a reasonable concentration of amine that is unprotonated and thus reactive. A mildly acidic pH is also favorable in the next step, where the hemi-aminal intermediate must be protonated to facilitate elimination of water and the formation of the iminium ion (step 3, Figure 7.12). Under neutral or more basic conditions this second step may not occur and the intrinsically unstable hemi-aminal will revert back to amine and aldehyde reactants.

In biological systems, hemi-acetals and imines can also form as a result of the oxidation of carbon atoms neighboring amines in drugs. Such oxidations are typically carried out by cytochrome P450 (CYP450) enzymes in the liver, as will be discussed in more detail in Chapter 8. The hemi-aminal products resulting from such oxidations will have a different fate depending on the pK_a of the amine function in the hemi-aminal. If the amine function is significantly protonated at pH ~7, the ammonium species will be a good leaving group and the hemi-aminal will break down to amine- and ketone- or aldehyde-containing drug metabolites (Figure 7.14). For less basic amines such as aromatic amines (anilines), the hemi-aminal will be protonated on the hydroxyl function and subsequent elimination of water produces an iminium ion. Such species are highly reactive

Imine Formation from Benzaldehyde and Methylamine

THE OVERALL REACTION:

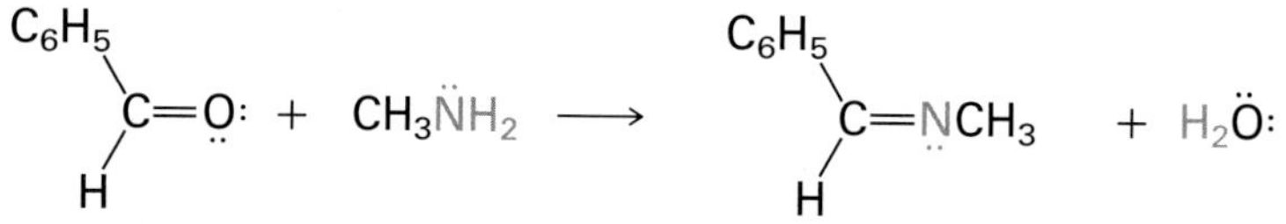

benzaldehyde   methylamine   *N*-benzylidenemethylamine   water

THE MECHANISM:

Step 1: The amine acts as a nucleophile, adding to the carbonyl group and forming a C–N bond.

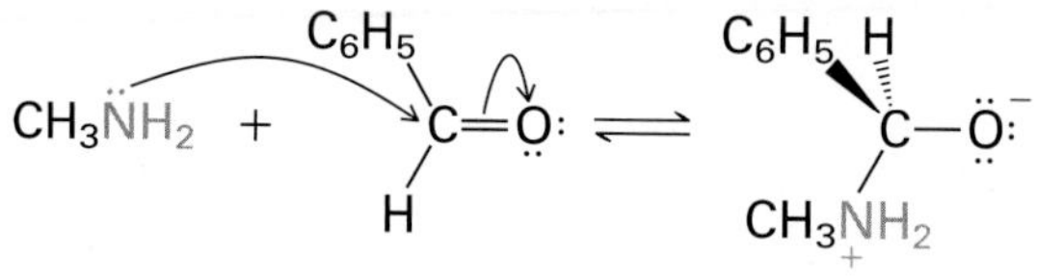

methylamine   benzaldehyde   first intermediate

Step 2: In a solvent such as water, proton transfers give the hemi-aminal.

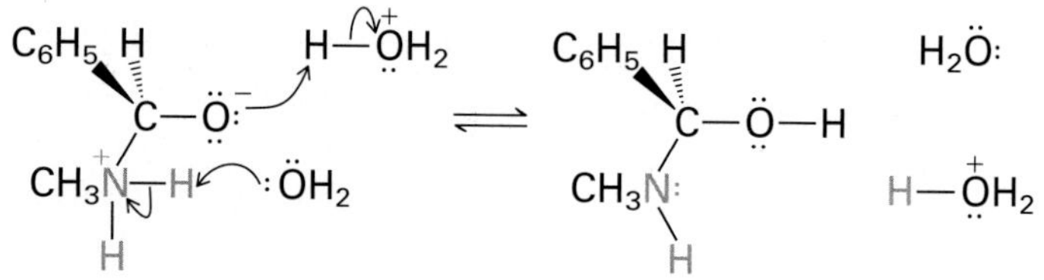

first intermediate   hemi-aminal

Step 3: The dehydration stage begins with protonation of the hemi-aminal on oxygen.

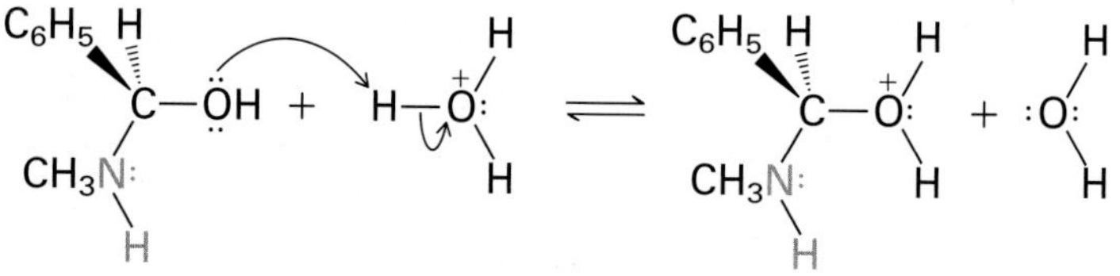

hemi-aminal   hydronium ion   *O*-protonated hemi-aminal   water

Step 4: The oxygen-protonated hemi-aminal loses water to give a nitrogen-stabilized carbocation.

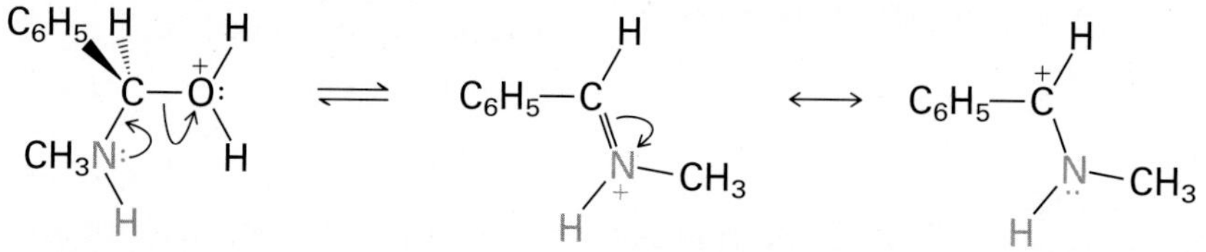

O-protonated hemi-aminal   nitrogen-stabilized carbocation

Step 5: The nitrogen-stabilized carbocation is the conjugate acid of the imine. Proton transfer to water gives the imine.

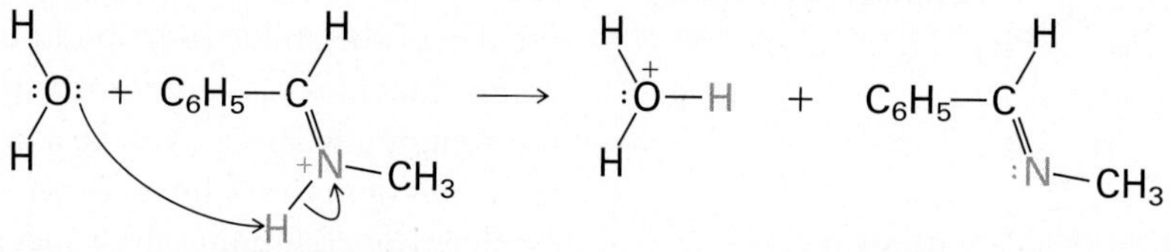

water   nitrogen-stabilized carbocation   hydronium ion   *N*-benzylidenemethylamine

Figure 7.12 Mechanism of imine formation in the reaction of benzaldehyde with methylamine. (Reproduced, with permission, from Carey FA, Giuliano RM. *Organic Chemistry.* 9th ed. New York: McGraw-Hill Education; 2014.)

Enamine Formation

THE OVERALL REACTION:

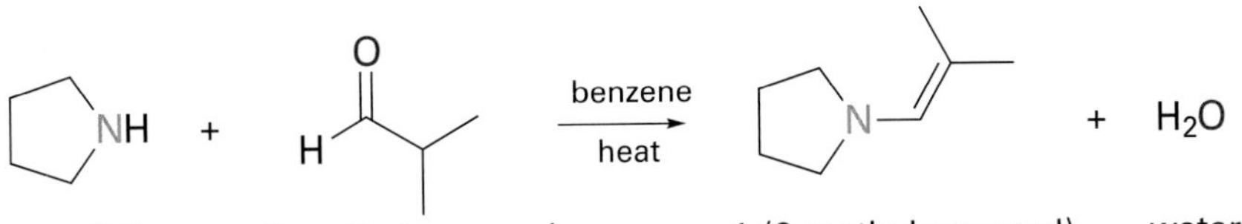

pyrrolidine   2-methylpropanal   benzene / heat → 1-(2-methylpropenyl)-pyrrolidine (94–95%)   + H_2O water

THE MECHANISM:

Step 1: Nucleophilic addition of pyrrolidine to 2-methylpropanal gives a hemi-aminal. The mechanism is analogous to the addition of primary amines to aldehydes and ketones (Figure 7.12).

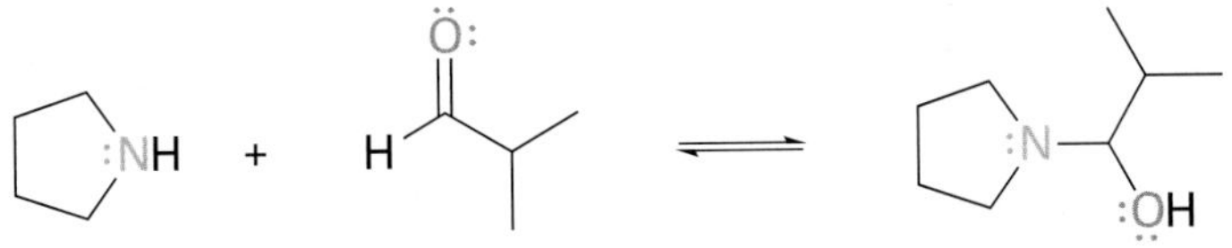

pyrrolidine   2-methylpropanal   hemi-aminal intermediate

Step 2: With assistance from the nitrogen lone pair, the hemi-aminal expels hydroxide to form an iminium ion.

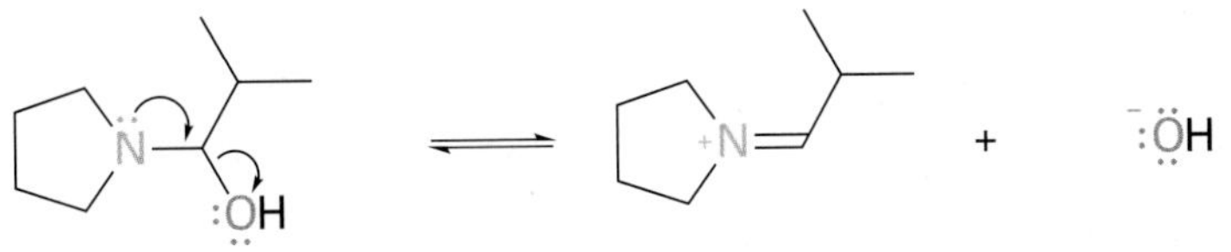

hemi-aminal intermediate   iminium ion   hydroxide ion

Step 3: The iminium ion is then deprotonated in the direction that gives a carbon–carbon double bond.

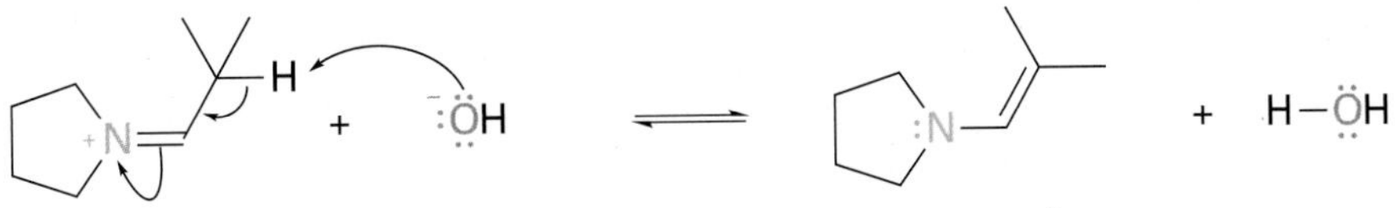

iminium ion   hydroxide ion   1-(2-methylpropenyl)-pyrrolidine   water

Figure 7.13 Mechanism of enamine formation in the reaction of the secondary amine pyrrolidine with 2-methylpropanal. (Reproduced, with permission, from Carey FA, Giuliano RM. *Organic Chemistry*. 9th ed. New York: McGraw-Hill Education; 2014.)

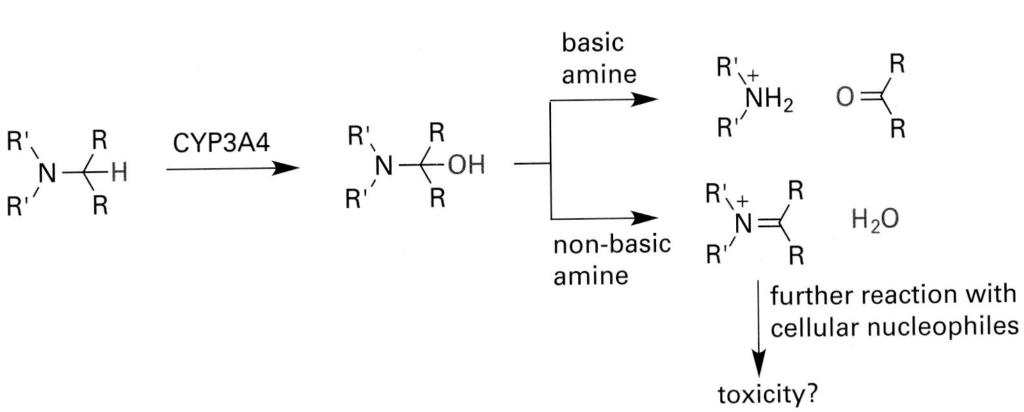

Figure 7.14 Oxidation of amine-containing drugs by liver CYP enzymes can produce a hemi-aminal. The fate of the hemi-aminal depends on the basicity of the amine function as described in the text.

Box 7.2 Imines in drug-protein conjugates.

The NSAID drug zomepirac was approved in 1980 and achieved some success in the market, until it was found that a small and unpredictable subset of patients receiving the drug developed anaphylaxis, a serious allergic reaction. Zomepirac, like many carboxylate-containing drugs, is eliminated primarily via conversion to an acyl glucuronide (see Box 7.1). Some acyl glucuronides, however, can undergo further reactions that transfer the acyl group to neighboring hydroxy groups of the glucuronic acid ring,

as illustrated below. These species possess a cyclic hemi-acetal function that is in equilibrium with an acyclic hydroxyaldehyde form. Studies of the zomepirac glucuronide in humans and animals suggested that imine formation between these aldehyde intermediates and nucleophilic amines (e.g., the ε-amine of lysine) in serum proteins is likely responsible for the immunogenic responses observed in some patients. Zomepirac was withdrawn from the market only three years after its approval.

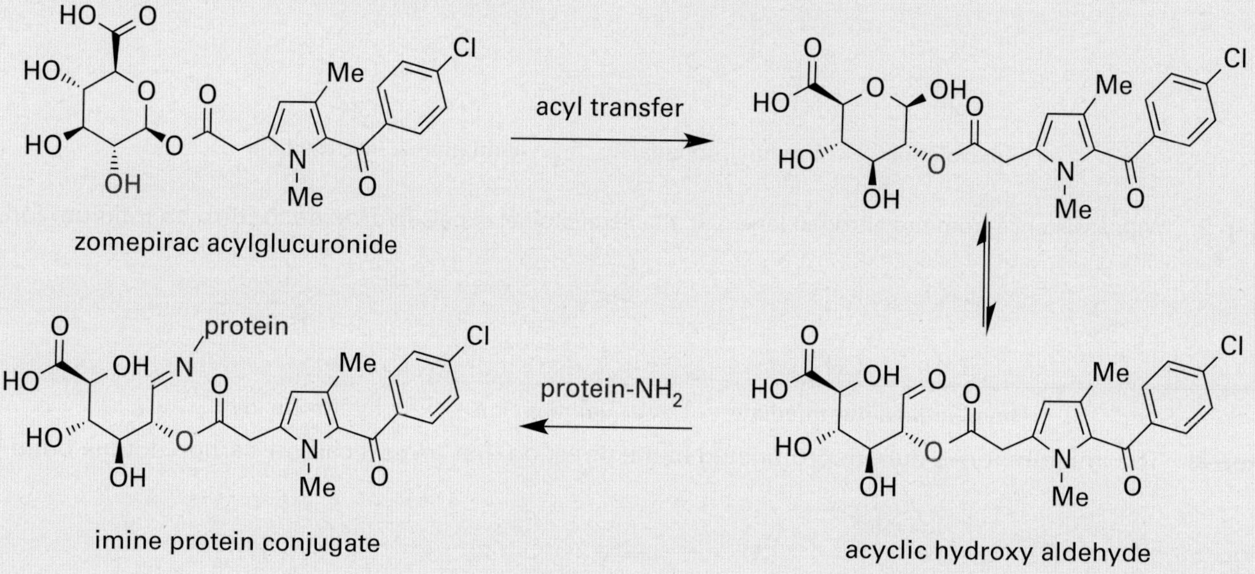

zomepirac acylglucuronide

acyl transfer →

protein-NH₂ ←

imine protein conjugate

acyclic hydroxy aldehyde

electrophiles that can react with cellular nucleophiles, potentially leading to undesirable side effects. The formation of imines under physiological conditions is illustrated for the case of specific metabolites of the drug zomepirac, an NSAID that was ultimately withdrawn from the market due to serious allergic reactions in some patients (Box 7.2).

7.7 Oximes and Hydrazones

In this section we examine the formation and reactivity of **oximes** and **hydrazones**. Like imines, oximes and hydrazones are formed by the reaction of a carbonyl species with an amine nucleophile. Oximes are formed when a ketone or an aldehyde reacts with a hydroxylamine, while hydrazones are formed in analogous reactions of hydrazines or an hydrazides (Figure 7.15). Note that the nucleophilic nitrogen atom in these species is not bonded to carbon but to a more electronegative oxygen or nitrogen atom. The electron-withdrawing effect

of the neighboring oxygen or nitrogen atom means that hydroxylamines and hydrazines will be less basic than similar aliphatic amines. Another difference is that hydrazines have *two* nitrogen atoms that could potentially react with the carbonyl electrophile. In unsymmetrical hydrazines, it is usually the less hindered nitrogen atom that is most nucleophilic. This difference in reactivity between nitrogen atoms is especially pronounced in the case of aryl hydrazines (Ar–NH–NH₂) or acyl hydrazides (Ac–NH–NH₂), where the lone pair of the central nitrogen atom is significantly delocalized into the π system of the aryl ring or acyl group.

At this point it is useful to examine the relative reactivity of the amine nucleophiles discussed so far, and also to consider the relative stability of their imine, oxime, or hydrazone products under physiological conditions. A good way to do this is to consider the pK_a values of the conjugate acids of the sp^3 hybridized nucleophiles and their sp^2 hybridized products (Table 7.2). Using this approach, we can predict that hydroxylamines and acyl hydrazines

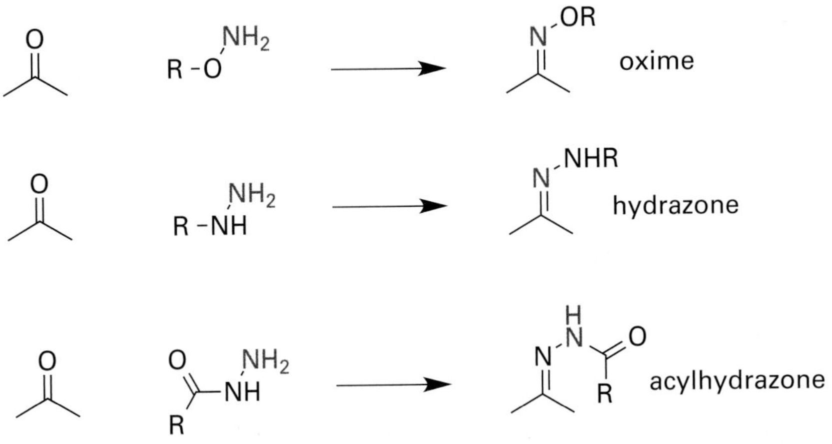

Figure 7.15 Reactions of hydroxylamines, hydrazines and hydrazides to form oximes and hydrazones.

Table 7.2 Relative Basicity of Amine Nucleophiles and their Corresponding Carbonyl Derivatives, Expressed as the pK_a of the Conjugate Acid.

Amine	pK_a of conjugate acid (BH+)	Carbonyl derivative	pK_a of conjugate acid (BH+)
R–NH$_2$	~7–11	Imine	~2–8
R–O–NH$_2$	~5–7	Oxime	~3–5
R–NH–NH$_2$	~7–8.5	Hydrazone	~4–6
RC(=O)NHNH$_2$	<3	Acylhydrazone	<1

with their lower pK_a values will remain unprotonated and thus nucleophilic at lower pH values. We can also see from the pK_a data in the table that the sp^2 hybridized reaction products have lower pK_a values than the amines from which they are derived. The pK_a values of the sp^2 hybridized carbonyl analogs can similarly tell us about the relative stability of imine, oxime, and hydrazone functions under physiological conditions. The hydrolysis reaction of these groups begins with protonation on nitrogen to form iminium-like species that are activated for reaction with water. Accordingly we would predict that acyl hydrazones, being essentially non-basic, should be very stable at physiological pH, while oximes and hydrazones would be more stable than imines, all else being equal.

Examples of drugs containing imine or oxime functional groups include clonazepam, a benzodiazepine anticonvulsant, and the topical antifungal agent oxiconazole (Figure 7.16). Note that in these drugs, the imine or oxime is conjugated to a larger aromatic ring system and thus the pK_a value for the conjugate acid will be low (<4). This ensures that the imine and oxime functions in these drugs will remain unprotonated at physiological pH and should be stable to hydrolysis. The antituberculosis drug isoniazid is one of the few drugs to contain a reactive hydrazide function. The propensity of the hydrazide to form acyl hydrazone adducts with biological aldehydes is behind some of the adverse side effects associated with isoniazid use. As one example, isoniazid can deplete stores of the cofactor pyridoxal phosphate (a reactive aldehyde), thereby impacting the biosynthesis of heme in red blood cells and leading to anemia.

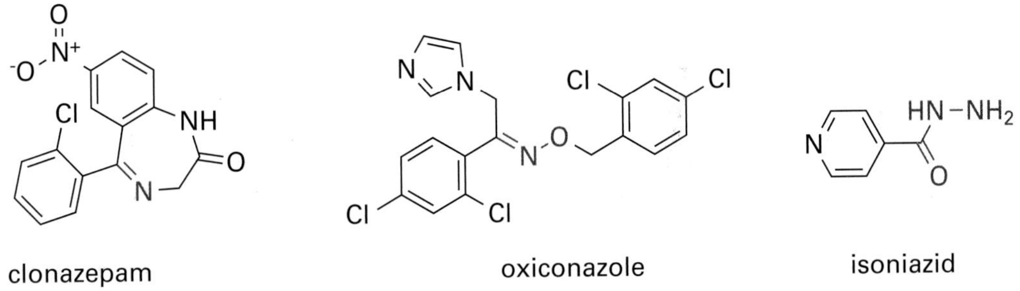

clonazepam   oxiconazole   isoniazid

Figure 7.16 Examples of drugs containing oxime and hydrazide functions.

7.8 Chemical Hydrolysis of Ester and Amide Bonds

The reaction of water with carboxylic acid derivatives such as esters or amides is called hydrolysis and is an important process in biology. The hydrolysis reaction is accelerated under either acidic or basic conditions, just as is the case with nucleophilic additions of water to aldehydes and ketones (Section 7.4). Because the hydrolysis reaction is slow at physiological pH, biology performs these reactions with the help of enzymes—esterases to cleave ester bonds and proteases to cleave amide (peptide) bonds. Hydrolysis of the neurotransmitter acetylcholine by acetylcholine esterase is an important mechanism by which signaling across synapses is terminated. Similarly, the hydrolysis of peptide bonds by proteases underlies a vast array of biological processes, from signaling cascades in coagulation and programmed cell death (apoptosis) to cellular housekeeping and the recycling of amino acids. Before discussing enzyme-catalyzed hydrolysis in the next section, we first examine the mechanisms of amide and ester bond hydrolysis under acidic and basic conditions.

We begin with a discussion of esters and their hydrolysis in aqueous solutions. Recall from Section 7.3 that esters are significantly weaker electrophiles than aldehydes or ketones. This is due to the electron-donating effect of the −OR substituent, which reduces polarization of the carbonyl bond. The reaction is slower than the hydration of aldehydes or ketones, but is promoted under acidic or basic conditions. Hence, under acidic conditions the oxygen of the ester carbonyl can become protonated, activating it toward nucleophilic water (Figure 7.17). Rapid proton transfer between oxygen atoms in the tetrahedral intermediate sets the stage for the loss of ROH and re-formation of a carbonyl bond in the carboxylic acid product.

Under basic conditions the ester electrophile is unactivated (unprotonated) but the hydroxide ion nucleophile is much more reactive than water. In this case the tetrahedral intermediate collapses to form, after proton transfer, carboxylate and alcohol products (Figure 7.18). Note that whereas the acid catalyst is regenerated in the ester hydrolysis reaction, base catalysis involves the consumption of a strong base (hydroxide) and the formation of a weak base (carboxylate).

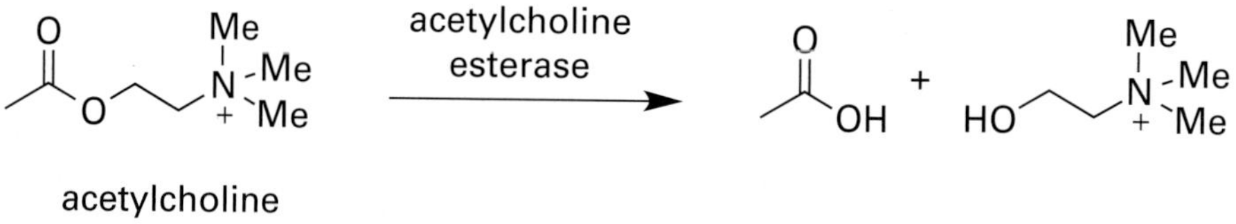

acetylcholine

Acid-Catalyzed Ester Hydrolysis

THE OVERALL REACTION:

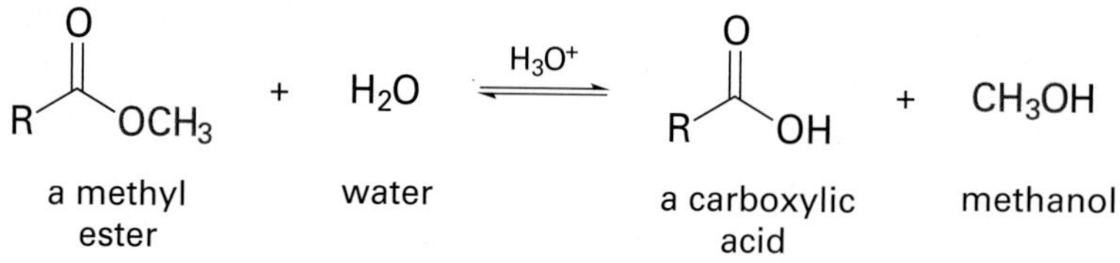

a methyl ester + water $\xrightarrow{H_3O^+}$ a carboxylic acid + methanol

THE MECHANISM:

First Stage: Formation of the tetrahedral intermediate   Steps 1–3 are analogous to the mechanism of acid-catalyzed hydration of an aldehyde or ketone.

Step 1:   Protonation of the carbonyl oxygen of the ester

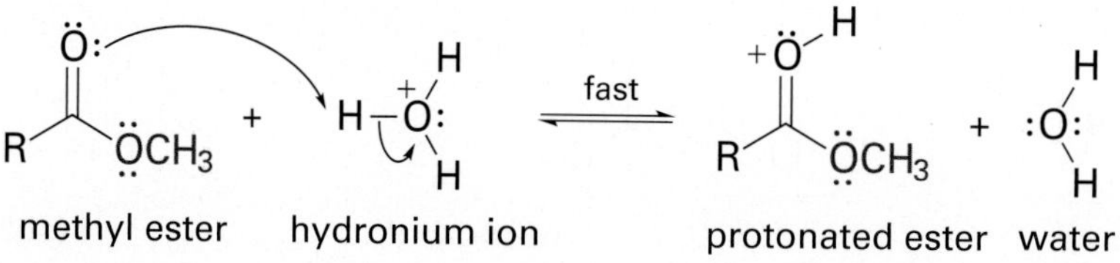

methyl ester   hydronium ion   ⇌ (fast)   protonated ester   water

Figure 7.17 Mechanism of ester hydrolysis under acidic conditions. (Reproduced, with permission, from Carey FA, Giuliano RM. *Organic Chemistry*. 9th ed. New York: McGraw-Hill Education; 2014.) (*Continued*)

Step 2: Nucleophilic addition of water to the protonated ester

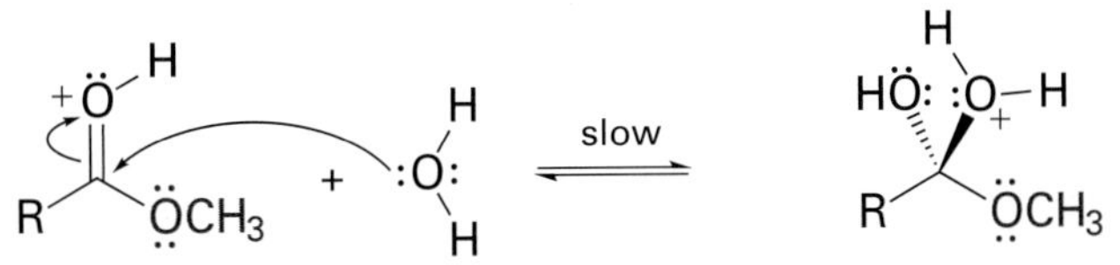

protonated ester   water

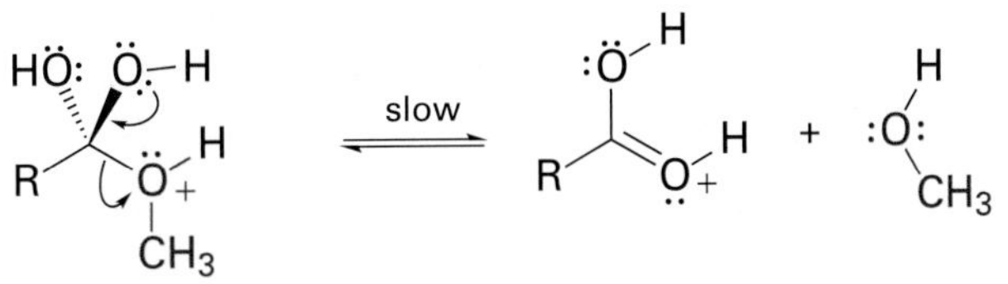

slow

conjugate acid of tetrahedral
intermediate (TI–H⁺)

Step 3: Deprotonation of TI—H⁺ to give the neutral form of the tetrahedral intermediate (TI)

conjugate acid of
tetrahedral intermediate
(TI–H⁺)

water

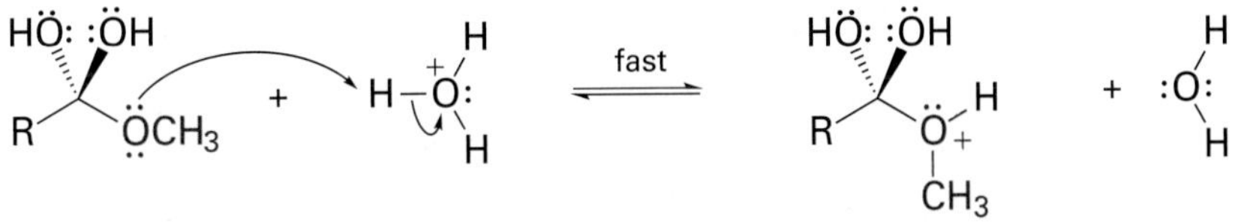

fast

tetrahedral
intermediate (TI)

hydronium ion

Second Stage: Dissociation of the tetrahedral intermediate Just as steps 1–3 corresponded to addition of water to the carbonyl group, steps 4–6 correspond to elimination of an alcohol, in this case methanol, from the TI and a restoration of the carbonyl group.

Step 4: Protonation of the alkoxy oxygen of the tetrahedral intermediate

tetrahedral
intermediate (TI)

hydronium ion

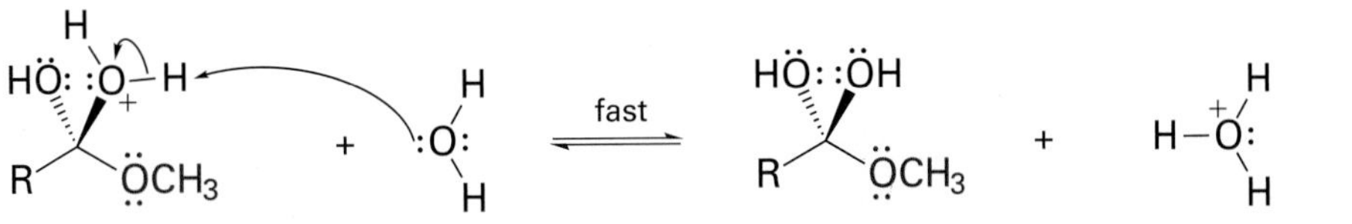

fast

conjugate acid of
tetrahedral intermediate
(TI–H⁺)

water

Step 5: Dissociation of the protonated form of the tetrahedral intermediate gives the alcohol and the protonated form of the carboxylic acid

conjugate acid of
tetrahedral intermediate
(TI–H⁺)

slow

protonated
carboxylic acid

methanol

Step 6: Deprotonation of the protonated carboxylic acid completes the process

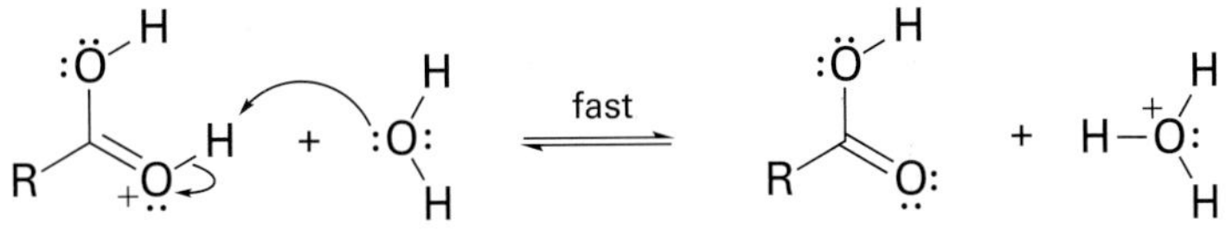

protonated
carboxylic acid

water

fast

carboxylic acid

hydronium
ion

Figure 7.17 (*Continued*)

Ester Hydrolysis in Basic Solution

THE OVERALL REACTION:

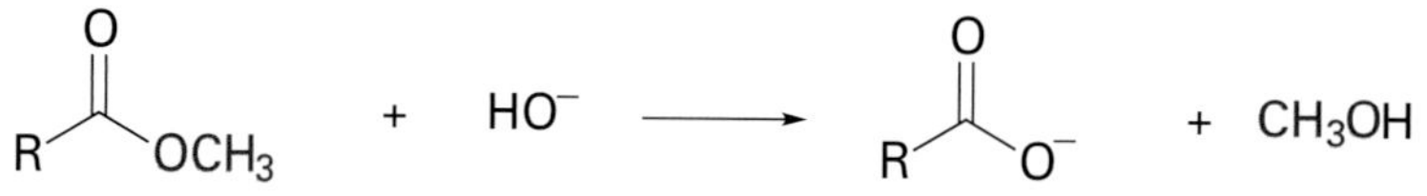

| a methyl ester | hydroxide ion | a carboxylate ion | methanol |

THE MECHANISM:

Step 1: Nucleophilic addition of hydroxide to the carbonyl group

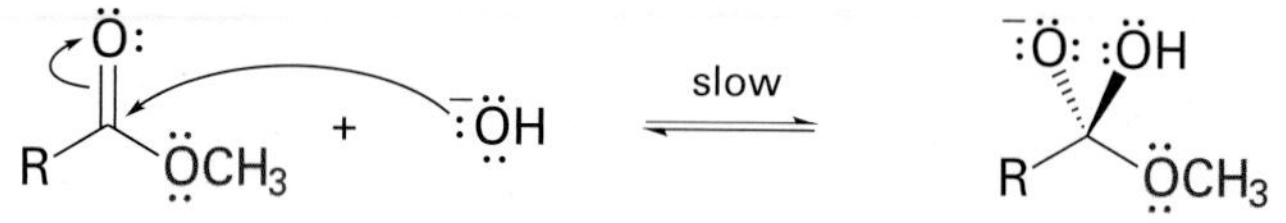

methyl ester   hydroxide ion   conjugate base of tetrahedral intermediate (TI⁻)

Step 2: Dissociation of the anionic tetrahedral intermediate TI⁻

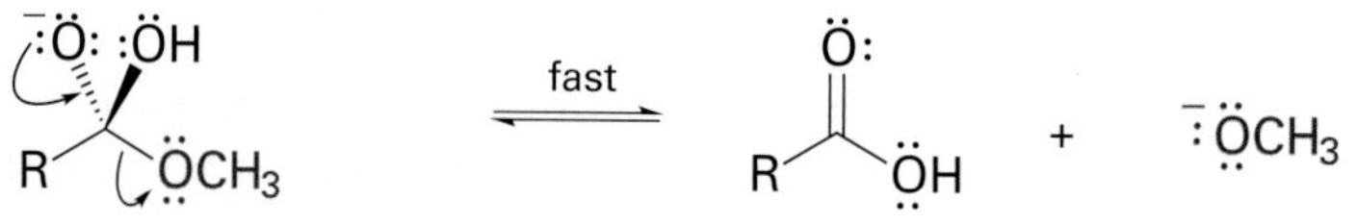

conjugate base of tetrahedral intermediate (TI⁻)   carboxylic acid   methoxide ion

Step 3: Proton transfers yield an alcohol and a carboxylate ion

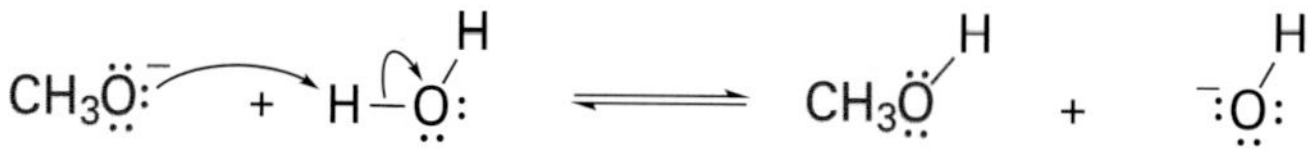

methoxide ion   water   methanol   hydroxide ion

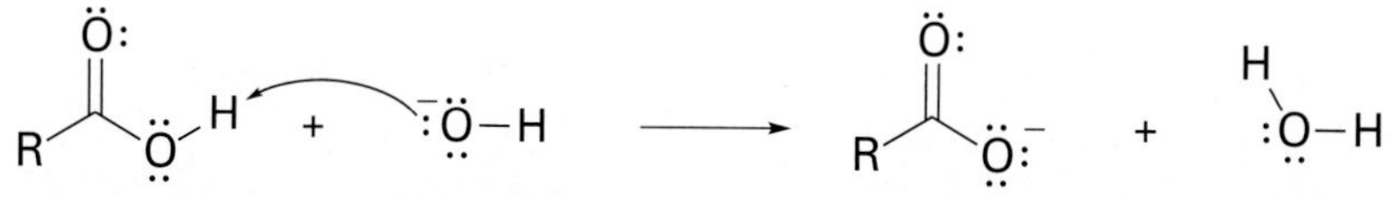

carboxylic acid (stronger acid)   hydroxide ion (stronger base)   carboxylate ion (weaker base)   water (weaker acid)

Figure 7.18 Mechanism of ester hydrolysis under basic conditions. (Reproduced, with permission, from Carey FA, Giuliano RM. *Organic Chemistry.* 9th ed. New York: McGraw-Hill Education; 2014.)

The hydrolysis of amides is even slower than esters on account of the delocalization of the nitrogen lone pair electrons into the carbonyl bond. This is most readily appreciated by considering the contribution of the resonance forms B and C shown below.

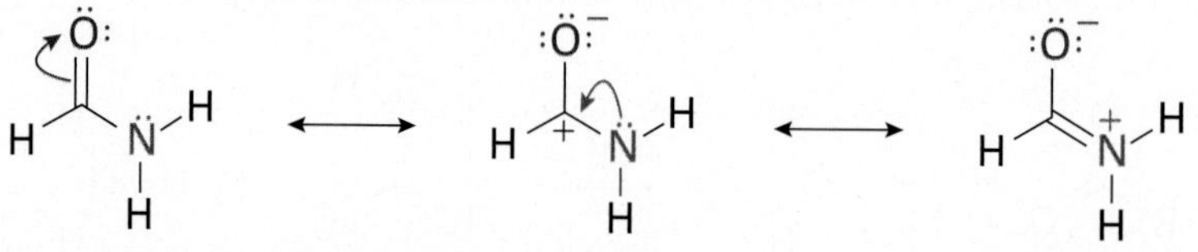

A   B   C

(Reproduced, with permission, from Carey FA, Giuliano RM. *Organic Chemistry.* 9th ed. New York: McGraw-Hill Education; 2014.)

The base-promoted mechanism of amide hydrolysis is especially slow because the amine that must be lost on collapse of the tetrahedral intermediate is a very poor leaving group. The acid catalyzed hydrolysis reaction (Figure 7.19) is more favorable for two reasons. First, the amino function in the tetrahedral intermediate is likely to be protonated, making it a better leaving group. Second, the amine product that is released following hydrolysis will most likely be protonated and thus cannot participate in the reverse reaction to re-form an amide. This helps drive the reaction toward the hydrolysis product under acidic conditions.

Amide Hydrolysis in Acid Solution

THE OVERALL REACTION:

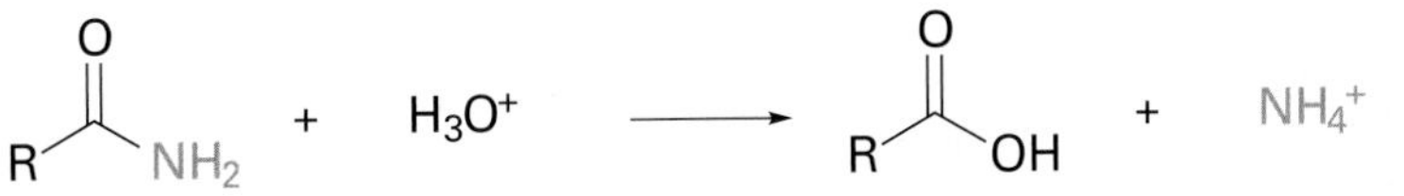

THE MECHANISM:

First Stage: Formation of the tetrahedral intermediate
Steps 1–3 are analogous to the mechanism of acid-catalyzed hydration of aldehydes and ketones and acid-catalyzed hydrolysis of esters.

Step 1: Protonation of the carbonyl oxygen of the amide

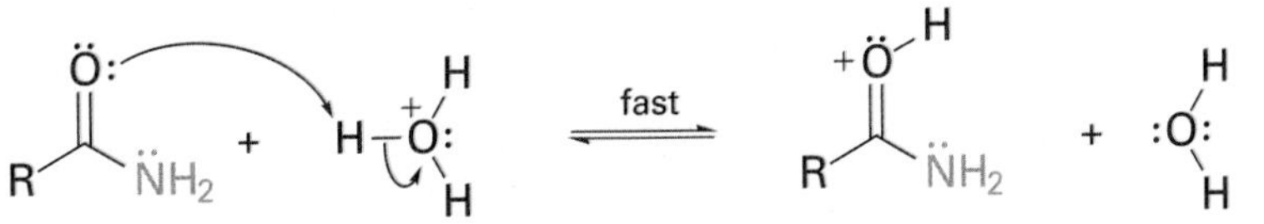

Step 2: Nucleophilic addition of water to the protonated amide

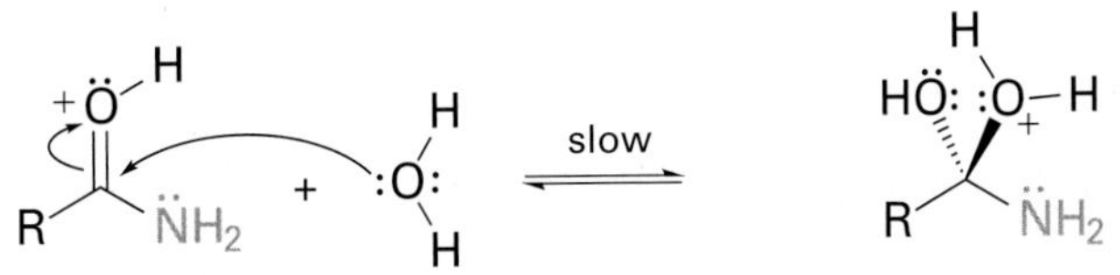

Step 3: Deprotonation of TI—H$^+$ to give the neutral form of the tetrahedral intermediate (**TI**)

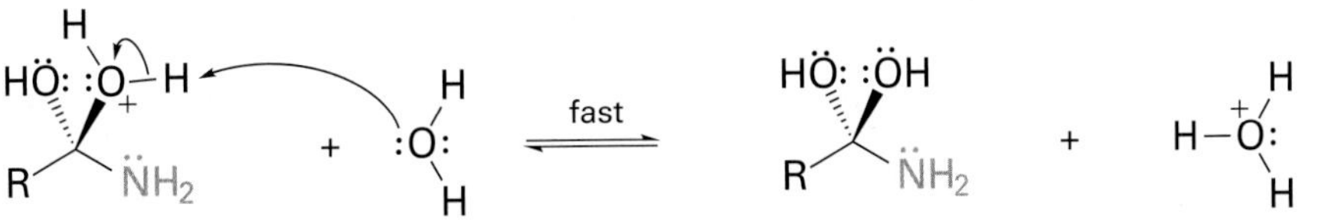

Figure 7.19 Mechanism of amide hydrolysis under acidic conditions. (Reproduced, with permission, from Carey FA, Giuliano RM. *Organic Chemistry*. 9th ed. New York: McGraw-Hill Education; 2014). (*Continued*)

Second Stage: Dissociation of the tetrahedral intermediate Just as steps 1–3 corresponded to addition of water to the carbonyl group, steps 4–6 correspond to elimination of ammonia or an amine from TI and restoration of the carbonyl group.

Step 4: Protonation of TI at its amino nitrogen

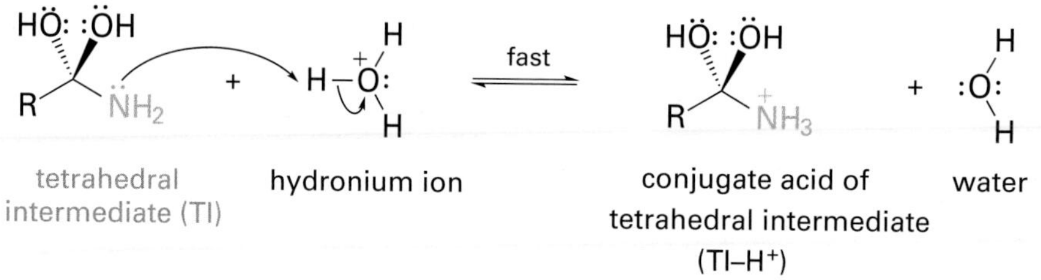

tetrahedral   hydronium ion
intermediate (TI)

conjugate acid of   water
tetrahedral intermediate
(TI–H$^+$)

Step 5: Dissociation of the *N*-protonated form of the tetrahedral intermediate to give ammonia and the protonated form of the carboxylic acid

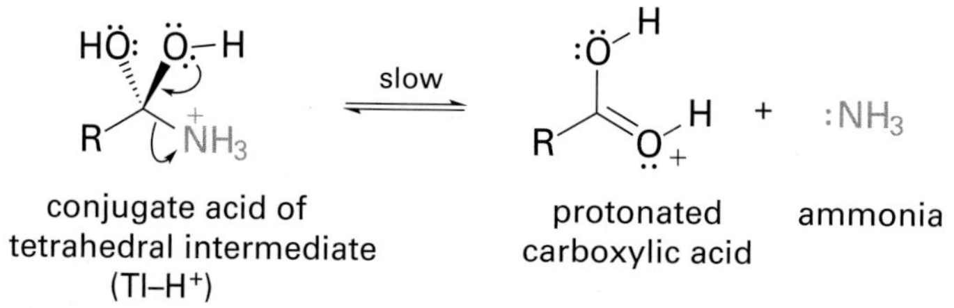

conjugate acid of
tetrahedral intermediate
(TI–H$^+$)

protonated   ammonia
carboxylic acid

Step 6: Proton transfer processes give the carboxylic acid and ammonium ion

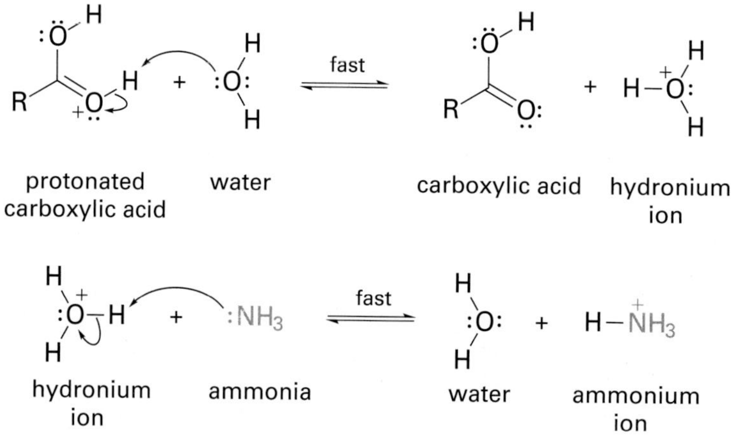

protonated   water
carboxylic acid

carboxylic acid   hydronium
ion

hydronium   ammonia
ion

water   ammonium
ion

Figure 7.19 (*Continued*)

7.9 Enzymatic Hydrolysis of Peptide Bonds by Proteases

If amide hydrolysis is slowest at neutral pH, how is it that protease enzymes are able to rapidly hydrolyze peptide bonds under physiological (neutral) conditions. As it turns out, nature has arrived at multiple solutions to this problem, using different amino acid residues and/or metal ions to promote what is an intrinsically slow reaction. All proteases share some general features, which include binding their substrates with high specificity in an **active site** removed from bulk solvent, and precisely

positioning the amide bond to be hydrolyzed in close proximity to the amino acid side chains that will serve as a **general acid**, **general base**, or nucleophile to assist in the hydrolysis reaction.

Proteases are subdivided into four main subtypes distinguished by the particulars of how they catalyze the amide hydrolysis reaction. Serine and cysteine proteases employ **nucleophlic catalysis** in which the peptide substrate reacts with an alcohol (from serine) or thiol (from cysteine) nucleophile in the active site of the protease. The resulting **acyl-enzyme intermediate** then reacts further with a nucleophilic water molecule to complete the

(1)

H   O
| ||
R₁—N—C—R₂

O=C—O⁻ ⋯ H—N⌒N ⋯ H—O

Asp 102   His 57   Ser 195

(2)

H   O⁻
| |
R₁—N—C—R₂

O—O—H ⋯ N⌒N—H   O

Asp 102   His 57   Ser 195

(3)

R₁—NH₂   O
         ||
         C—R₂

O—O⁻ ⋯ H—N⌒N   O

Asp 102   His 57   Ser 195

(4)

H   O
| ||
O   C—R₂

O—O⁻ ⋯ H—N⌒N ⋯ H   O

Asp 102   His 57   Ser 195

(5)

H   O⁻
| |
O   C—R₂

O—O—H ⋯ N⌒N—H ⋯ O

Asp 102   His 57   Ser 195

HOOC—R₂

(6)

O—O⁻ ⋯ H—N⌒N ⋯ H—O

Asp 102   His 57   Ser 195

hydrolysis reaction and regenerate the active enzyme. Aspartyl proteases in contrast employ water directly as the nucleophile and use a pair of aspartate residues as general acid/base to facilitate both nucleophilic attack of water on the substrate and breakdown of the tetrahedral intermediate. Finally, metalloproteases employ an active site metal ion such as Zn^{2+} to both activate the amide carbonyl and lower the pK_a of a water molecule that serves as nucleophile.

The active sites of serine and cysteine proteases possess a "catalytic triad" of amino acid side chains that perform the requisite nucleophilic and proton transfer functions of the enzyme. These include the nucleophile residue (serine or cysteine), a general acid/base (histidine), and an asparate (in serine proteases) or glutamine (in cysteine proteases) residue that properly orients the histidine residue. The mechanism of the hydrolysis reaction for the serine protease chymotrypsin is detailed in Figure 7.20. Note that the histidine residue serves as either acid or base at various points in the reaction. This is possible because the imidazole ring has a $pK_a \sim 7$ and can be either basic (when neutral) or acidic (when protonated) depending on the protonation state of the surrounding residues and substrate in the active site. An important region of the active site not shown in the figure is the so-called oxyanion hole. This site typically comprises backbone amide functions that donate hydrogen bonds to the carbonyl of the amide substrate, serving both to polarize and activate the carbonyl for reaction and to stabilize the negative charge on oxygen in the tetrahedral intermediate.

As the name suggests, aspartyl proteases employ active-site aspartate residues to promote the peptide hydrolysis reaction. Unlike serine and cysteine proteases, aspartyl proteases employ water directly as the nucleophile that attacks the amide carbonyl. The active

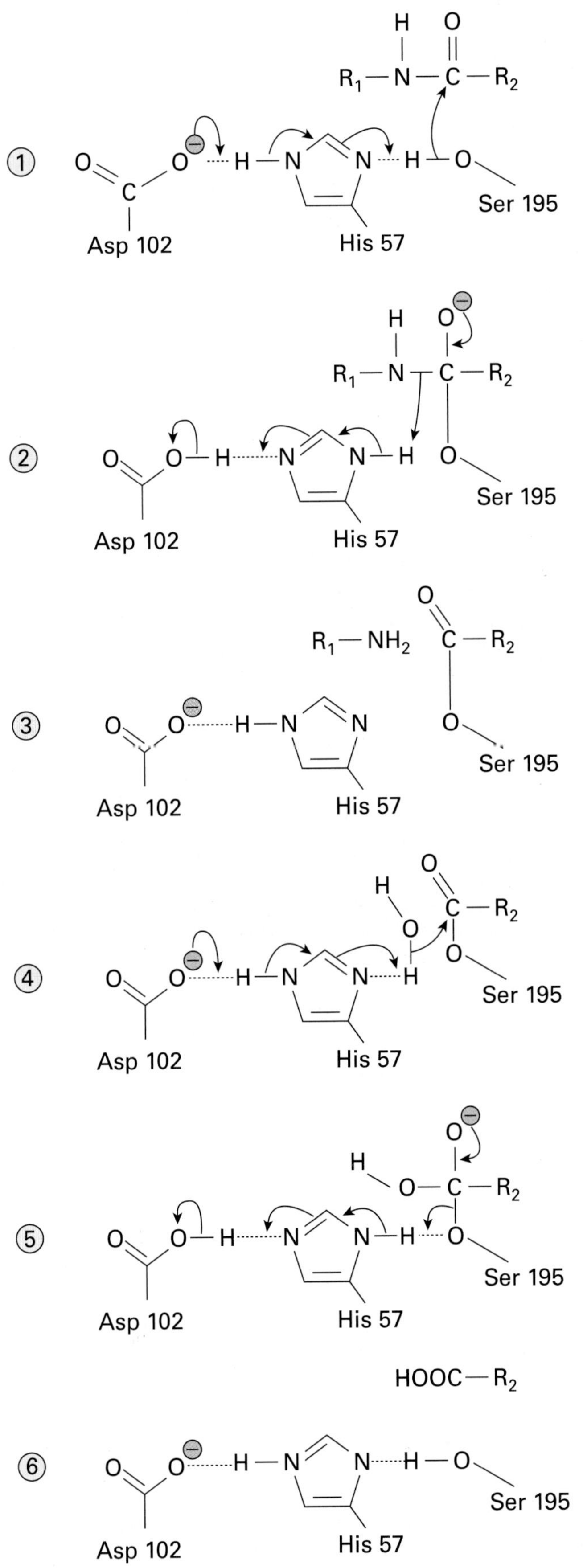

Figure 7.20 Mechanism of proteolysis by the serine protease chymotrypsin. In step 1, His 57 acts as general base to extract a proton from Ser 195. Following nucleophilic attack of Ser 195 on the substrate, the His residue shuttles a proton to the now-basic amine of the tetrahedral intermediate (step 2), thus facilitating formation of the acyl-enzyme intermediate (step 3). In step 4, His 57 again serves as general base to accept a proton from the catalytic water molecule as it attacks the acyl-enzyme intermediate. Finally, His 57 shuttles a proton back to Ser 195 as the tetrahedral intermediate breaks down (step 5), releasing the hydrolyzed product and regenerating the enzyme (step 6). (Reproduced, with permission, from Murray RK, Bender D, Botham KM, Kennelly PJ, Rodwell VW, Weil PA. *Harper's Illustrated Biochemistry*. 29th ed. New York: McGraw-Hill Education; 2012.)

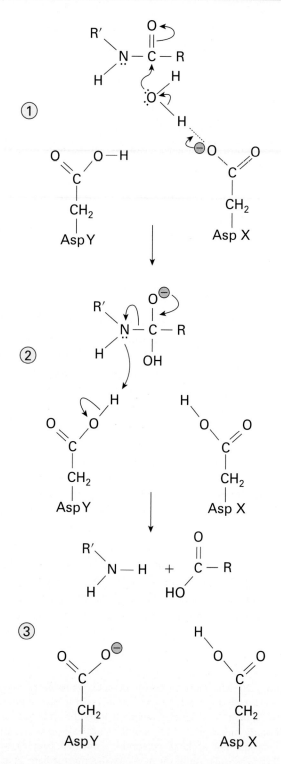

① ② ③

site contains two aspartate residues with pK_a values of ~6.5–7 and ~5–5.5, each designed to perform its specific function. The hydrolytic activity of aspartyl proteases is maximal at around pH 6, which provides a hint as to how these proteases function. At pH 6, one aspartate will be substantially protonated while the other will be substantially deprotonated. One Asp will thus serve as a general base to activate and accept a proton from the nucleophilic water. The other Asp serves as a general acid to protonate the amine of the tetrahedral intermediate and facilitates cleavage of the C–N bond. The mechanism of the hydrolysis reaction promoted by an aspartyl protease is shown in Figure 7.21.

The final class of protease are the metalloproteases. These enzymes employ a metal ion such as Zn^{2+} that is often positioned in the active site by histidine and/ or glutamate residues. The active-site residues of the metalloprotease carboxypeptidase A bound to a peptide substrate is shown in Figure 7.22. Note that the metal ion coordinates to the carbonyl of the peptide bond, polarizing the bond and activating it for reaction. The catalytic cycle begins when a water molecule coordinates to the metal center, displacing the Glu side chain

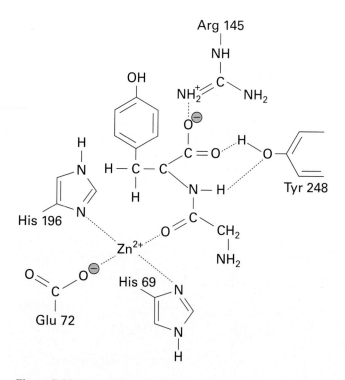

Figure 7.21 Mechanism of amide bond hydrolysis by an aspartyl protease. Two Asp residues in the active site with different pK_a values serve as either general base or general acid to promote the nucleophilic addition of water and breakdown of the tetrahedral intermediate. A final transfer of a proton between Asp X and Asp Y returns the protease to its initial state. (Reproduced, with permission, from Murray RK, Bender D, Botham KM, Kennelly PJ, Rodwell VW, Weil PA. *Harper's Illustrated Biochemistry*. 29th ed. New York: McGraw-Hill Education; 2012.)

Figure 7.22 Key residues in the active site of the metalloprotease carboxypeptidase A. The N-terminal amino acids of a protein substrate are shown bound to the active site Zn^{2+} ion. (Reproduced, with permission, from Murray RK, Bender D, Botham KM, Kennelly PJ, Rodwell VW, Weil PA. *Harper's Illustrated Biochemistry*. 29th ed. New York: McGraw-Hill Education; 2012.)

from the metal. The Glu residue can then serve as general base to deprotonate the metal-bound water, the pK_a of which is lowered on binding to the metal center. Coordination of both the substrate and nucleophile also serves to bring the reactants into close proximity for reaction. Following nucleophilic attack, the metal-bound

tetrahedral intermediate is protonated on nitrogen by Glu, now serving as a general acid. This leads to collapse of the tetrahedral intermediate and dissociation of the hydrolysis products from the active site. Examples of drugs that inhibit each of the three types of proteases described in this section are provided in Box 7.3.

Box 7.3 Drugs designed to inhibit proteases.

The important role proteases play in biology and in the progression of some diseases makes these enzymes promising drug targets. The different mechanisms by which proteases cleave amide bonds, as discussed in this chapter, can be exploited in the design of drugs intended to inhibit them. Likewise, knowledge about the specific amino acid sequences recognized by a protease is useful in the design of selective protease inhibitors. The diverse structures of the protease inhibitors shown below reflect the very different proteases they were designed to inhibit. Indinavir is an inhibitor of HIV protease (an aspartyl protease) and its structure includes a central hydroxyl function that mimics the tetrahedral intermediate formed during peptide bond cleavage.

The lymphoma drug vorinostat is an inhibitor of the enzyme histone deacetylase (HDAC). HDACs are metalloenzymes that bind acetylated lysines and remove the acetyl group. Vorinostat therefore mimics an acetylated lysine substrate but possesses a hydroxamic acid function in place of the amide bond of the biological substrate. The hydroxamic acid can form a bidentate interaction with the zinc ion in the HDAC active site, thus inhibiting the enzyme. Finally, odanacatib was designed to inhibit the cysteine protease cathepsin K for the treatment of osteoporosis (for more details see the case study at the end of this chapter). The nitrile function in odanacatib serves as an electrophile that reacts with the nucleophilic cysteine thiol function in the active site of cathepsin K.

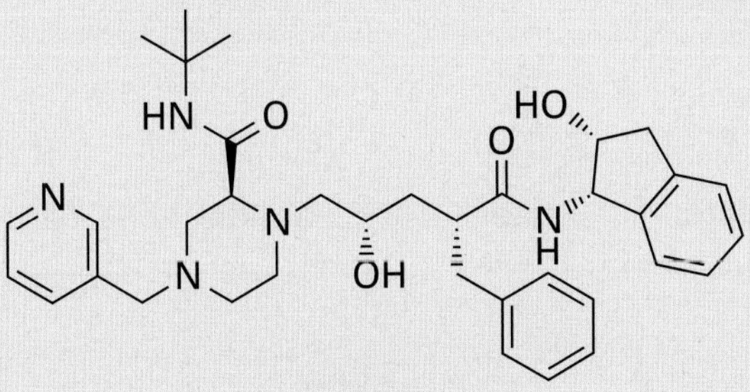

indinavir

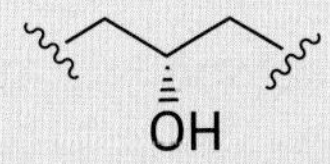

mimics tetrahedral
intermediate

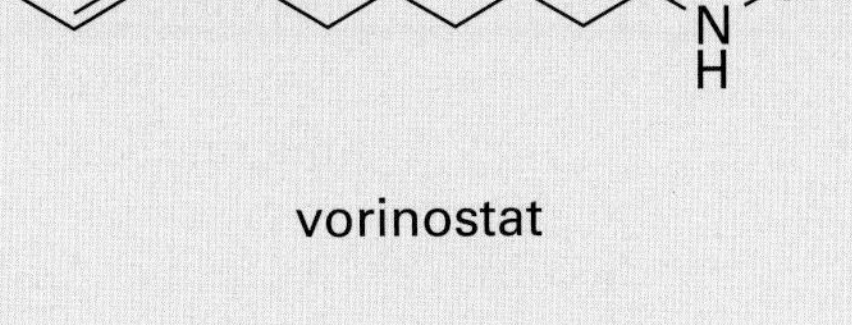

vorinostat

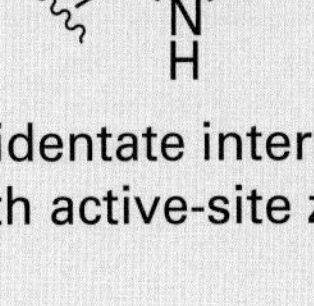

bidentate interaction
with active-site zinc ion

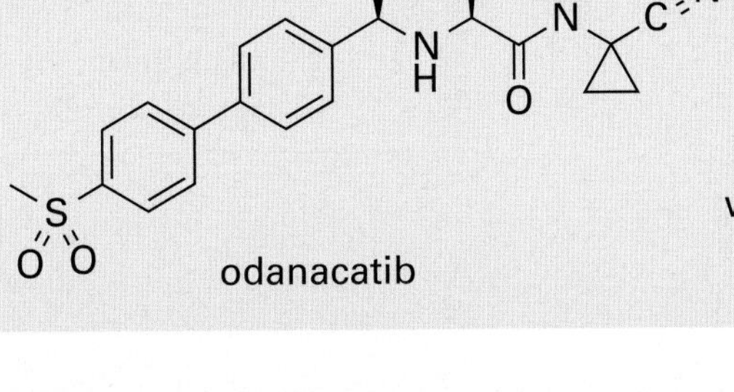

odanacatib

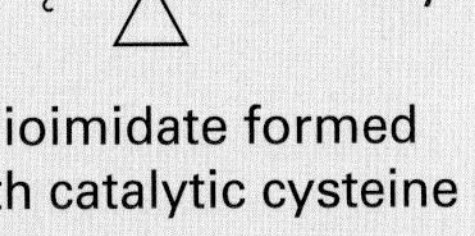

thioimidate formed
with catalytic cysteine

7.10 Summary

Section 7.1 Carbonyl-containing functional groups play important structural and functional roles in biological macromolecules and in drugs.

Section 7.2 A carbonyl (C=O) bond is composed of a σ bonding component and a π bonding component and is analogous to the C=C bond in ethylene. Carbonyl bonds are electrophilic and their relative reactivity is impacted by both electronic and steric factors.

Section 7.3 Electronic effects on carbonyl reactivity are mediated through **inductive** and **resonance** effects. The reactivity of carbonyl-containing functional groups varies widely depending on the nature of the substituent on carbon. Biologically relevant examples are shown below in order of their reactivity with nucleophlies.

Section 7.4 The hydration reactions of **aldehydes** and **ketones** proceed via distinct mechanisms at acidic, neutral, or basic pH. In general, C–O bond formation is slow compared to proton transfer (acid-base) reactions.

Section 7.5 The reaction of aldehydes and ketones with alcohols is similar to hydration but can involve a second addition step to afford an **acetal** or **ketal**. A special type of acetal is that found in the **glycosidic bond** that links sugars into di-, tri-, or polysaccharides.

Section 7.6 Reactions of amines with carbonyl species leads to **imines** or **enamines** depending on whether a primary or secondary amine is undergoing reaction. Imine and enamine formation proceeds through tetrahedral intermediates.

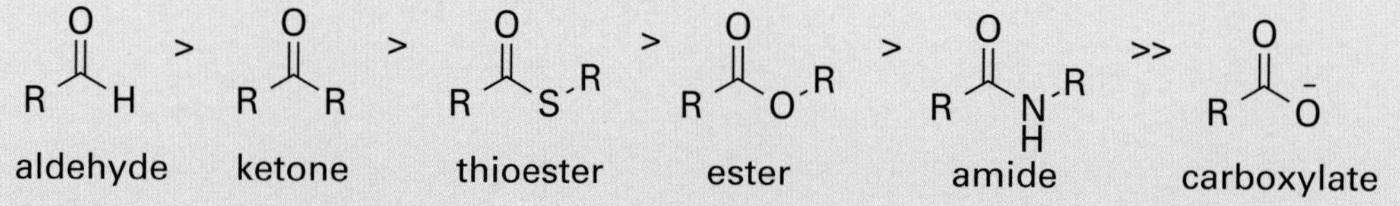

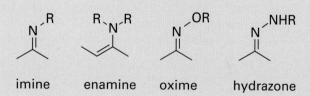

Section 7.7 **Oximes** and **hydrazones** are formed from the reaction of a hydroxylamine or hydrazine with an aldehyde or ketone. Close cousins of imines, oximes and hydrazones are generally more stable to hydrolysis due to their reduced basicity as compared to imines.

imine · enamine · oxime · hydrazone

Section 7.8 Ester hydrolysis can be promoted under either acidic or basic conditions. Protonation of the ester carbonyl is required under acidic conditions where neutral water is the nucleophile. Amide hydrolysis is most favorable under acidic conditions where amine protonation favors breakdown of the tetrahedral intermediate.

Section 7.9 Proteases are enzymes that perform peptide (amide) bond hydrolysis under physiological conditions. Proteases are classified as serine, cysteine, aspartyl, or metallo proteases depending on the mechanism by which they hydrolyze peptide bonds.

7.11 Case Study—Odanacatib

Cathepsin K is one member of a family of cysteine proteases that employ an active-site cysteine residue to promote peptide bond cleavage. Cathepsin K is highly expressed in the osteoclast cells of bone, which are responsible for bone remodeling during development or following a bone fracture. The strength and resilience of bone is a consequence of its composite structure—formed of a matrix of type I collagen (a structural protein) and the inorganic mineral hydroxyapatite. Osteoclast cells secrete acid to dissolve the inorganic component of bone, and produce cathepsin K to degrade the collagen by hydrolysis of its peptide bonds. In patients with osteoporosis, there is an imbalance of bone resorption and bone formation, leading to a net decrease in bone mass and susceptibility to bone fracture. Inhibition of cathepsin K has thus emerged as a promising new therapeutic strategy to reduce bone density loss in patients with osteoporosis.

A common approach to designing cysteine protease inhibitors is to combine a peptidic (substrate-like) structure with an electrophilic group that forms a covalent bond to the active-site cysteine thiol. The electrophilic group should react with the thiol function to form a stable intermediate that does not undergo further reactions that would regenerate the active protease. Various electrophilic carbonyl groups have been evaluated for this purpose (Figure 7.23). Ketones with a leaving group at the alpha position react to form a stable ketone that cannot undergo further hydrolysis reactions. Other ketone electrophiles lacking a leaving group will react reversibly to form hemi-thioacetals that can revert to starting materials but may be kinetically stable, acting as reversible-covalent inhibitors.

The electrophilic nitrile function in odanacatib was selected because it forms just such a reversible-covalent bond with the catalytic thiol function of cathepsin K (Figure 7.24). The reversible nature of reaction

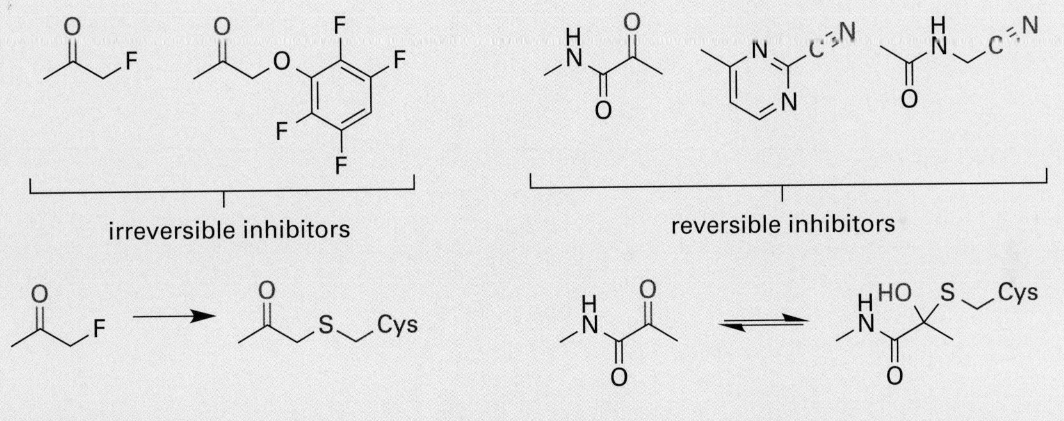

Figure 7.23 Examples of carbonyl and related electrophilic groups employed as cysteine-reactive "warheads" in protease inhibitors. As illustrated at bottom, warhead groups can react irreversibly or reversibly with cysteine proteases.

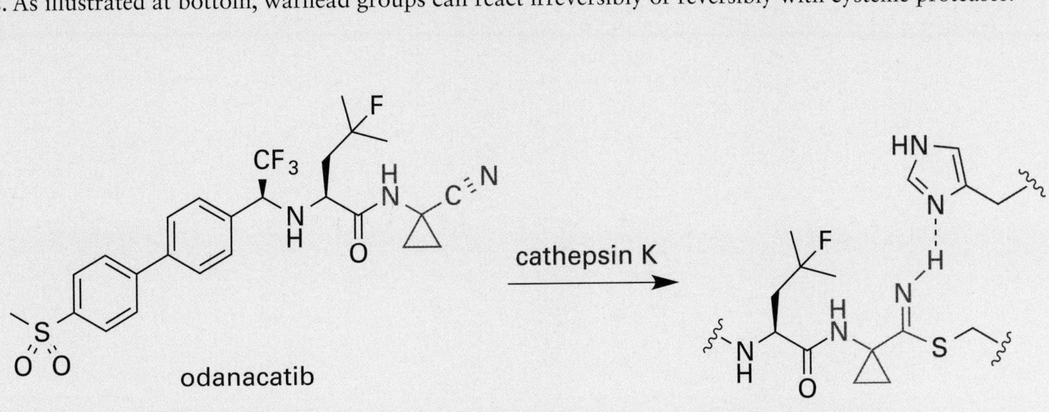

Figure 7.24 Reaction of odanacatib to form a stable thioimidate function.

with thiol was expected to minimize the possibility of immunogenicity arising in response to covalent drug-protein conjugates that might be formed with non-targeted proteins in the body. Minimizing the potential for such side effects is essential when developing a drug intended to treat a chronic condition in a large and generally healthy population.

Several additional features of the odanacatib structure merit mention. The cyclopropyl ring adjacent to the nitrile function was found to limit the extent of amide bond hydrolysis by serum proteases, leading to more sustained drug exposure in the body. This same amide bond forms important hydrogen bonding interactions in the cathepsin K active site that serve to position the nitrile group in proximity to the reactive thiol function. The fluorine atom in the leucine-like side chain of odanacatib was introduced to block the oxidative metabolism of the isopropyl group. In odanacatib analogs lacking the fluorine atom, metabolism resulted in greatly reduced concentrations of circulating drug. Finally, the trifluoromethyl group reduces the basicity of the amine function, allowing the N–H bond to donate a hydrogen bond to the backbone carbonyl of Gly66 in the cathepsin K active site.

Cysteine proteases have long been recognized as attractive drug targets for cancer, inflammation, and neurodegenerative diseases. However, developing safe and effective drugs that inhibit cysteine proteases has been extremely challenging. Should odanacatib ultimately win regulatory approval, it would represent a first-in-class treatment of osteoporosis and a rare example of a covalent (albeit reversible) drug developed for a chronic indication.

7.12 Exercises

Problem 7.1 Under mildly acidic conditions, the compound shown below is hydrolyzed to products I and II. Under more strongly acidic conditions, products I and II are formed initially but I is further converted to products III and IV. What are the structures of compounds I–IV?

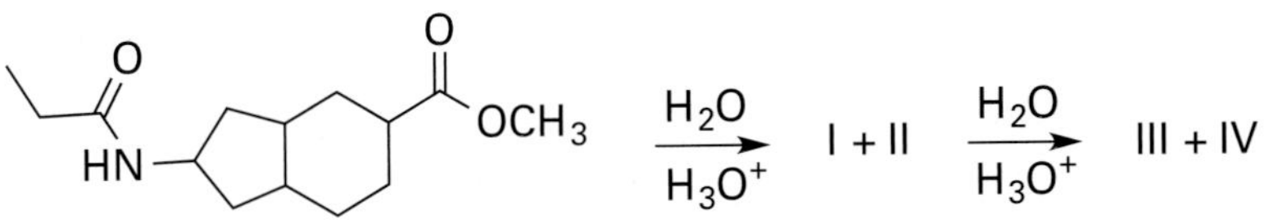

Problem 7.2 In each of the reactions below, two related starting materials are shown. In each case, which of the two starting materials will react more rapidly? What is the structure of the product of the reaction?

(a)

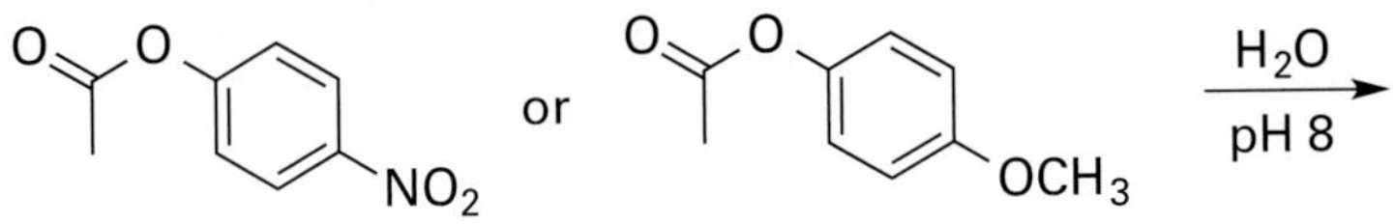

(b)

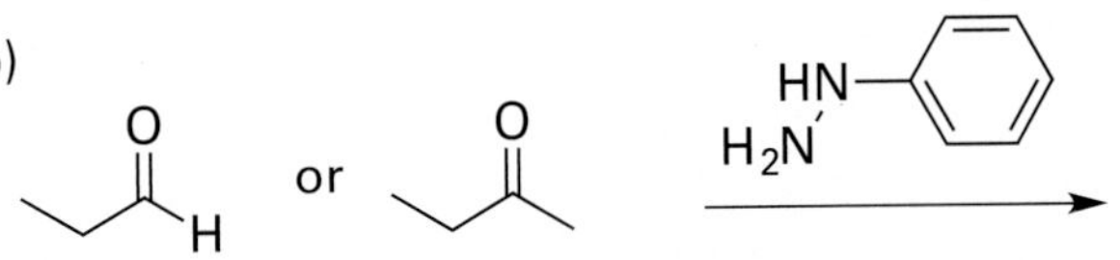

(c)

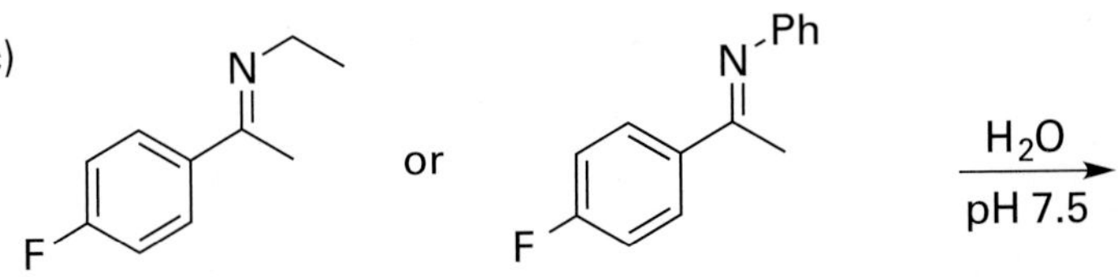

(d)

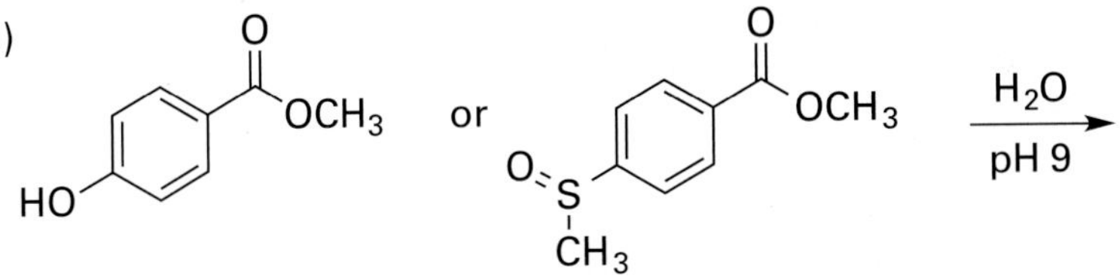

Problem 7.3 On the left below is the partial structure of azilsartan medoxomil, a prodrug of azilsartan shown on the far right. A simple methyl ester of the drug is too sterically hindered to undergo hydrolysis by esterases, but the more accessible cyclic carbonate in the prodrug is readily hydrolyzed. Write a mechanism for the hydrolysis of the cyclic carbonate at the indicated pH.

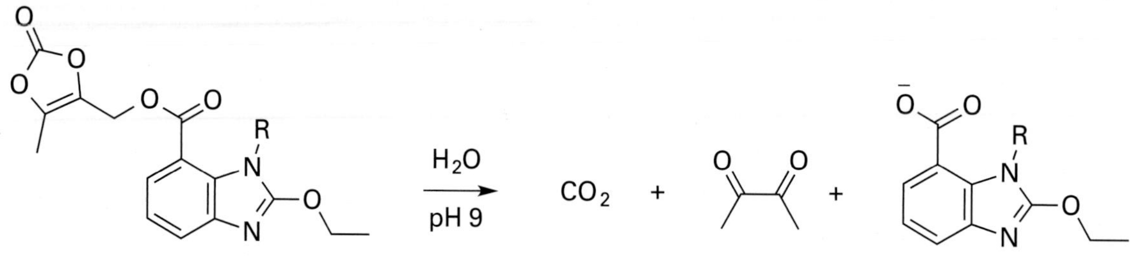

$$H_2O, \quad pH\ 9$$

$$CO_2 \ + \quad + $$

azilsartan medoxomil
(prodrug)

azilsartan

Problem 7.4 The hydroxyketone shown below is in equilibrium with two different hemiketals. What are the structures of these two hemiketals and what is the stereochemical relationship between them? Write a detailed mechanism for their formation.

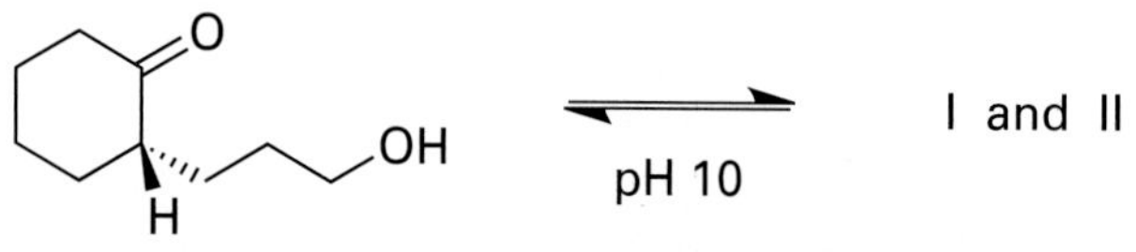

pH 10   I and II

Problem 7.5 The diastereomeric esters shown below undergo hydrolysis at dramatically different rates at neutral pH. Write a mechanism that illustrates how the neighboring carboxylate function accelerates the rate of the lower reaction. Why is the rate of reaction so much faster in this case? It may help to draw chair conformations of the two starting materials.

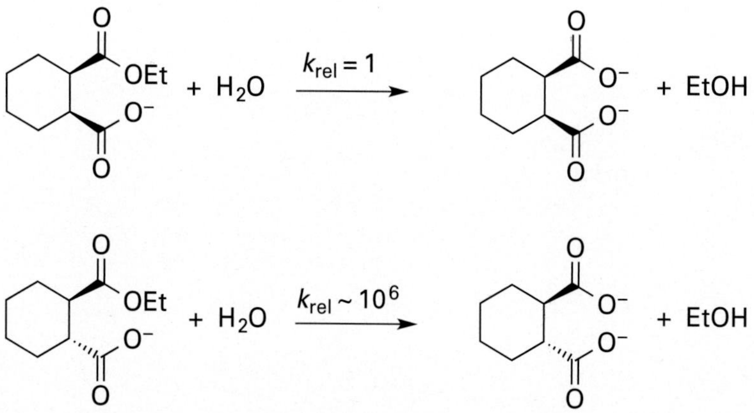

$$k_{rel} = 1 \qquad + \ EtOH$$

$$k_{rel} \sim 10^6 \qquad + \ EtOH$$

Problem 7.6 Bacampicillin is a prodrug of ampicillin that possesses improved oral bioavailability. Once absorbed from the gut, bacampicillin is hydrolyzed by serum esterases to afford ampicillin. Considering steric and electronic effects, which carbonyl function in bacampicillin should be more readily hydrolyzed by serum esterases? Draw a mechanism for the hydrolysis of bacampicillin to ampicillin at pH 9. Show all intermediates with formal charges and use arrows to show the movement of electrons.

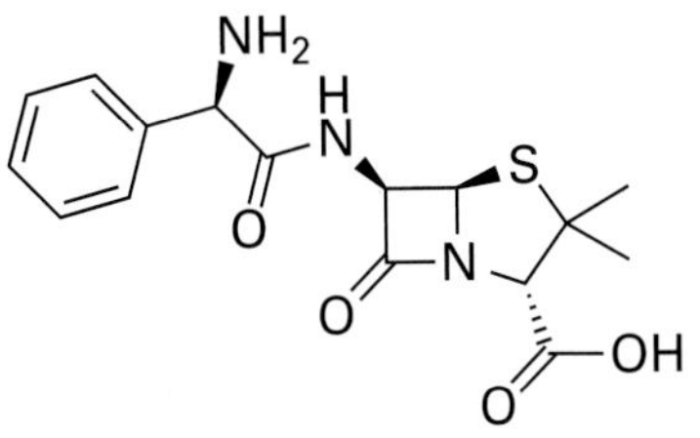

ampicillin 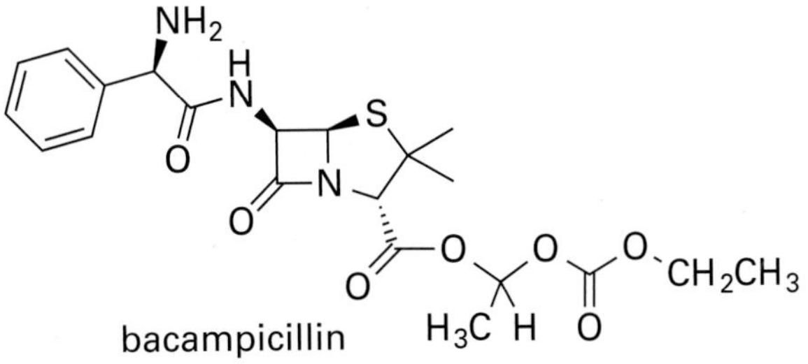   bacampicillin

Problem 7.7 The hydrolysis of a cyclic sugar yields the acyclic compound shown below. Propose a mechanism for this reaction. Show all intermediates with formal charges and use arrows to show the movement of electrons.

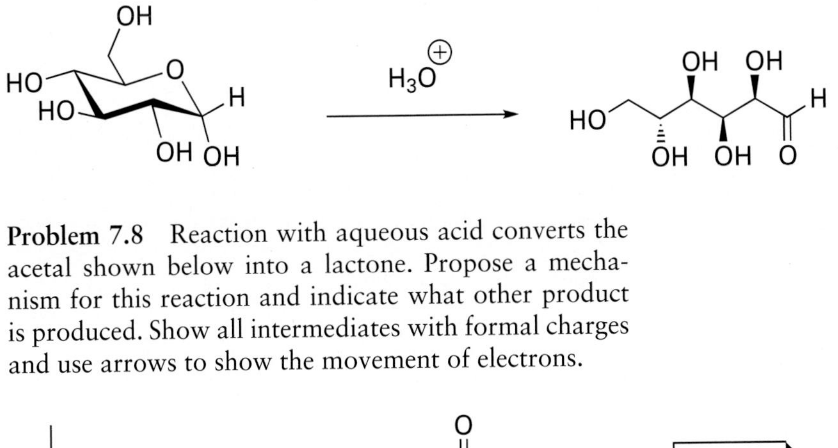

Problem 7.8 Reaction with aqueous acid converts the acetal shown below into a lactone. Propose a mechanism for this reaction and indicate what other product is produced. Show all intermediates with formal charges and use arrows to show the movement of electrons.

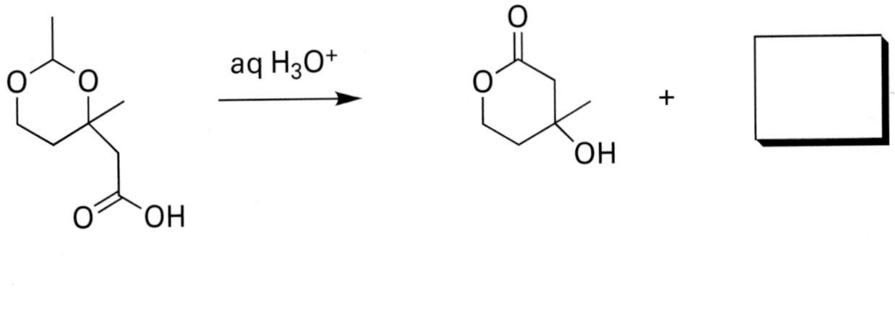

Chapter 8
Radical Chemistry

John Flygare & Adam Renslo

CHAPTER OUTLINE

8.1 Introduction
8.2 Formation, Stability, and Molecular Orbital View of Radicals
8.3 Radical Reactions
8.4 Reactions of Molecular Oxygen
8.5 Iron-Mediated Radical Reactions in Drug Metabolism
   Box 8.1—Fenton chemistry in the action of antimalarial drugs

8.6 Summary
8.7 *Case Study*—Calicheamicin γ_1
8.8 Exercises

8.1 Introduction

In this chapter we will examine the **homolysis** (homolytic cleavage) of σ bonds to form highly reactive **radical** species. When a bond breaks homolytically, the two electrons of the breaking bond end up on different atoms. The resulting radical species possess a single unpaired electron on an atom lacking a full octet of electrons. This makes radicals very electron deficient and unstable. They are often formed in low concentrations and are rarely stable enough to isolate, though they can serve as intermediates in chemical processes, as we will see. Biological systems take advantage of the high reactivity and transient nature of radicals to mediate a host of transformations required for life. Molecular oxygen exists as a diradical and we will see how it acts as a powerful oxidant, attacking organic molecules to initiate radical reactions. These oxygen-mediated radical reactions cause cellular damage and we will take a close look at how the antioxidant vitamins E and C (Figure 8.1) prevent this damage by acting as radical scavengers.

8.2 Formation, Stability, and Molecular Orbital View of Radicals

The homolysis of a covalent bond to form two radicals is illustrated using two single-headed ("fishhook") arrows, each of which indicates the movement of a single electron (Figure 8.2). Note that fishhook arrows are reserved for keeping track of electron count in radical reactions and are not interchangeable with the standard

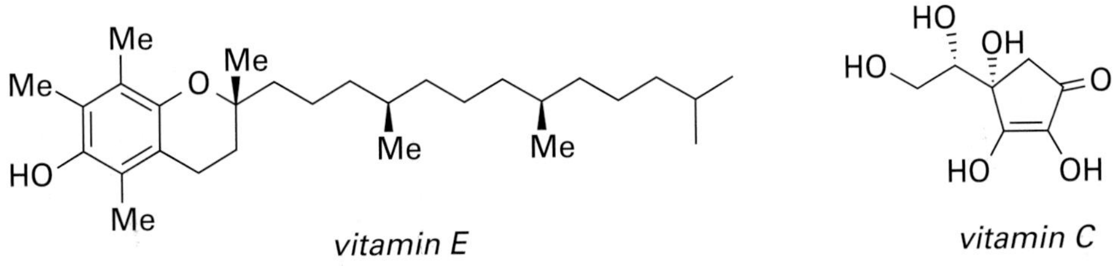

vitamin E

vitamin C

Figure 8.1 The antioxidant vitamins E and C.

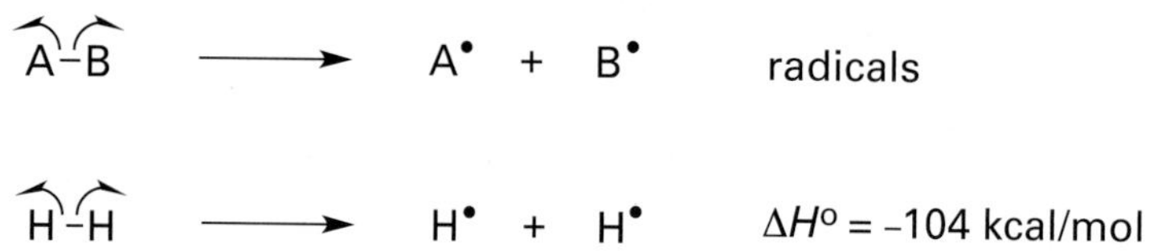

$$A\overset{\frown}{-}B \longrightarrow A^\bullet + B^\bullet \qquad \text{radicals}$$

$$H\overset{\frown}{-}H \longrightarrow H^\bullet + H^\bullet \qquad \Delta H^\circ = -104 \text{ kcal/mol}$$

Figure 8.2 Homolytic cleavage of a bond is illustrated using "fishhook" arrows, which indicate the movement of a single electron. The homolysis of molecular hydrogen (H_2) yields two hydrogen atom radicals.

arrows used to indicate the movement of pairs of electrons in acid/base or nucleophile/electrophile chemistry. The homolysis of molecular hydrogen (H_2) yields two free atoms of hydrogen. The process requires an amount of heat (104 kcal/mol) that is equal to the amount of heat produced when two free atoms of hydrogen combine to form a covalent bond. This is referred to as the bond dissociation energy. We will use bond dissociation energies to help understand the strength of bonds and the relative reactivity of radicals.

Homolysis of the C–H bond in methane yields a methyl radical in a process that requires 105 kcal/mol of energy (Figure 8.3). The homolysis of a C–H bond at a primary (101 kcal/mol), secondary (98.5 kcal/mol), or tertiary (96.5 kcal/mol) substituted carbon atom requires sequentially less energy. This trend in dissociation energies corresponds to the relative stability of the resulting primary, secondary, and tertiary radicals, with the tertiary radical being the most stable.

Let us examine this stability trend in more detail by comparing methyl and *tert*-butyl radicals (Figure 8.4). In forming either radical, homolysis of the C–H bond converts the carbon center from tetrahedral to trigonal planar geometry. The carbon radical is sp^2 hybridized with the unpaired electron located in the unhybridized p orbital. Replacing H atoms on the methyl radical with additional carbon substituents increases stability of the radical (Figure 8.3). The increasing stability is related to both steric and conjugative effects. For example, the methyl groups in 2-methylpropane will feel steric

crowding to a much greater extent than the hydrogen atoms in methane. This steric crowding is relieved as bond angles increase in the transition from tetrahedral to planar geometry. The second effect relates to stability of the unpaired electron in the p orbital of the radical, which is electron deficient and thus looking to add some electron density. In the *tert*-butyl radical, the sp^3 orbital of a neighboring C–H bond can donate electron density into the p orbital of the radical in a process called **hyperconjugation**. With three adjacent methyl groups, the *tert*-butyl radical can benefit from three such interactions. Although the additional stability provided is rather small (roughly 2 kcal/mol per methyl group), it adds up and results in the tertiary radical being the most stable radical in the series.

Electron-deficient carbon radicals can also be stabilized by resonance delocalization. This fact is evident in the lower bond dissociation energy for a C–H bond located adjacent to a π bond (Figure 8.5). In terms of the orbitals involved, the electron-deficient p orbital of the radial is delocalized into the more electron rich p orbitals of the π bond. Resonance delocalization of allylic and benzylic radicals can be illustrated using resonance structures, as shown in Figure 8.5. Note that we must use fishhook arrows to keep track of electrons when drawing resonance structures of radical species. The stability of the allylic radical is roughly equal to that of the benzylic radical in spite of the benzylic radical having access to more resonance structures. The loss of some aromatic character in the benzylic radical explains this.

Figure 8.3 The formation of methyl radical and the relative stability of carbon radicals.

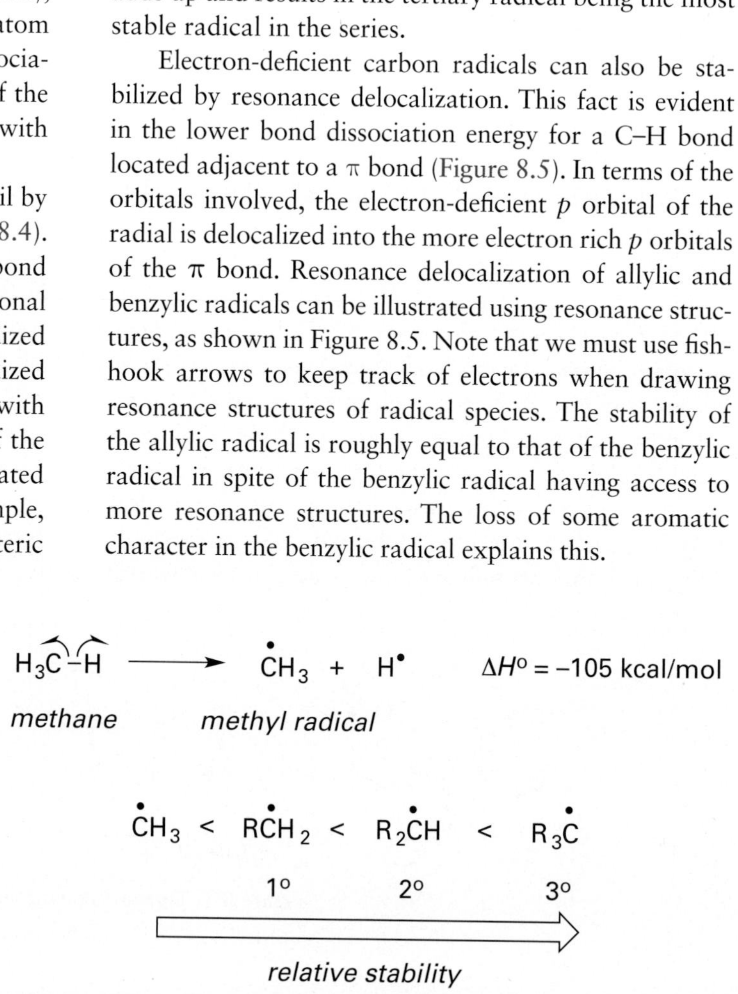

$$H_3C\overset{\frown}{-}H \longrightarrow {}^\bullet CH_3 + H^\bullet \qquad \Delta H^\circ = -105 \text{ kcal/mol}$$

methane   *methyl radical*

$${}^\bullet CH_3 < R\overset{\bullet}{C}H_2 < R_2\overset{\bullet}{C}H < R_3\overset{\bullet}{C}$$

$$\qquad\qquad 1^\circ \qquad\qquad 2^\circ \qquad\qquad 3^\circ$$

relative stability

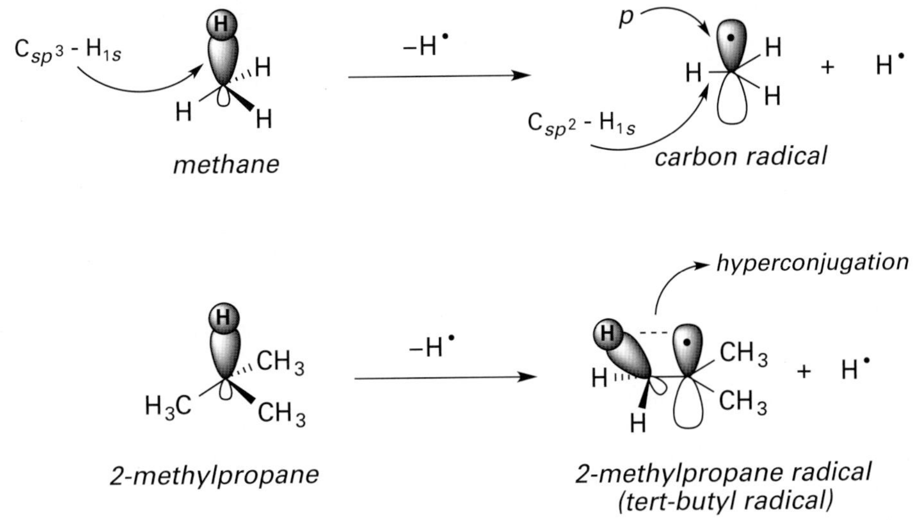

methane C_{sp^3} - H_{1s} $-H^{\bullet}$ C_{sp^2} - H_{1s} *carbon radical*

2-methylpropane $-H^{\bullet}$ *hyperconjugation* *2-methylpropane radical (tert-butyl radical)*

Figure 8.4 The electronic structure of carbon radicals.

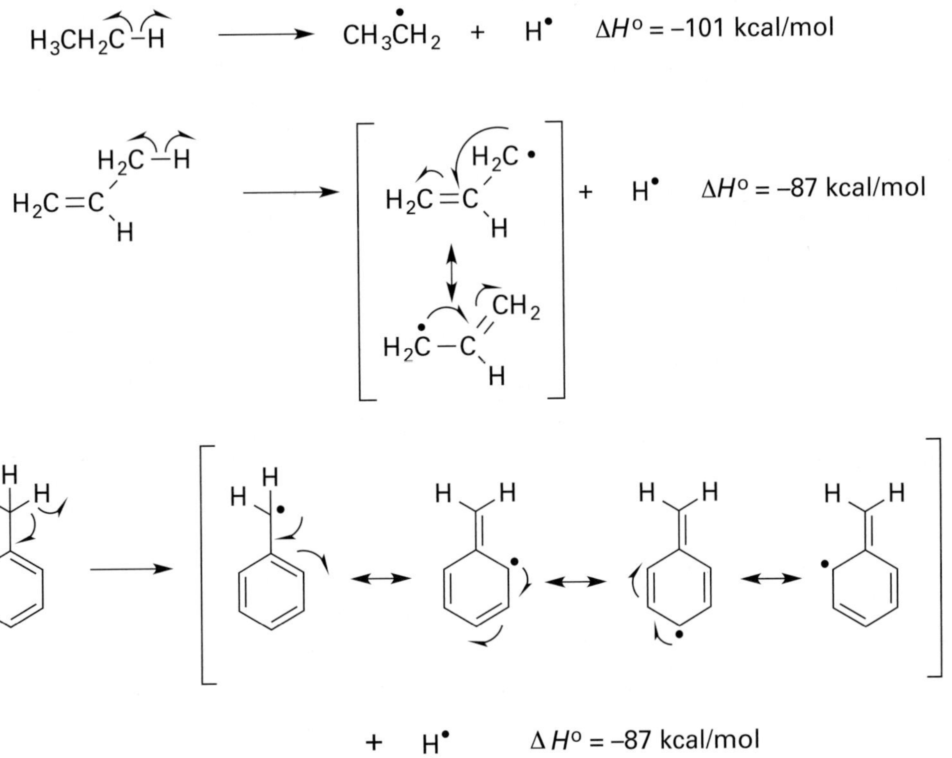

$H_3CH_2C-H \longrightarrow CH_3\overset{\bullet}{C}H_2 + H^{\bullet}$ $\Delta H^o = -101$ kcal/mol

$+ \quad H^{\bullet}$ $\Delta H^o = -87$ kcal/mol

$+ \quad H^{\bullet}$ $\Delta H^o = -87$ kcal/mol

Figure 8.5 Formation of ethyl, allyl, and benzylic radicals with the corresponding bond dissociation energies shown.

8.3 Radical Reactions

In this section we will describe the three stages of a radical reaction, which include **initiation, propagation, and termination**. The chemical behavior of radicals is dominated by their high reactivity and electron-deficient character. Radicals will often react with the closest atom available, and can involve reaction with a σ or π bond

(Figure 8.6). One common radical reaction is the abstraction of a hydrogen atom from a C–H σ bond of a nearby molecule. This produces a new radical species and is one of the ways a radical reaction can be propagated. A second important reaction of radicals is addition to a π bond to form a new C–C bond and a new radical species. On rare occasions, two radicals will be in close enough proximity to combine and form a new σ bond.

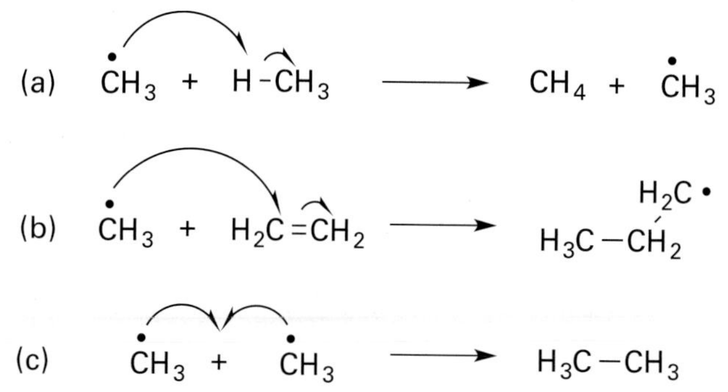

(a) $\overset{\bullet}{C}H_3$ + H$-\overset{\frown}{C}H_3$ $\longrightarrow$ CH$_4$ + $\overset{\bullet}{C}H_3$

(b) $\overset{\bullet}{C}H_3$ + H$_2$C$=\overset{\frown}{C}H_2$ $\longrightarrow$ H$_2$C$\bullet$ / H$_3$C$-\overset{\prime}{C}H_2$

(c) $\overset{\bullet}{C}H_3$ + $\overset{\bullet}{C}H_3$ $\longrightarrow$ H$_3$C$-$CH$_3$

Figure 8.6 Radical reactions involving (a) breaking a C–H σ bond, (b) addition to a π bond, and (c) reaction with another radical.

X$_2$ + H$-$CH$_3$ $\xrightarrow{\text{heat or light}}$ X$-$CH$_3$ + HX

X = Cl$_2$ or Br$_2$

Figure 8.7 General reaction scheme for the halogenation of methane.

The product of this process is no longer a radical and is representative of a termination step in a radical reaction sequence.

As we will see in the following sections, radical reactions are important in a variety of biological processes, including the metabolism and clearance of many drugs. Before describing these more complex processes, let us examine in detail a relatively simple radical reaction—the chlorination of methane with Cl$_2$ (Figure 8.7). As with most radical reactions, radical chlorination of an alkane proceeds through distinct initiation, propagation, and termination steps. We examine each of these steps separately below.

The initiation step in the chlorination of methane involves homolysis of the Cl–Cl bond in molecular chlorine (Cl$_2$). This bond is a weak one (bond dissociation energy of just −58 kcal/mol) and will be more prone to homolytic cleavage than the stronger C–H bonds of methane. Homolysis can be promoted with either heat or light to produce a small concentration of chlorine atom radicals (Figure 8.8). This initiation step thus generates

:$\overset{\cdot\cdot}{\underset{\cdot\cdot}{C}}l-\overset{\cdot\cdot}{\underset{\cdot\cdot}{C}}$l: $\xrightarrow{\text{heat (}\Delta\text{) or light(}\lambda\upsilon\text{)}}$:$\overset{\cdot\cdot}{\underset{\cdot\cdot}{C}}l\bullet$ + $\bullet\overset{\cdot\cdot}{\underset{\cdot\cdot}{C}}$l: $\Delta H° = -58$ kcal/mol

Figure 8.8 Homolysis of a Cl–Cl bond to form two chlorine atoms. This reaction represents the initiation step in the chlorination of methane.

the reactive chlorine radical species that allows the rest of the steps in the overall process to proceed. Only a small fraction of the total Cl$_2$ present need be converted to chlorine radicals in the initiation step, for reasons that will become clear as we examine the propagation stage of the reaction.

During the propagation stage of a radical reaction, the initial radical species produced during initiation reacts to form a new bond and in the process generate a new radical species. There are two propagation steps to consider in the chlorination of methane, the first being when a chlorine atom abstracts a hydrogen atom from methane (step 1, Figure 8.9). The resulting methyl radical then attacks a Cl$_2$ molecule yielding the chloromethane product and a chlorine atom radical (step 2). Note that the second step produces the reaction product while also generating a chlorine radical that can feed back into propagation step 1. This perpetual formation of chlorine radicals during propagation explains why very little homolysis of chlorine (by heat or light) is needed to initiate the reaction. It also explains why radical reactions are often referred to as chain reactions.

Termination occurs when two radicals combine to form a new covalent bond. These are called termination steps because they do not produce a new radical species to carry on the chain reaction (propagation). There are several possible termination reactions in the chlorination of methane (Figure 8.10). Note that the termination reaction of a chlorine and methyl radical produces the same

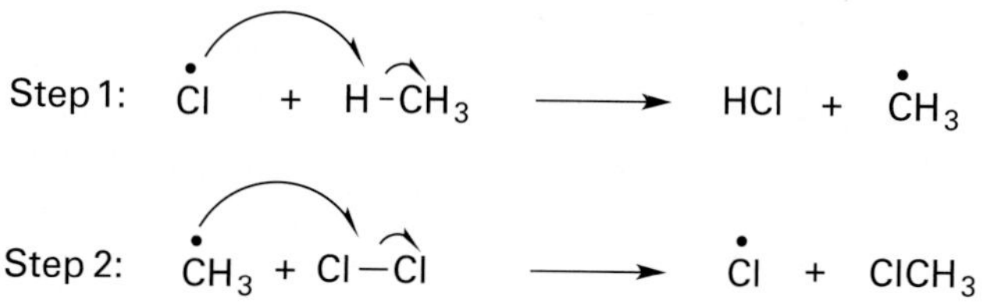

Step 1: $\overset{\bullet}{C}$l + H$-\overset{\frown}{C}H_3$ $\longrightarrow$ HCl + $\overset{\bullet}{C}H_3$

Step 2: $\overset{\bullet}{C}H_3$ + Cl$-\overset{\frown}{C}$l $\longrightarrow$ $\overset{\bullet}{C}$l + ClCH$_3$

Figure 8.9 The two propagation steps in a radical chlorination reaction.

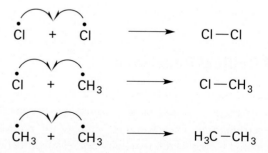

$\overset{\bullet}{C}$l + $\overset{\bullet}{C}$l $\longrightarrow$ Cl$-$Cl

$\overset{\bullet}{C}$l + $\overset{\bullet}{C}H_3$ $\longrightarrow$ Cl$-$CH$_3$

$\overset{\bullet}{C}H_3$ + $\overset{\bullet}{C}H_3$ $\longrightarrow$ H$_3$C$-$CH$_3$

Figure 8.10 Radical reaction termination steps in the chlorination of methane.

chloromethane product that is also formed in step 2 of the propagation stage. Recombination of two methyl radicals on the other hand will produce a different reaction product (ethane). Remember, however, that the concentration of radical species remains very low over the course of a radical reaction. Once formed, a methyl radical is much more likely to react with Cl_2 to form the desired product (and propagate the reaction) than it is to encounter and react with another methyl radical. The low concentration of radial species present allows the chain reaction to propagate and restricts the number of termination reactions.

8.4 Reactions of Molecular Oxygen

The most stable form of molecular oxygen (O_2) has two unpaired electrons occupying two degenerate molecular orbitals. These electrons have the same spin and are unable to form a bond, thus making oxygen a diradical. This diradical form of oxygen is referred to as triplet oxygen. Higher in energy by roughly 20 kcal/mol is singlet oxygen, which is much more reactive than triplet oxygen. Since the air you breathe is triplet oxygen and this diradical is what drives the biochemical processes of aerobic systems, we will focus our further discussion on triplet oxygen (Figure 8.11).

The diradical nature of oxygen allows it to drive many oxidation reactions ranging from the spoilage of food to oxidative damage in cells. A close look at how oxygen oxidizes unsaturated lipids will help us understand the role oxygen plays in these oxidative processes. Linoleic acid is a polyunsaturated fatty acid used in the biosynthesis of many bioactive compounds (arachidonic acid, prostaglandins) and is found in the lipids of cell membranes. As we have seen earlier (Figure 8.5), an allylic radical is stabilized by resonance delocalization with the adjacent π bond. We might therefore predict that the C–H bonds lying between the two double bonds of linoleic acid will be most prone to homolytic cleavage. Indeed, in the initiation step of the oxidation process, oxygen abstracts a hydrogen atom from the doubly allylic methylene group in linoleic acid to form an allylic radical that is stabilized by two neighboring double bonds (Figure 8.12).

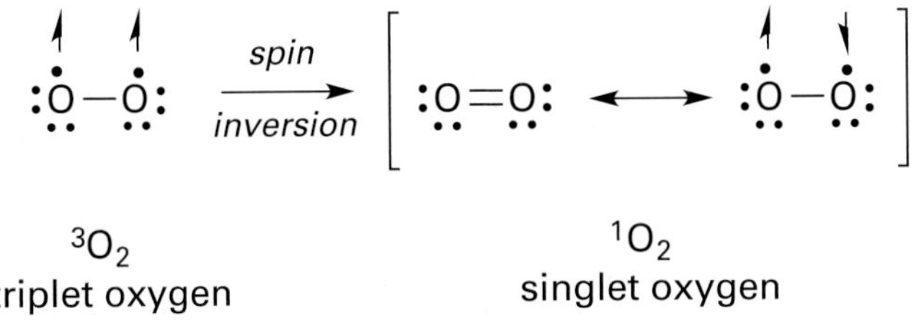

In a propagation step, this resonance-stabilized radical combines with another molecule of oxygen to form a peroxy radical. The peroxy radical abstracts a hydrogen atom from another molecule of linoleic acid to propagate the chain reaction and produce linoleic acid hydroperoxide. The weak O–O bond in the hydroperoxide species can cleave homolytically to yield an alkoxy radical (Figure 8.12). The alkoxy radical further decomposes to form an unsaturated aldehyde and other decomposition products that can wreak havoc on the integrity of a cell.

The reason that these products of lipid oxidation are toxic to cells is that they are reactive electrophiles. We have seen in Chapters 6 and 7 that the side chains of certain amino acids such as cysteine (protein—SH) and lysine (protein—NH_2) are potentially nucleophilic. Thus, the electrophilic products of lipid oxidation can covalently modify the nucleophilic side chains of proteins in nonspecific and detrimental ways. The biological function of these proteins becomes compromised and this contributes to the development of heart disease, cancer, emphysema, and many other chronic disease states.

You will note that the mechanism of oxygen-mediated lipid oxidation involves the three steps of initiation, propagation, and termination we outlined earlier for the chlorination of methane. Thus, a large amount of cellular damage can be initiated with a tiny amount of oxygen attacking a lipid molecule. Wouldn't it be nice if your body had access to some "terminator" molecules that could help stop this damaging process before it had a chance to get going? In fact it does—our bodies use vitamins E and C in concert to help minimize the harmful effects of radical intermediates. Let us take a look at the structures of these vitamins to understand how they work.

Looking at the structure of vitamin E you might note that the long hydrocarbon chain is similar to that in linoleic acid. It is not surprising then that, like linoleic acid, large amounts of vitamin E are found in the lipid membrane. We also expect that the phenolic (OH) function of vitamin E should be quite acidic since the negative charge of the corresponding phenoxide anion will be delocalized into the aromatic ring. It is in fact the phenoxide form of vitamin E that is able to donate an electron to lipid radicals, reducing them to an anionic state (which is then rapidly protonated) and thereby interrupting the lipid degradation process that otherwise

$$^3O_2$$
triplet oxygen

$$^1O_2$$
singlet oxygen

Figure 8.11 Triplet and singlet oxygen.

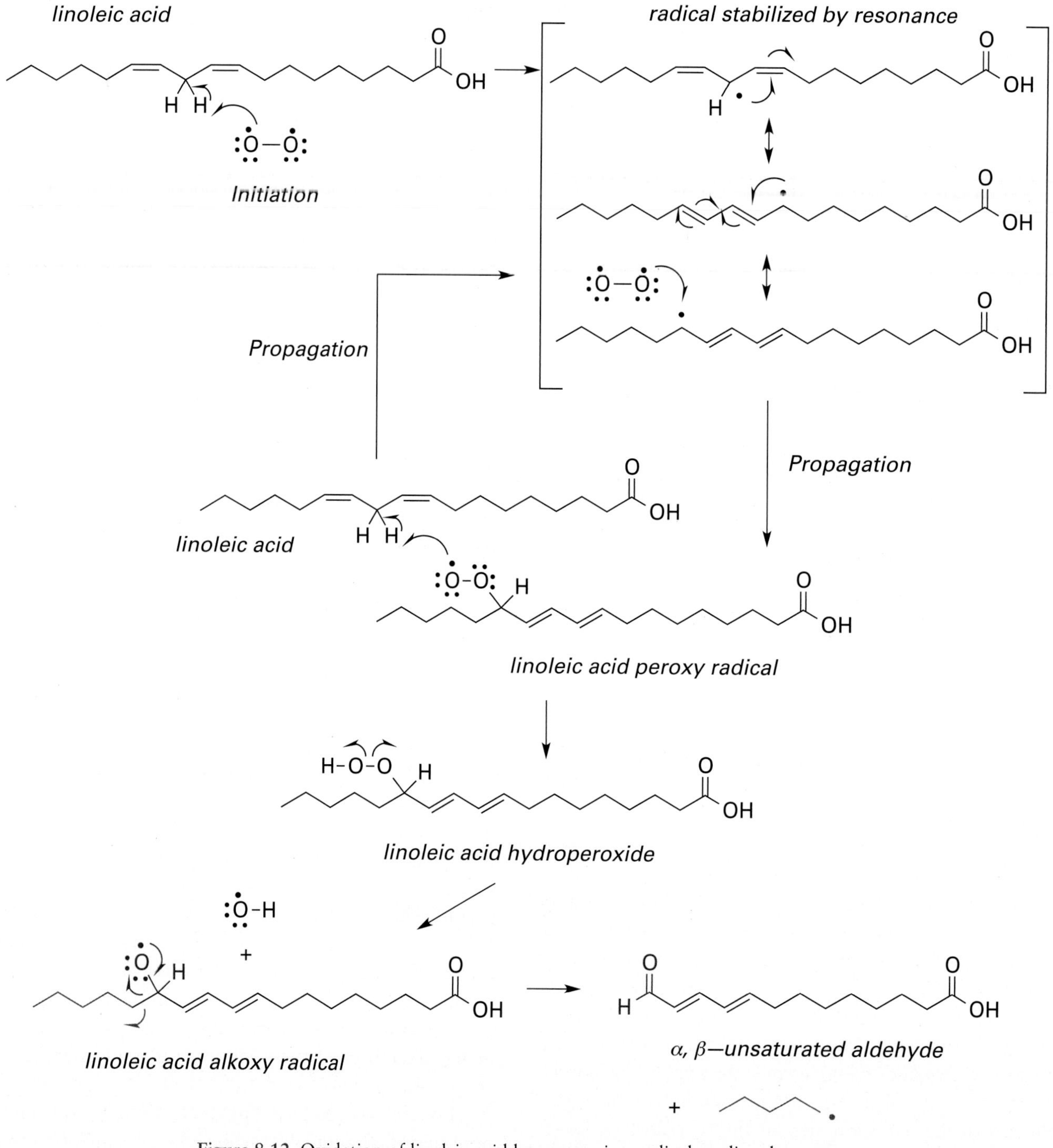

Figure 8.12 Oxidation of linoleic acid by oxygen is a radical-mediated process.

leads to reactive electrophilic species. Of course, in the process of donating one electron, vitamin E itself is converted to a radical. However, unlike the lipid radical, the vitamin E radical is much more stable and less reactive, due to the many resonance forms available to it (Figure 8.13). This radical form of vitamin E persists

until it encounters a water-soluble reducing agent such as vitamin C at the surface of the cell membrane.

As its other common name ascorbic acid suggests, vitamin C is an acid that exists significantly in an anionic form at physiological pH. This anion is able to donate an electron to the oxidized vitamin E radical, thus

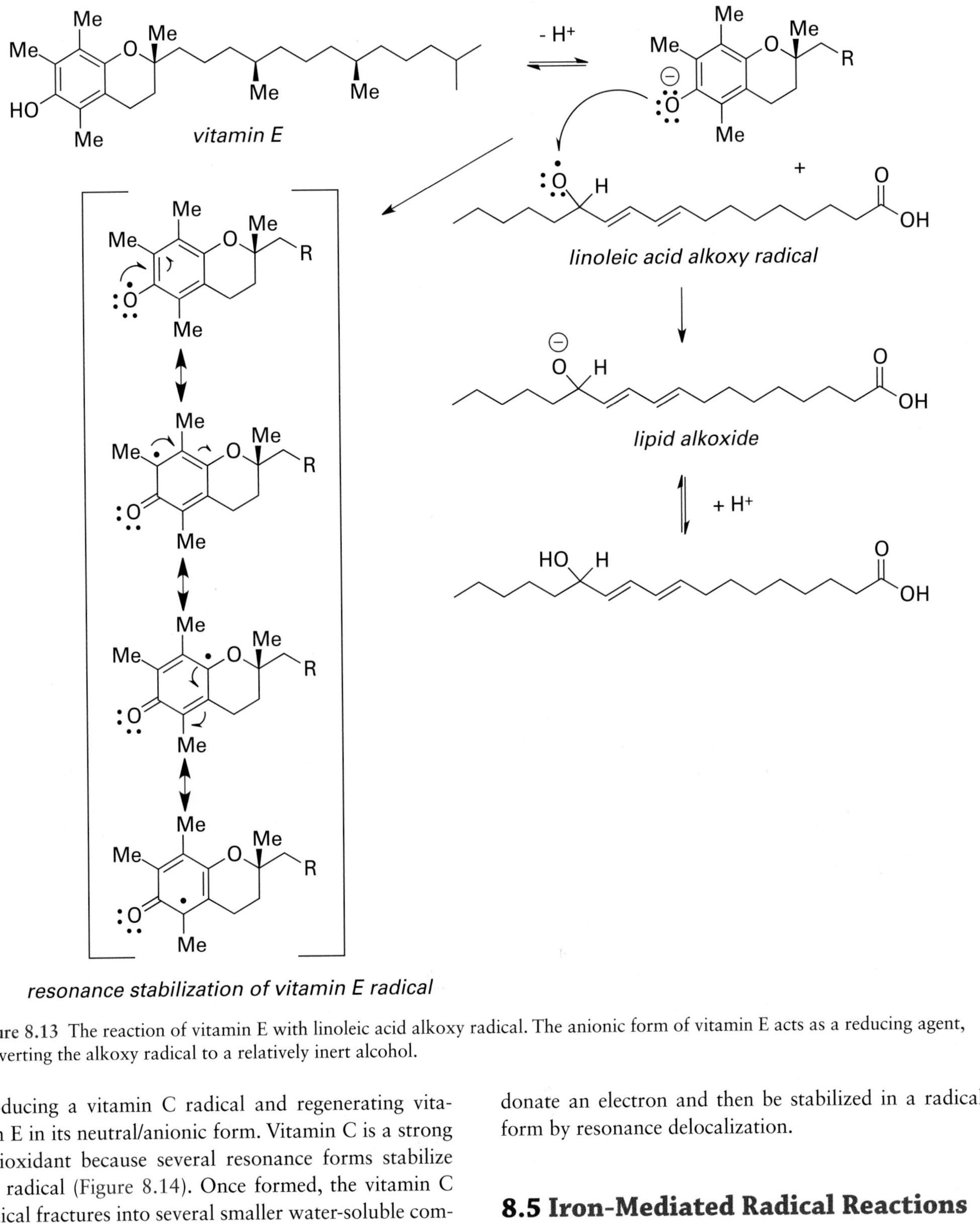

Figure 8.13 The reaction of vitamin E with linoleic acid alkoxy radical. The anionic form of vitamin E acts as a reducing agent, converting the alkoxy radical to a relatively inert alcohol.

producing a vitamin C radical and regenerating vitamin E in its neutral/anionic form. Vitamin C is a strong antioxidant because several resonance forms stabilize the radical (Figure 8.14). Once formed, the vitamin C radical fractures into several smaller water-soluble compounds that are quickly excreted by your body. In this way, vitamins E and C work together as radical scavengers to rid the cell of toxic radical intermediates. Note that the essential structural feature of these vitamins is an acidic function (phenol or phenol-like O–H) that can

donate an electron and then be stabilized in a radical form by resonance delocalization.

8.5 Iron-Mediated Radical Reactions in Drug Metabolism

Iron can be used to initiate a variety of radical reactions, both in the test tube and in biological systems. The reaction of hydrogen peroxide with ferrous sulfate is known

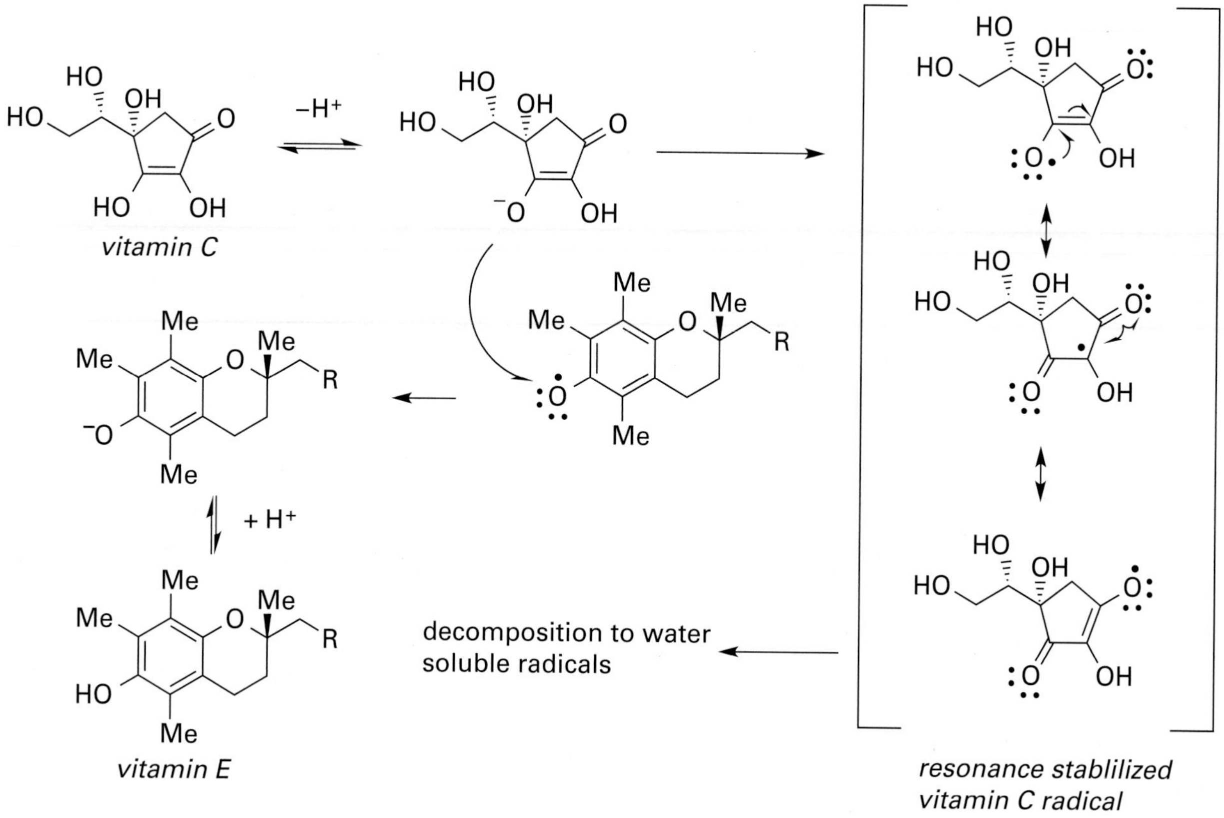

Figure 8.14 Formation of vitamin C radical by reduction of the vitamin E radical. Together vitamins E and C act as radical scavengers to protect the cell from potentially toxic radical species.

as the Fenton reaction. In this reaction ferrous iron (2+ oxidation state) is oxidized by hydrogen peroxide to ferric iron (3+), with the consequent production of hydroxyl radical and hydroxide anion (Figure 8.15). Ferric iron (3+) is in turn reduced back to ferrous iron (2+) in reaction with hydrogen peroxide to form a hydroperoxyl radical and a proton. The overall process leads to the **disproportionation** of two equivalents of hydrogen peroxide into two highly reactive radical species (hydroxyl and hydroperoxyl radicals) and water. Fenton chemistry is also implicated in the action of antimalarial drugs such as artemisinin and arterolane (Box 8.1).

The ferrous (2+) and ferric (3+) forms of iron involved in the Fenton reaction are also the two major forms of iron that exist under physiological conditions.

The ability of iron to undergo one-electron reduction or oxidation is central to the useful chemistry performed by biological macromolecules that employ iron. However, the potential of iron to generate oxygen radical species also means that the transport and storage of iron is highly regulated in biology. One large family of enzymes that exploit iron chemistry is the cytochrome P450 enzymes (CYP enzymes, for short). The CYP superfamily includes mitochondrial enzymes involved in cellular respiration, important biosynthetic enzymes such as steroid hydroxylases, and not least, the microsomal CYP enzymes involved in drug metabolism.

Microsomal CYPs are abundant in the liver, where they function to oxidize organic xenobiotics (including many drugs), leading to their elimination from the body.

Figure 8.15 The Fenton reaction of ferrous iron with hydrogen peroxide.

Box 8.1 Fenton chemistry in the action of antimalarial drugs.

Peroxide bonds are rarely seen in the structures of drugs, and for good reason. The reactive nature of peroxides and their potential to produce hydroxyl and hydroperoxyl radicals would seem to offset any possible advantages that might be realized by incorporating a peroxide bond into a drug. Nature, however, has provided a powerful counterpoint to this assumption. Artemisinin (or qinghaosu) is a biologically active component of sweet worm-wood (*Artemisia annua*), a medicinal plant used in traditional Chinese medicine. The compound was isolated and its structure assigned in the 1970s by Chinese scientists, and its effectiveness as an antimalarial was established in the ensuing decades. Today, semi-synthetic forms of artemisinin are employed in combination with other agents as frontline antimalarial therapy. So-called artemisinin combination therapy has saved millions of lives to date and has inspired the development of synthetic antimalarial peroxides such as arterolane. As you might have guessed by now, the action of these drugs is intimately connected to the peroxide embedded in their structures. It appears that the peroxide bond in artemisinin and arterolane undergoes a Fenton reaction promoted by unbound ferrous iron heme, a species that is produced in the parasite during its invasion of red blood cells. This homolytic cleavage of the peroxide bond leads to the formation of oxygen- and carbon-centered radicals, and possibly to the reaction of the radical with heme itself. These various radical and redox-active species subject the parasite to significant oxidative stress, and ultimately lead to cell death.

artemisinin   arterolane

Two of the most common reactions performed by microsomal CYPs are the oxidation of a C–H to a hydroxyl (C–OH) function and the epoxidation of an alkene or aromatic ring (Figure 8.16). Hydroxylation products of CYPs can be further converted to glucuronides (as introduced in Chapter 7), highly water-soluble conjugates that are rapidly eliminated from the body. Epoxidation products of CYPs can be converted to diols by epoxide hydrolase or can react as electrophiles in reaction with glutathione. In either case the result is a more hydrophilic metabolite that is more readily removed from the body.

To perform their oxidative functions, CYP enzymes possess a hydrophobic substrate-binding site situated in close proximity to an iron-heme cofactor that provides for the oxidizing capacity of the enzyme. The cofactor is a planar porphyrin ring made up of four pyrrole rings, with a single ferrous or ferric iron ion bound at the center (Figure 8.17). The porphyrin nitrogen atoms provide a planar coordination geometry that leaves available axial coordination sites above and below the plane of the porphyrin ring. One of these sites is typically occupied by a chelating imidazole (from histidine) or thiol (from cysteine) function that binds the cofactor to the

protein. The remaining axial position can be bound by water or, significantly, by oxygen during the catalytic cycle of the enzyme.

A detailed discussion of the catalytic cycle of CYP enzymes is beyond the scope of this text. Some important aspects of the catalytic cycle are, however, captured in cartoon format in Figure 8.18. The resting state of the enzyme finds the iron cofactor in the ferric (3+) state. The early stages of the catalytic cycle see the binding of substrate and reduction of heme to the ferrous (2+) state necessary to promote binding of oxygen. This reduction is carried out by an NADPH-dependent CYP reductase or similar reductase that works in concert with the oxidizing CYP. Following reduction, oxygen binds to the iron center and the resulting adduct is further reduced to the anionic peroxy species shown. Two protonation steps lead to cleavage of the O–O bond and loss of water. This produces a highly reactive iron oxo [Fe=O] species that has a radical character and is capable of performing oxidation chemistry on the bound substrate (a hydroxylation in the case shown).

In this chapter we have seen examples of natural small molecules such as vitamins C and E that protect cells and

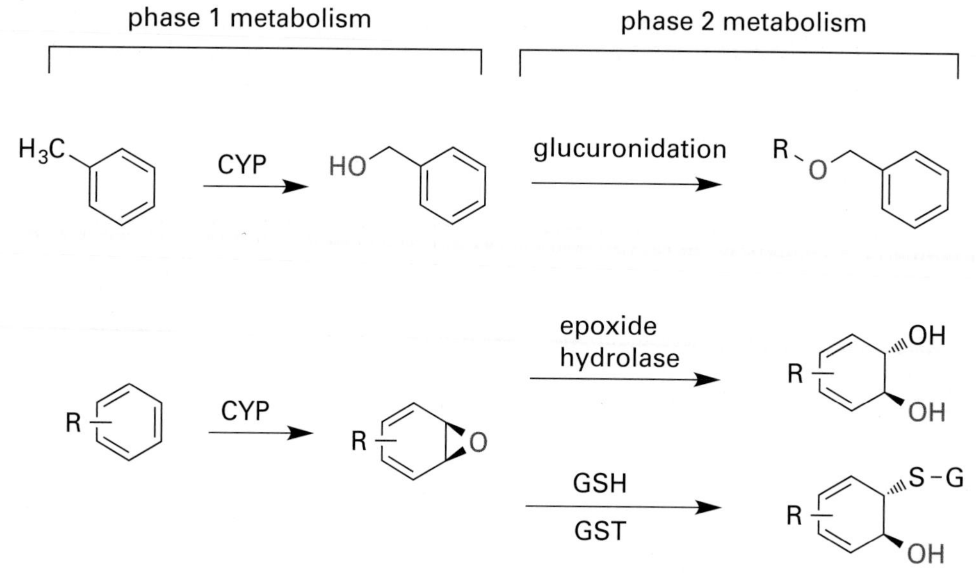

Figure 8.16 Examples of hydroxylation and epoxidation reactions carried out by iron-dependent CYP enzymes. These "phase 1" metabolic processes are often followed by phase 2 metabolism involving conjugation to hydrophilic groups such as glucuronic acid or glutathione.

Figure 8.17 Chemical structure of heme, in which an Fe ion is bound in the center of a porphyrin ring. A common shorthand notation for heme is shown at right.

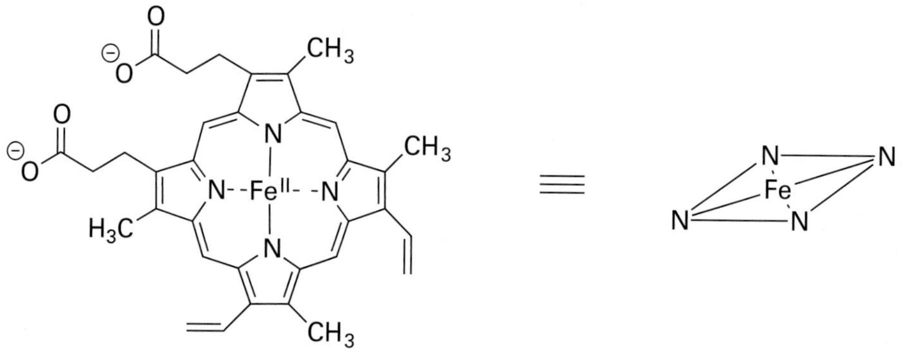

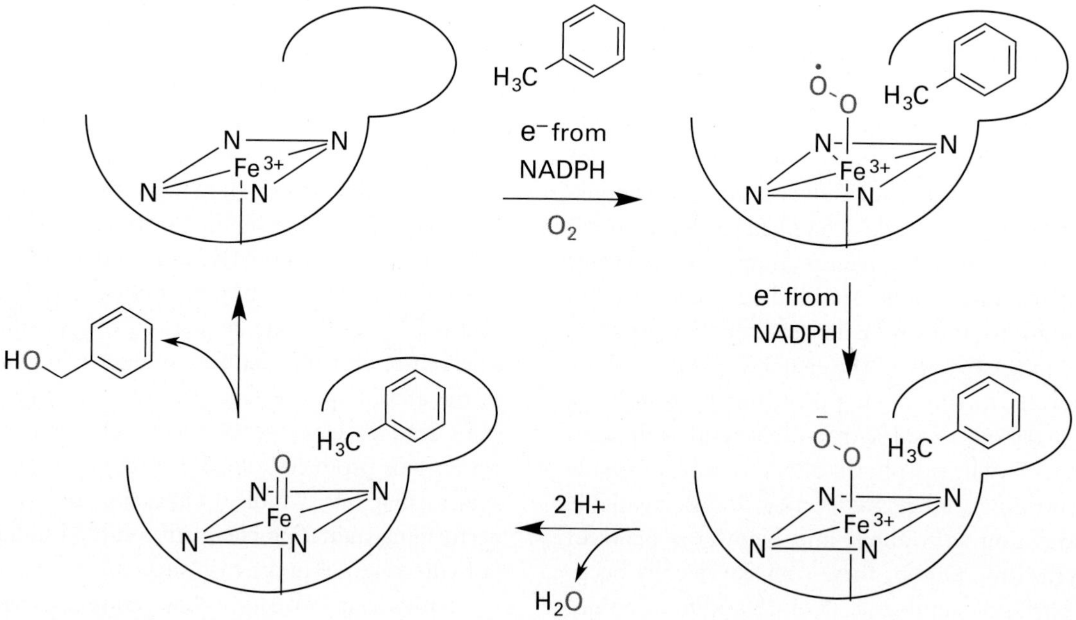

Figure 8.18 Abbreviated catalytic cycle for the hydroxylation reaction performed by heme-dependent microsomal CYP enzymes working in concert with NADPH-dependent reductases.

tissues from the harmful effects of oxidation by diradical oxygen. We have likewise seen how iron-dependent CYP enzymes detoxify organic xenobiotics using one-electron redox chemistry. These examples only hint at the larger role of radical chemistry in biology, which also includes the biosynthesis of steroids and DNA bases, oxygen transport and storage, and the process of oxidative phosphorylation whereby the energy of the reactive oxygen diradical is converted to a small-molecule energy source (ATP) that can be readily exploited by the molecules of life.

8.6 Summary

Section 8.1	A **radical** is a compound with a single unpaired electron on an atom that does not have a full octet of electrons.
Section 8.2	Radicals are formed by **homolysis** of a covalent bond. They are electron deficient and can be stabilized by neighboring σ or π bonds that are able to share electron density through conjugation or **hyperconjugation**.
Section 8.3	Radical reactions involve three distinct steps—**initiation**, **propagation**, and **termination**. Only a small amount of radical is present during the course of the reaction.
Section 8.4	Molecular oxygen (O_2) exists as a diradical and mediates a variety of radical-mediated biological processes. Vitamins E and C are used as radical scavengers to terminate these radical reactions.
Section 8.5	Iron plays an important role in initiating radical reactions. This includes the iron-dependent cytochrome P450 enzymes in the liver that are responsible for modifying and eliminating drugs from the blood system.

8.7 Case Study—Calicheamicin γ_1

Calicheamicin γ_1 is a naturally occurring antibiotic and one of the most potent cellular toxins known (Figure 8.19). A *single molecule* of calicheamicin γ_1, after entering a cell and cleaving a covalent bond in DNA, is capable of causing cell death. How is this possible? In Chapter 6 we have seen how some electrophilic chemotherapy drugs alkylate and cross-link strands of DNA. In contrast, calicheamicin causes *breaks* in the DNA strand employing a radical-mediated reaction. In a series of choreographed events, calicheamicin first binds to DNA and is then reduced and undergoes multiple structural rearrangements leading to a diradical species that attacks DNA. In this case study we will discuss some of the key reactions involved in this process.

The chemical structure of calicheamicin is remarkable and reflects the complexity of its mechanism of action. The highly substituted aryl ring and four sugars in the molecule are mainly responsible for specificity in binding of the molecule to the minor grove of DNA. The highly unsaturated enediyne function (an alkene flanked by two alkynes) is the "warhead" of calicheamicin, a chemical precursor to the diradical species that will ultimately do irreversible damage to DNA. If the enediyne is the warhead, then the three sulfur atoms and the electrophilic Michael acceptor together comprise a "trigger" that must be pulled to unleash the warhead.

After binding in the minor groove of DNA, a disulfide bond in calicheamicin is reduced in an

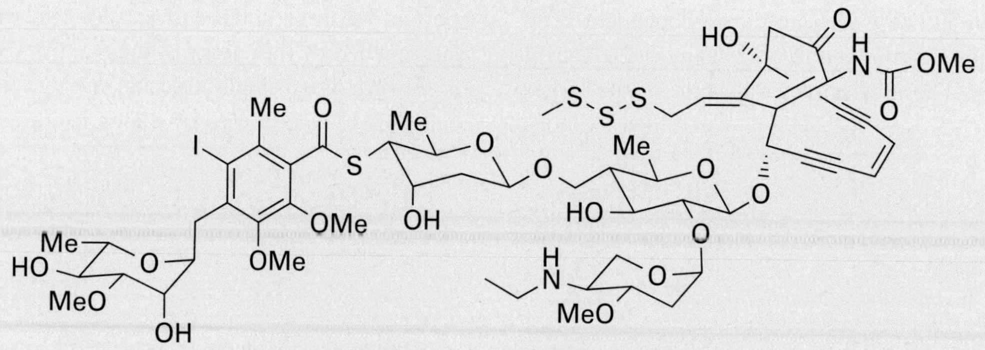

Figure 8.19 Structure of calicheamicin γ₁.

enzymatic process to yield a nucleophilic thiol side chain (Figure 8.20). The thiol undergoes intramolecular Michael addition to the cyclohexenone ring that is part of the bridged bicyclic ring system. An important consequence of this Michael reaction is that the two alkynes of the enediyne are brought slightly closer together in space. This in turn leads to an electrocyclization reaction (Bergman cyclization) that produces an aryl diradical intermediate.

The aryl diradical is the species that abstracts a hydrogen atom from the backbone of DNA. This can happen at various sites, one of which is the 5′ carbon directly adjacent to phosphate in the DNA backbone (Figure 8.21). Once generated, the 5′ carbon radical reacts with oxygen to form a peroxy radical and, after abstracting a hydrogen atom, a hydroperoxide intermediate. Note that these steps are similar to the propagation steps involved in the oxidation of linoleic acid (Figure 8.12). The DNA strand is broken via breakdown of the 5′ hydroperoxide acetal, with phosphate serving as the (excellent) leaving group. This is but one mechanism by which the calicheamicin diradical can cleave DNA; strand breaks can also occur following hydrogen abstraction from the 1′, 3′, or 4′ carbons. In each case the cell is unable to repair the strand breaks and this leads to cell death.

These potent cell-killing effects generated interest in using calicheamicin γ₁ to treat cancer. Not surprisingly, the compound was found to exhibit little selectivity between cancer cells and normal cells. However,

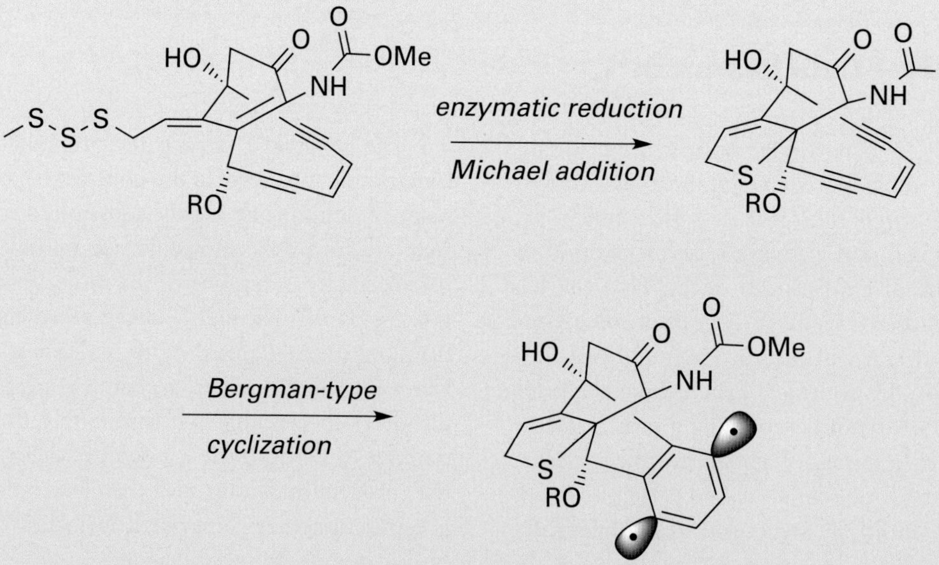

Figure 8.20 Reaction sequence leading to activation of the calicheamicin enediyne and Bergman cyclization to produce an aryl diradical intermediate. For clarity, the sugar moiety is not shown.

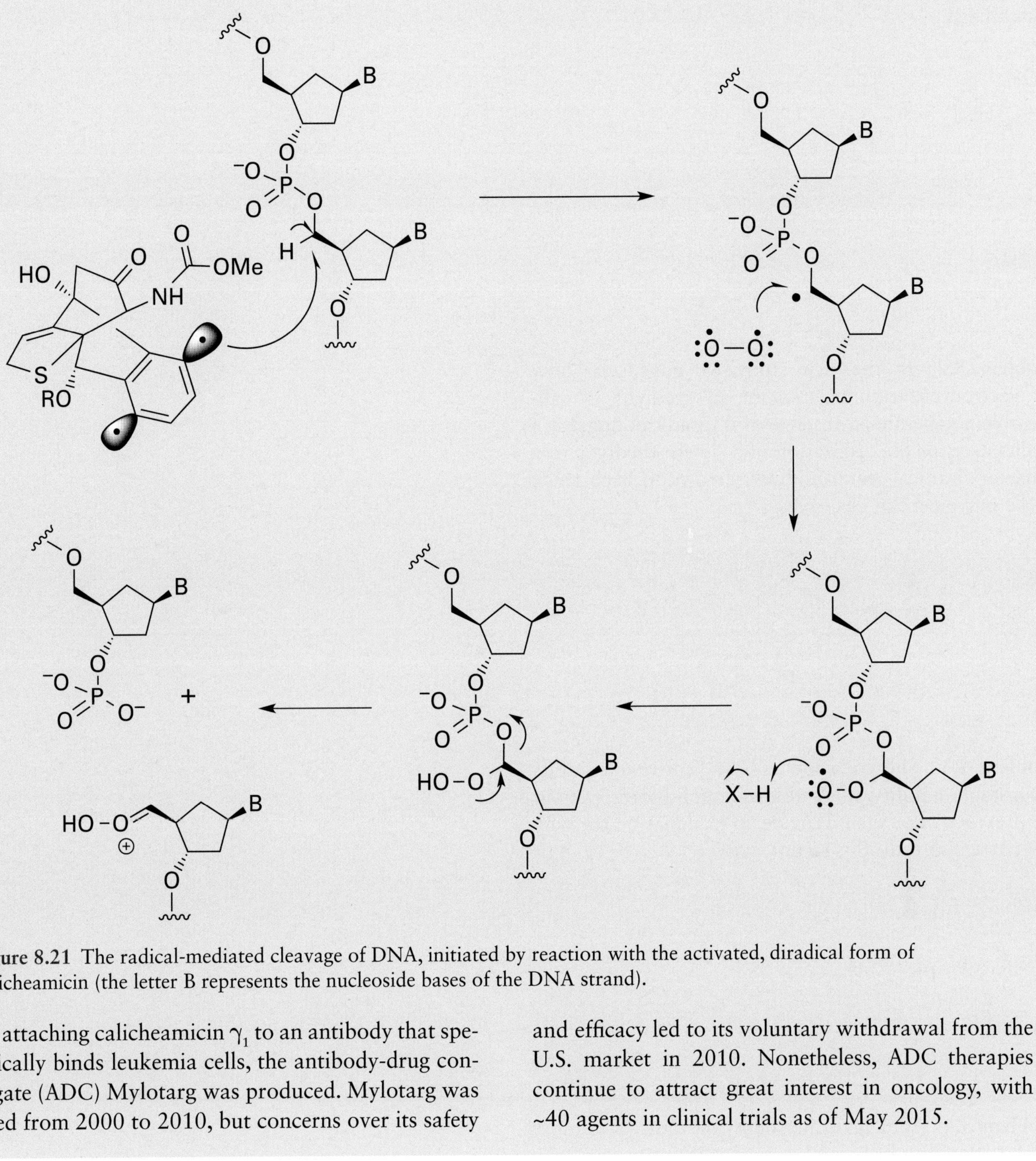

Figure 8.21 The radical-mediated cleavage of DNA, initiated by reaction with the activated, diradical form of calicheamicin (the letter B represents the nucleoside bases of the DNA strand).

by attaching calicheamicin γ_1 to an antibody that specifically binds leukemia cells, the antibody-drug conjugate (ADC) Mylotarg was produced. Mylotarg was used from 2000 to 2010, but concerns over its safety and efficacy led to its voluntary withdrawal from the U.S. market in 2010. Nonetheless, ADC therapies continue to attract great interest in oncology, with ~40 agents in clinical trials as of May 2015.

8.8 Exercises

Problem 8.1 The food additive BHA is a synthetic antioxidant that shares structural features with natural antioxidants like vitamin E. Explain how BHA might work to prevent food spoilage (exposure to oxygen), drawing resonance forms to show how the BHA radical is stabilized.

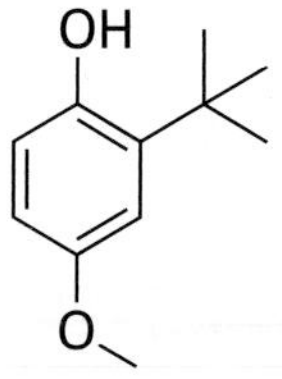

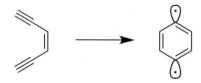

BHA

Problem 8.2 In the case study we have seen how an electrocyclization reaction of an enediyne in calicheamicin generates a reactive aryl diradical. Suggest a mechanism for the cyclization of a simple enediyne to a benzene diradical using fishhook arrows to keep track of the movement of electrons.

Problem 8.3 Shown below is a radical that exhibits remarkable stability. It is stable in its solid form, even in the presence of oxygen. Provide an explanation for why this particular radical is so unreactive.

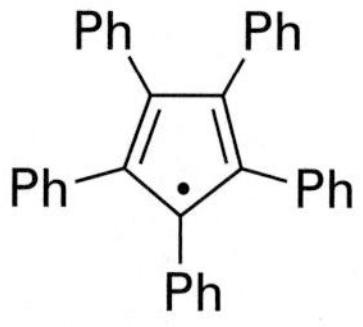

Problem 8.4 Which of the following radicals is most stable? Provide a brief explanation.

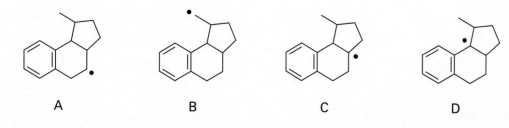

Problem 8.5 Which product do you predict will be the major bromination product formed in the following reaction?

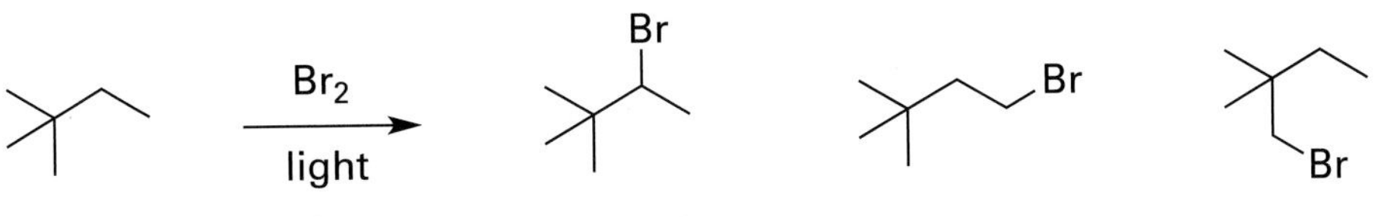

A   B   C

Problem 8.6 Explain why the following radical reaction produces the two products shown. In your explanation, use resonance forms of the relevant radical intermediate.

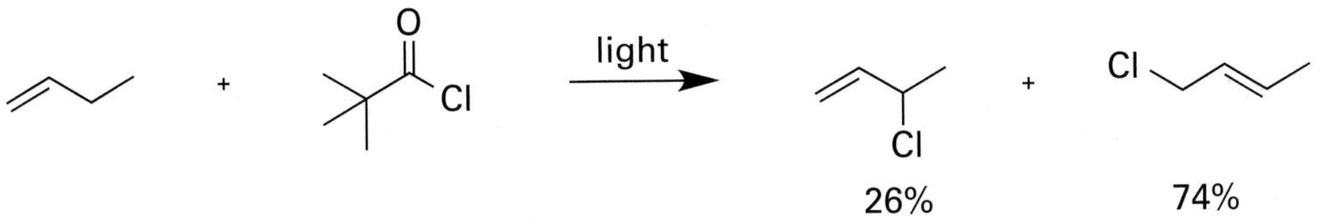

26%   74%

Problem 8.7 Shown below is the "auto-oxidation" reaction of a compound in the presence of oxygen. Write a mechanism for this radical reaction that includes initiation, propagation, and termination steps.

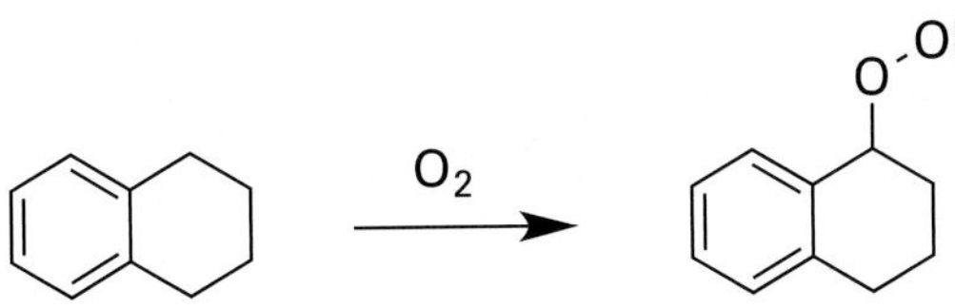

Problem 8.8 The addition of HBr across an alkene occurs with "anti-Markovnikov" regioselectivity when it is carried out in the presence of light or peroxides. Write mechanisms for the polar and radical reactions shown below that explain the change in regioselectivity.

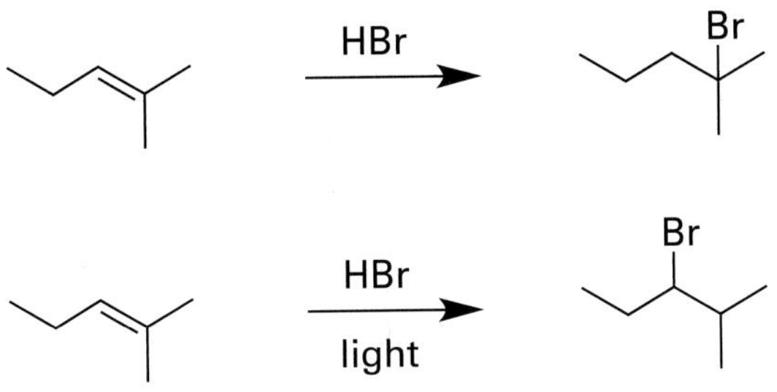

Solutions to Exercises

Chapter 1

Solution 1.1

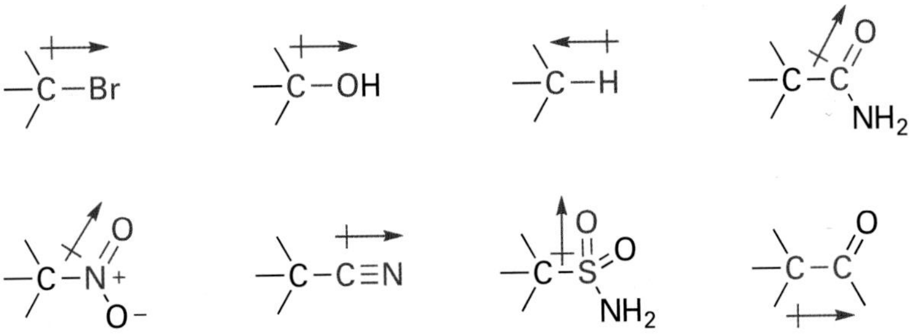

Solution 1.2

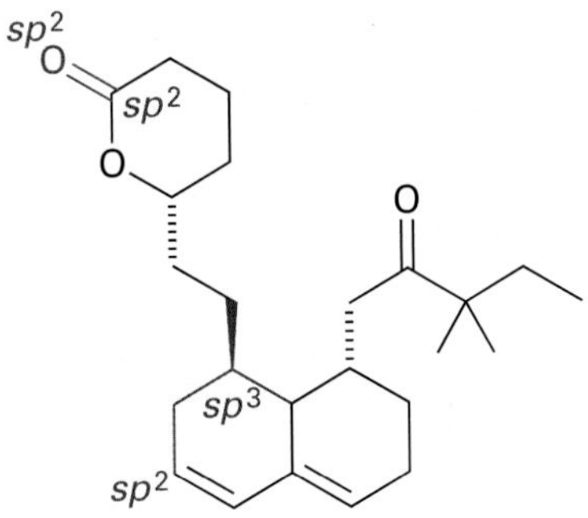

simvastatin

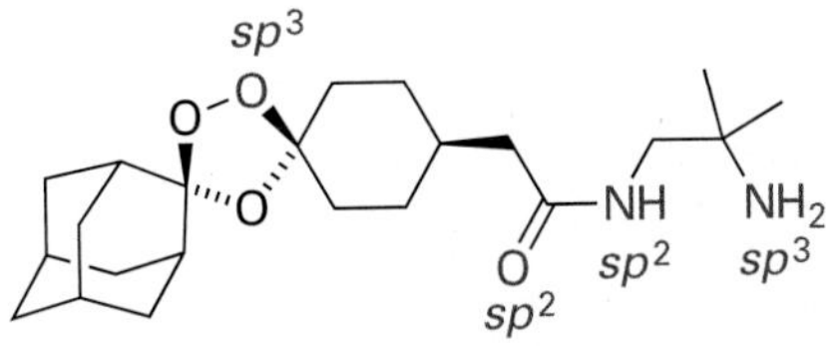

arterolane

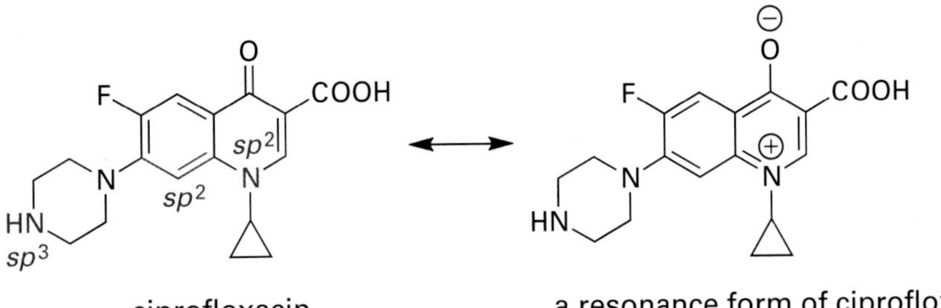

ciprofloxacin

a resonance form of ciprofloxacin

Explanation: Recall that nitrogen atoms in amides have partial double bond character (Section 1.6) and are best thought of as sp^2-hybridized atoms. In ciprofloxacin, the nitrogen atom in the bicyclic ring is conjugated via a double bond to a carbonyl (C=O) function and to the aromatic ring (as illustrated in the resonance form shown above). Thus, this nitrogen atom contributes its lone pair electrons to an aromatic ring system containing 10 π electrons. The planar arrangement of p orbitals required for aromaticity is possible only if the nitrogen atom is sp^2-hybridized.

Solution 1.3

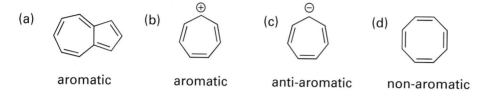

| (a) aromatic | (b) aromatic | (c) anti-aromatic | (d) non-aromatic |

Explanation: The ring systems in examples (a) and (b) possess a planar, contiguous array of p orbitals with 10 and 6 π electrons, respectively, and thus are aromatic. The ring system in (c) is planar and contains 8 π electrons and is thus anti-aromatic. The eight-membered ring in (d) cannot form a planar structure and so is a non-aromatic ring system.

Solution 1.4

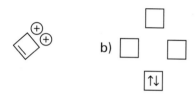

Explanation: The correct answer is (b). To construct the relevant Frost circle we first draw the cyclic ring system with one of its vertices pointing down (as illustrated above and in Figure 1.21). The cyclobutadienyl dication has a co-planar array of p orbitals and has only 2 π electrons. These two electrons will fill the single bonding π molecular orbital and produce an aromatic π system ($4n + 2$ where $n = 0$).

Solution 1.5

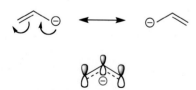

Explanation: The allyl anion is more stable since the negative charge is shared by multiple atoms. This can be illustrated with a resonance hybrid as shown above. In molecular orbital terms, the negative charge is delocalized into the π bond by overlap of the p orbitals on the three sp^2-hybridized carbon atoms in the allyl anion.

Solution 1.6

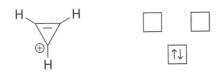

Explanation: The cation is aromatic since it is composed of a cyclic, co-planar array of p orbitals containing 2 π electrons ($4n + 2$ when $n = 0$).

Solution 1.7

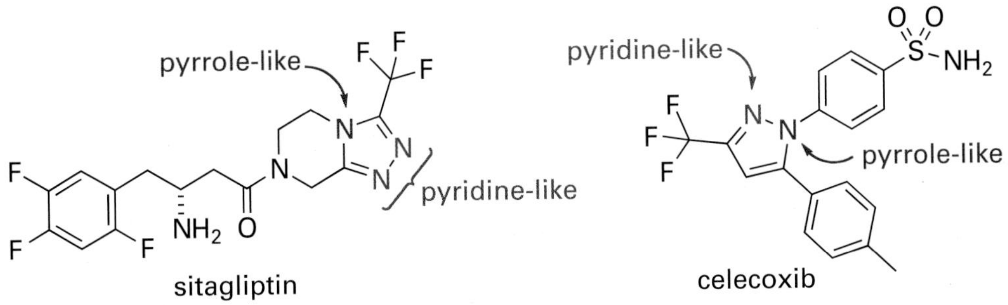

pyrrole-like

pyridine-like

sitagliptin

pyridine-like

pyrrole-like

celecoxib

Chapter 2

Solution 2.14: Shown below are some possible solutions to problems 2.1–2.6. There are other reasonable solutions since certain amino acid side chains can make different types of intermolecular contacts, as discussed in Chapter 2.

Solution 2.1

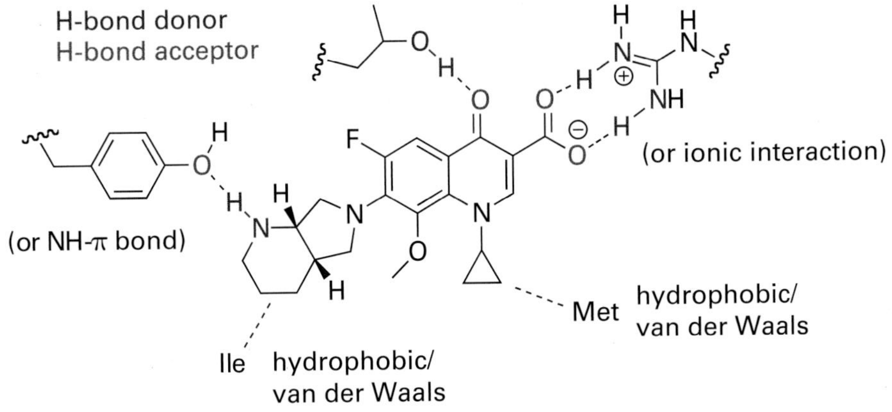

H-bond donor
H-bond acceptor

(or ionic interaction)

(or NH-π bond)

Met   hydrophobic/
van der Waals

Ile   hydrophobic/
van der Waals

Solution 2.2

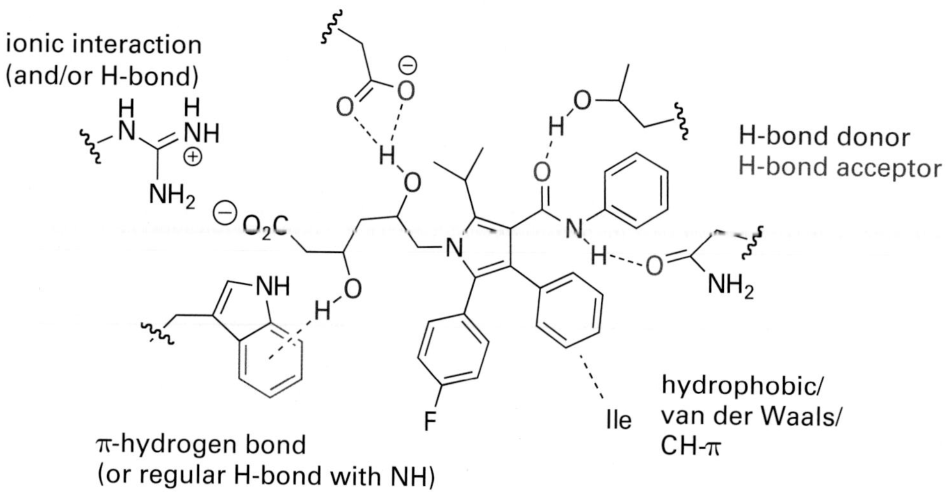

Solution 2.3

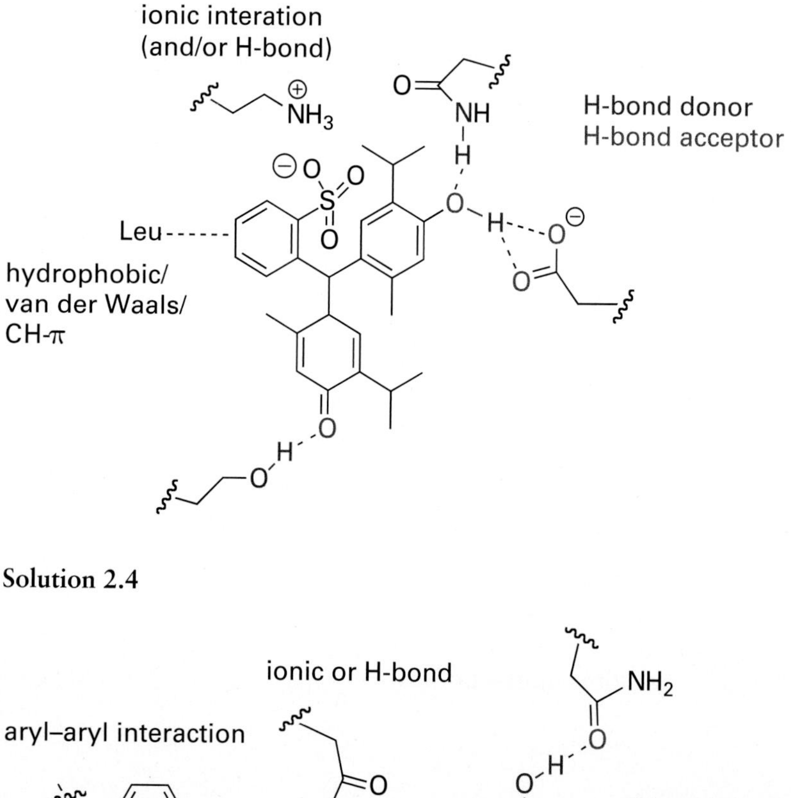

Solution 2.4

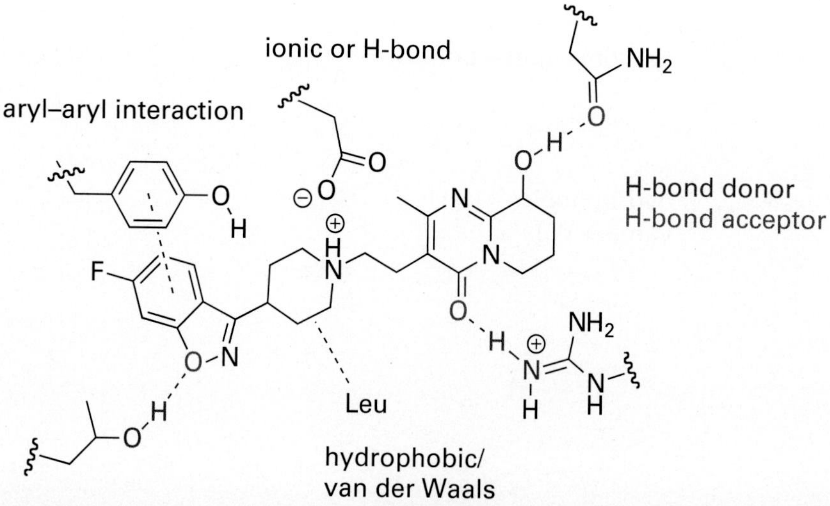

Solution 2.5

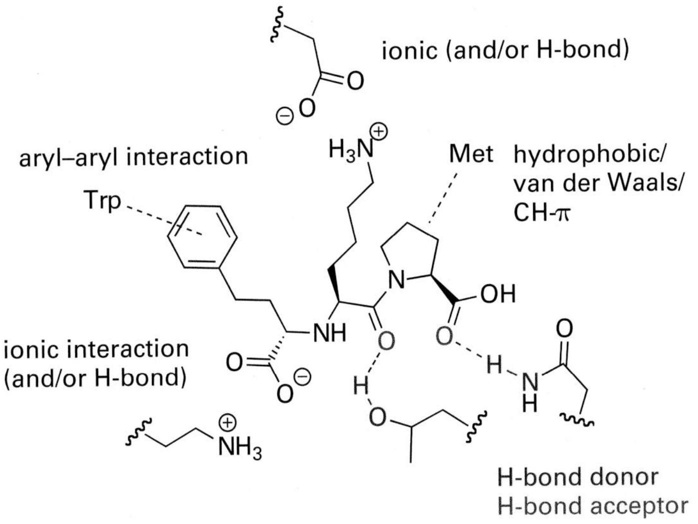

Solution 2.6

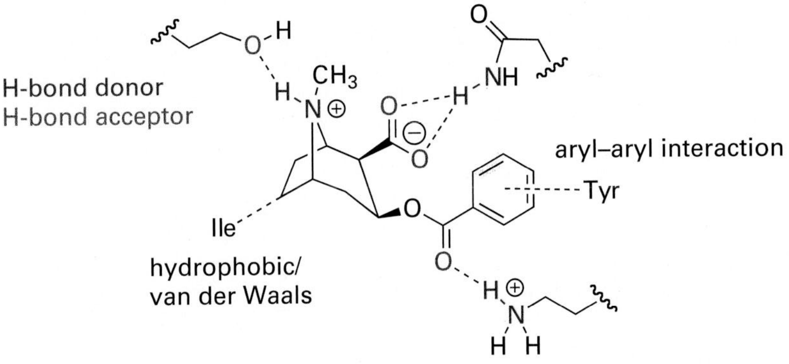

Chapter 3

Solution 3.1

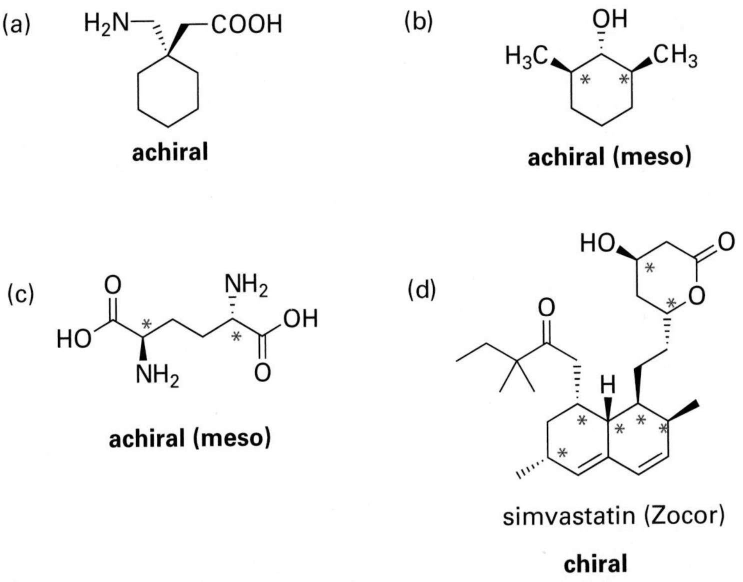

(a)

H₂N—⟨ ⟩—COOH

achiral

(b)

achiral (meso)

(c)

achiral (meso)

(d)

simvastatin (Zocor)

chiral

Explanation: Chirality centers are indicated with blue asterisks. Examples (b) and (c) are achiral due to the presence of a bisecting mirror plane. The mirror plane is more apparent for (c) if one draws the molecule after a rotation of 180 degrees about the central C–C bond, as illustrated below. Both (b) and (c) are also meso compounds since they are achiral members of a larger set of stereoisomers that contain chiral members. Example (a) does not have a chirality center and thus cannot be chiral or have any chiral diastereomers. It therefore cannot be a meso compound.

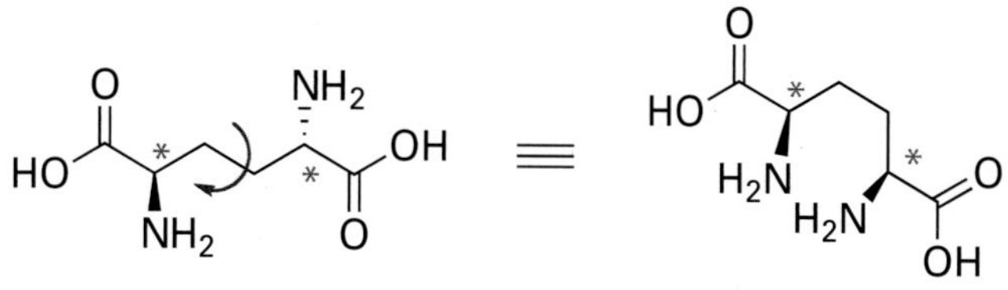

Solution 3.2

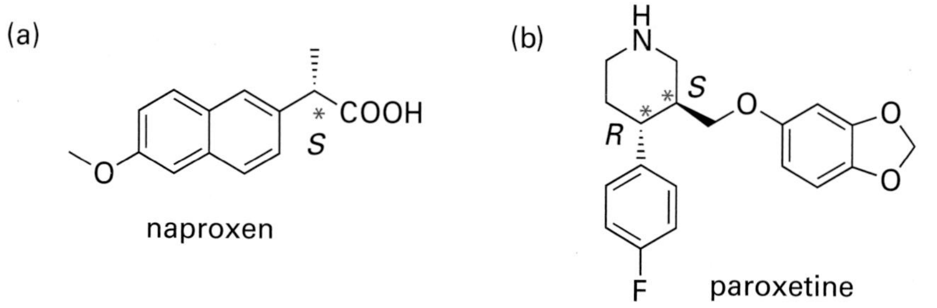

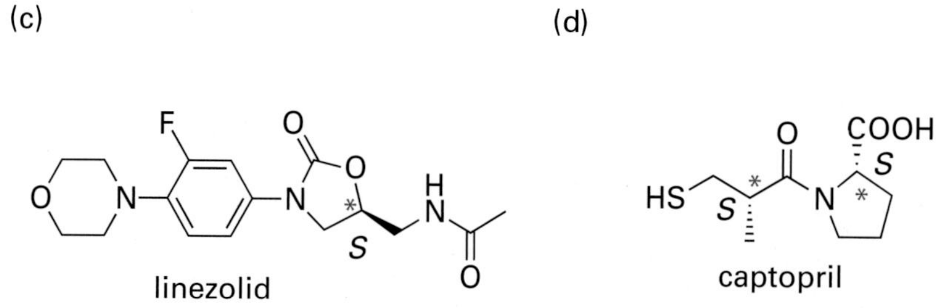

(a)

naproxen

(b)

paroxetine

(c)

linezolid

(d)

captopril

Solution 3.3

(a)

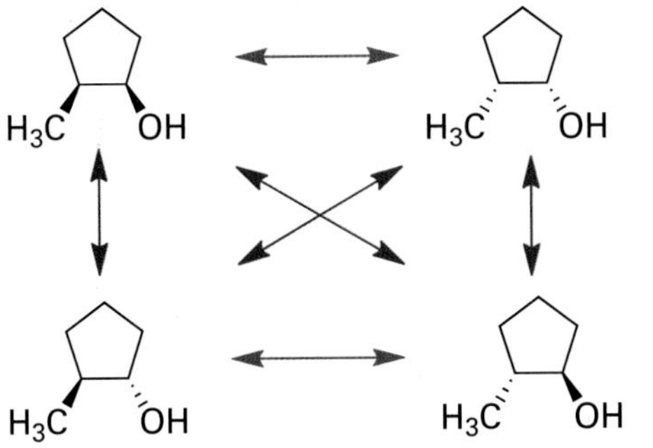

enantiomers

diastereomers

(b)

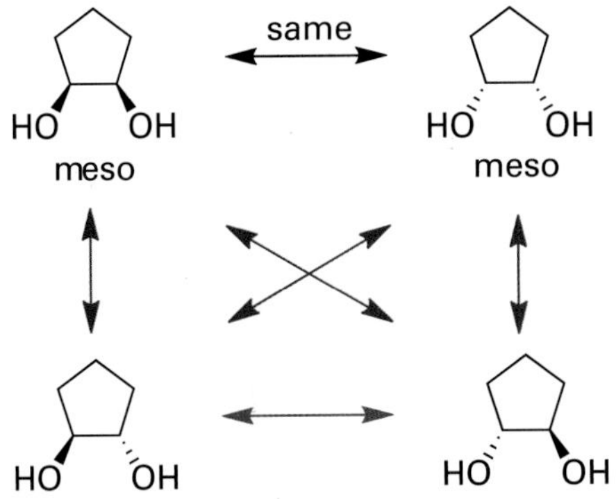

enantiomers

diastereomers

(c)

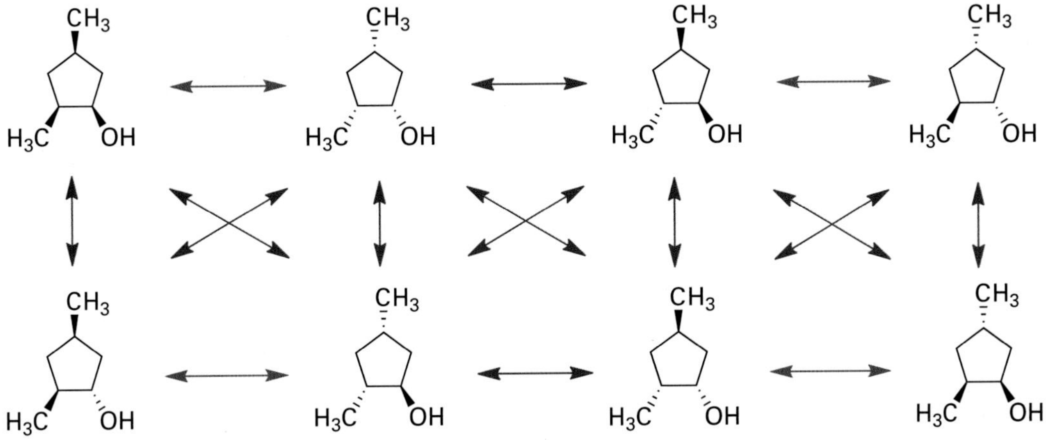

enantiomers

diastereomers

Solution 3.4

(a)

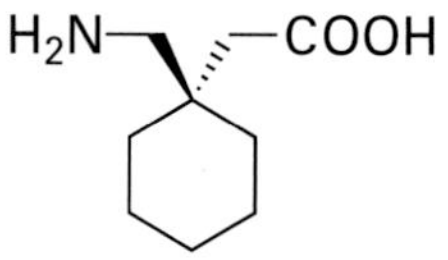

identical

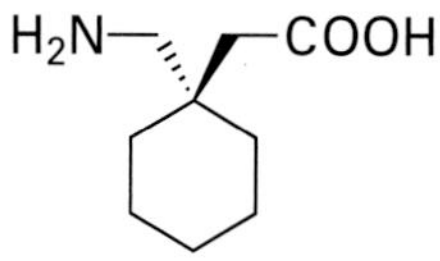

(b)

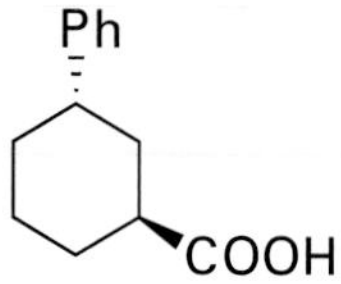

none of the above

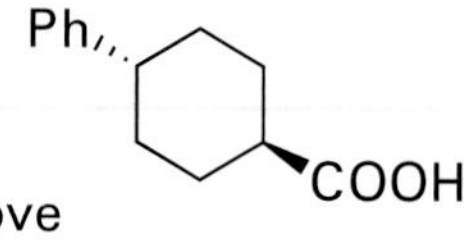

(c)

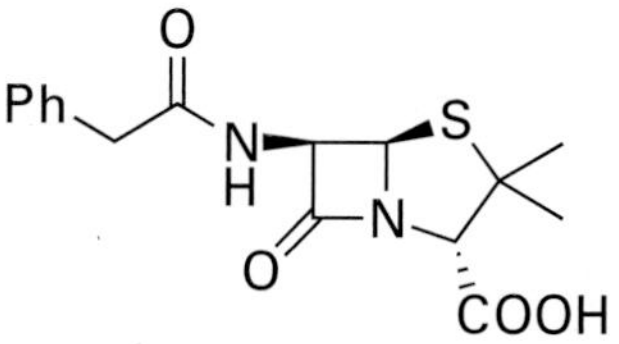

enantiomers

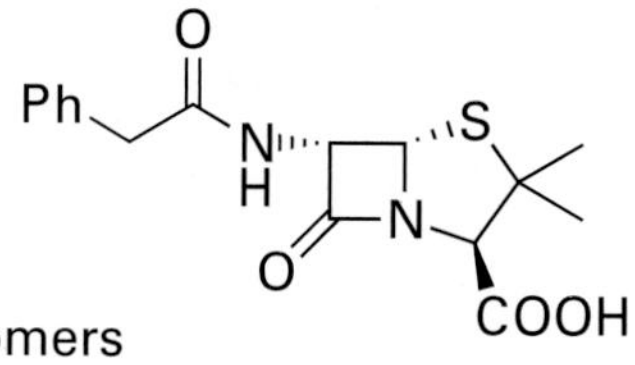

(d)

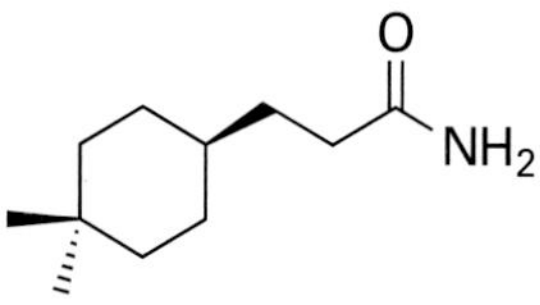

identical

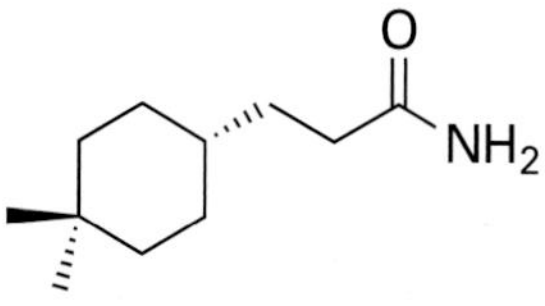

(e)

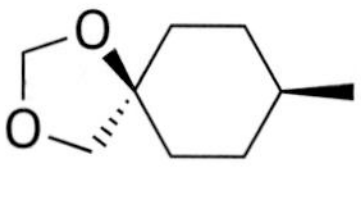

diastereomers

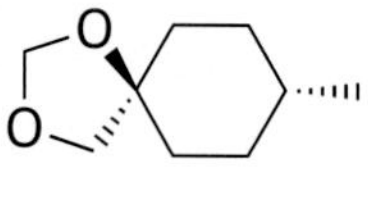

(f)

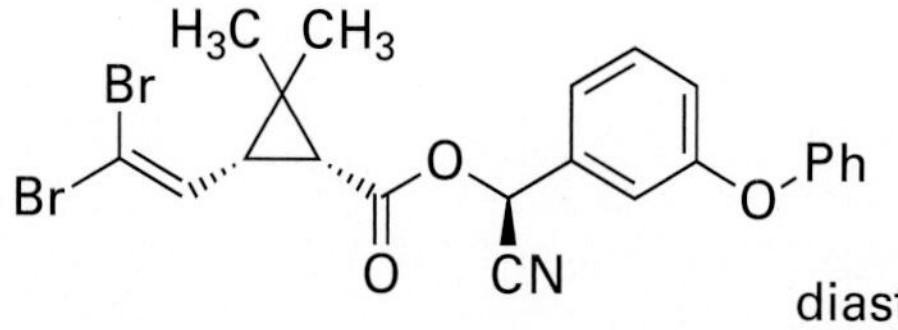

diastereomers

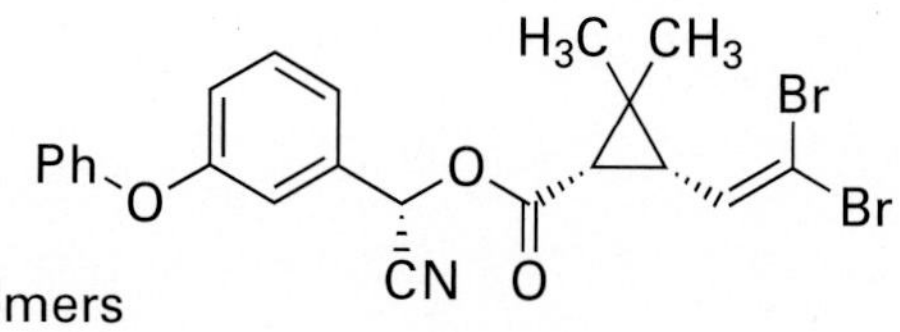

Solution 3.5

(a)

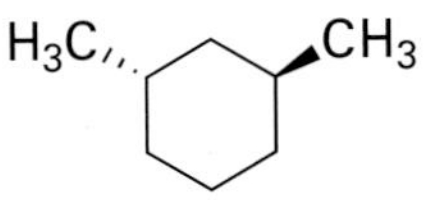

(b)

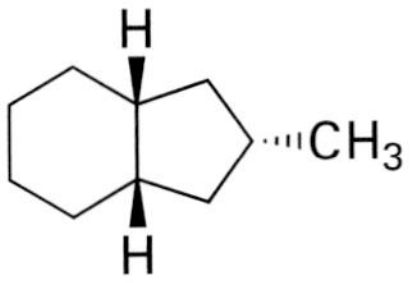

meso

(c)

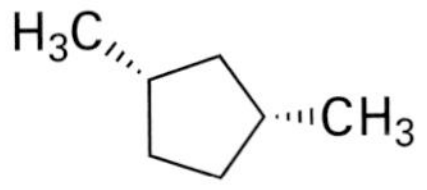

meso

(d)

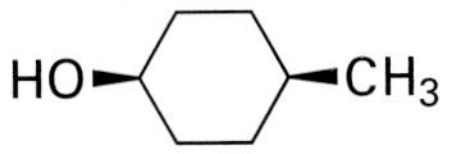

Chapter 4

Solution 4.1

Explanation: For each example below, the second molecule in the pair has been redrawn so as to facilitate the comparison with the first.

(a)

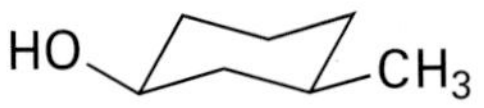

enantiomers

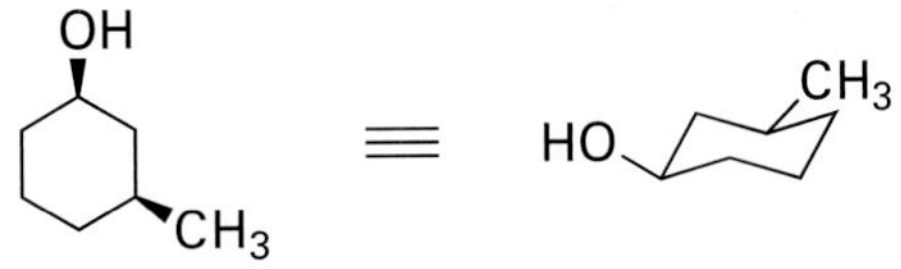

(b)

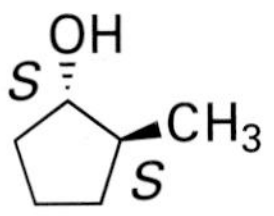

identical

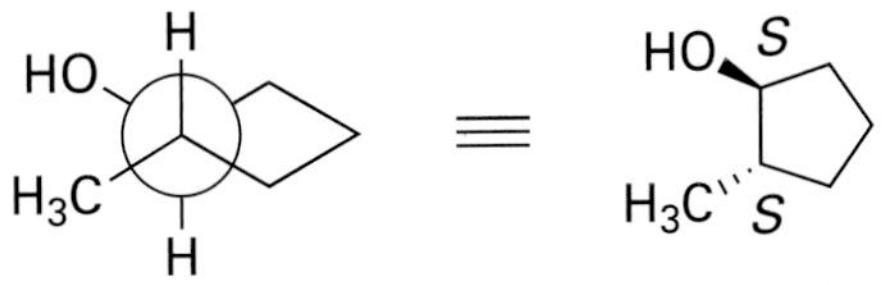

(c)

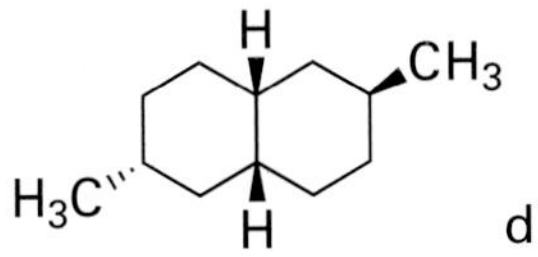

diastereomers

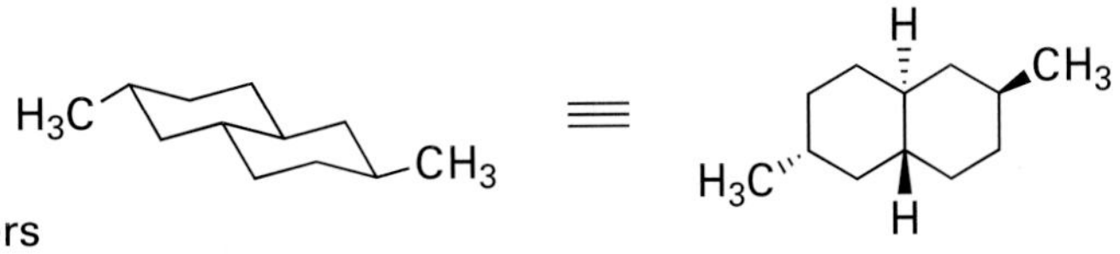

(d)

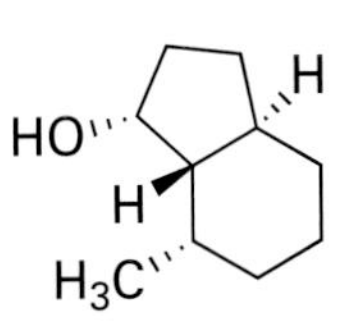

diastereomers

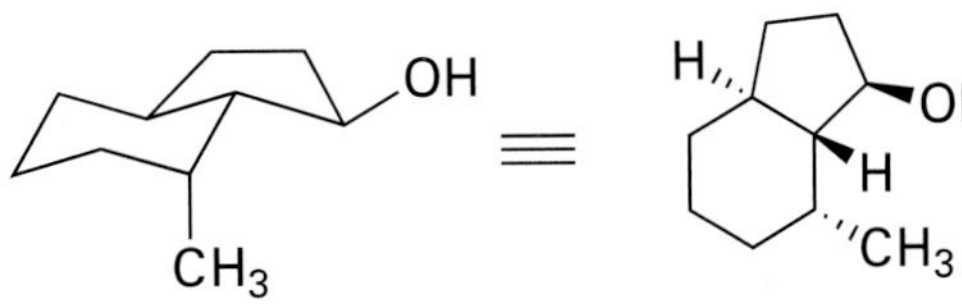

(e)

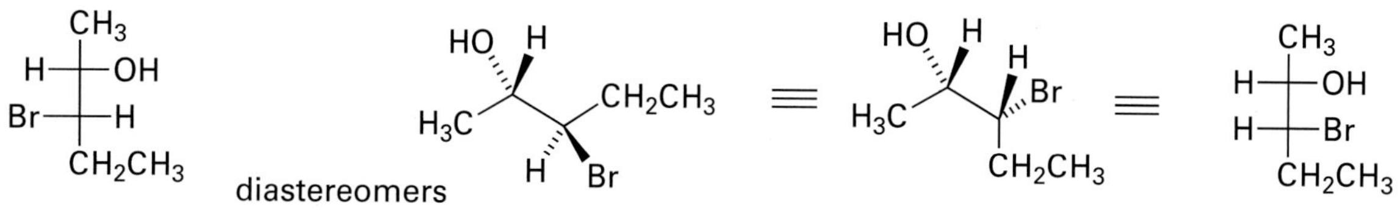

diastereomers

(f)

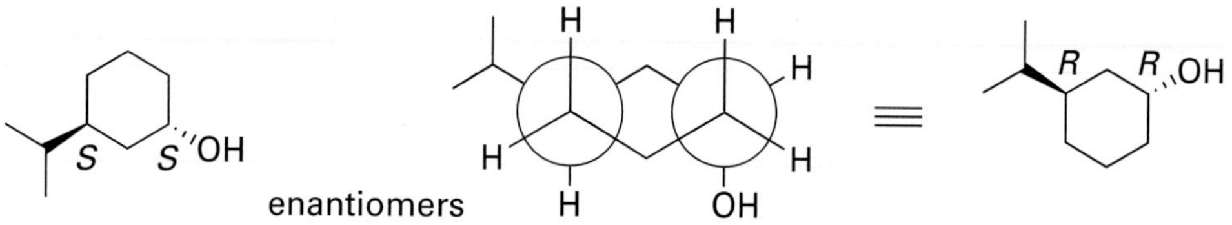

enantiomers

(g)

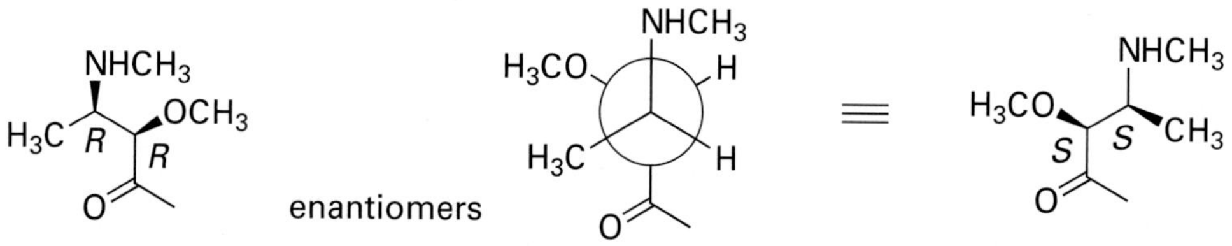

enantiomers

Solution 4.2

(a)

lower in energy

(b)

lower in energy

(c)

lower in energy

Explanation: For (a) the gauche/staggered conformer is preferred over syn/eclipsed due to reduced torsional strain and reduced through-space interaction of the two methyl groups. For (b) the chair-like conformation of the cyclohexane ring in the conformer at left is preferred over the boat-like conformation at right. For (c) both conformers are gauche but that on left is preferred since it has only one through-space methyl–methyl interaction, whereas the conformer at right has two such through-space interactions.

Solution 4.3

(a)

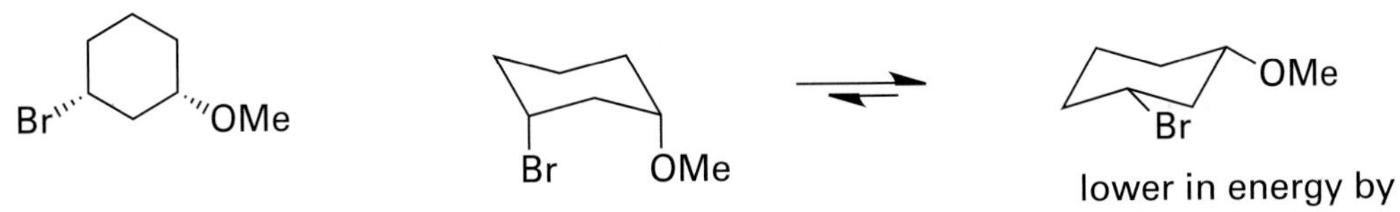

lower in energy by ~1.1 kcal/mol

(b)

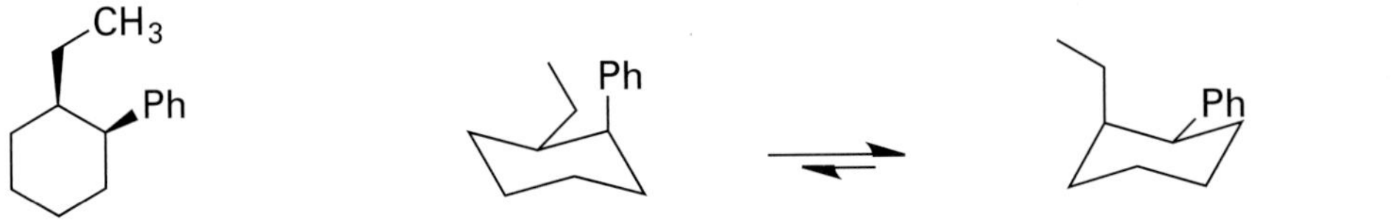

lower in energy by ~1.1 kcal/mol

(c)

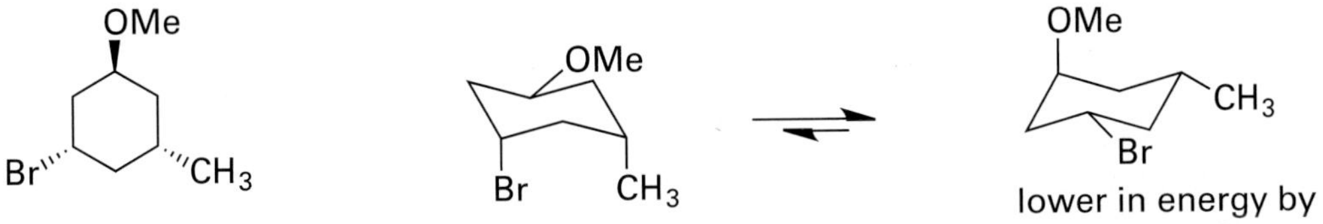

lower in energy by ~1.7 kcal/mol

(d)

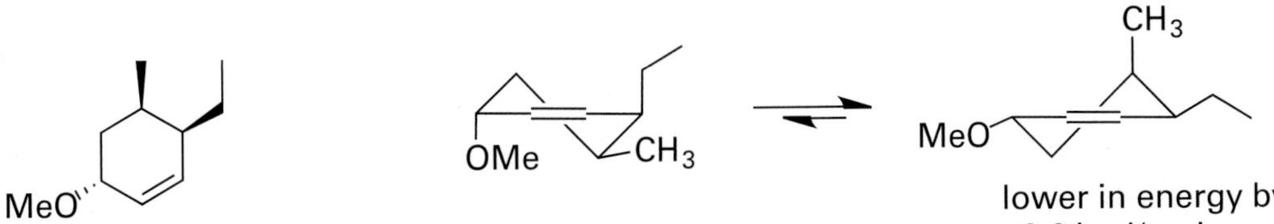

lower in energy by ~0.6 kcal/mol

(e)

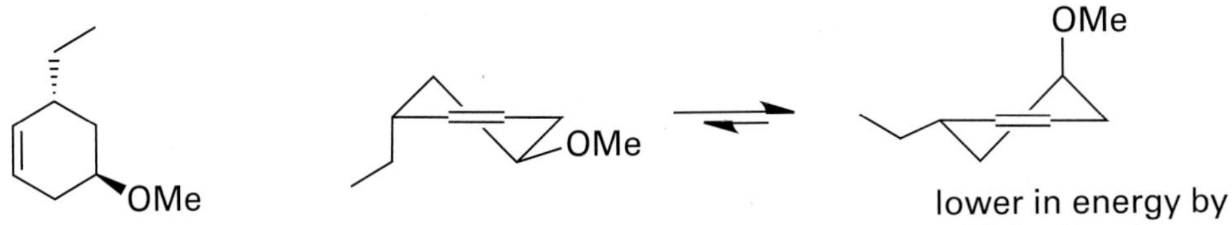

lower in energy by ~1.2 kcal/mol

Explanation: The two relevant chair conformers are drawn above for each example, with the lower energy conformer shown on the right. For each conformer, $-\Delta G°$ values for axial substituent(s) are summed and the difference in $-\Delta G°$ values provides an estimate of the energy difference between conformer pairs.

Chapter 5

Solution 5.1

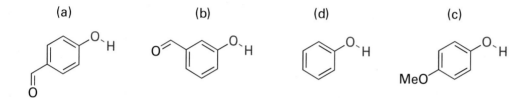

(a) (b) 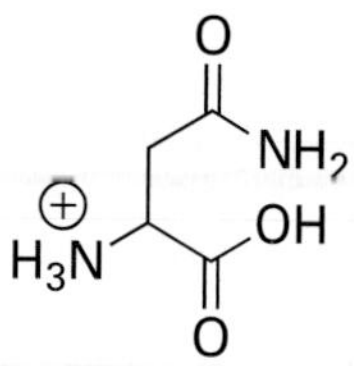 (c)

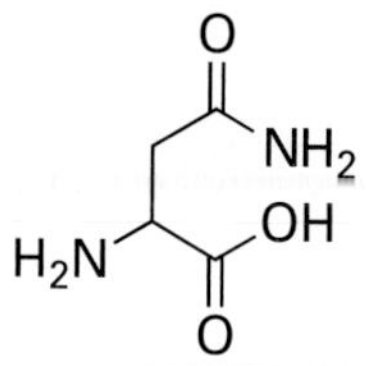

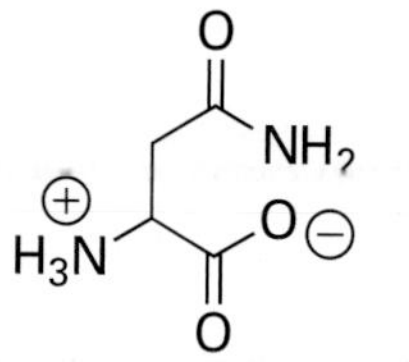

Solution 5.2

(a) (b) (d) (c)

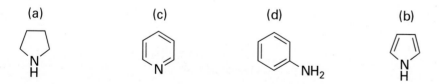

Explanation: The acidic bond is the phenolic O−H, shown in blue. The aldehyde function is electron-withdrawing by a resonance and/or inductive effect depending on its position relative to the O−H function. Compound (a) is the most acidic since with *para* substitution both the inductive and resonance-withdrawing effects of the aldehyde are conferred to the O−H bond. The *para*-methoxy compound (c) is least acidic of the set and slightly less acidic than phenol (d) due to a resonance electron-donating effect of *para*-methoxy that is slightly stronger than the inductive withdrawing effect.

Solution 5.3

(a) (c) (d) (b)

Explanation: Recall that pyrrole-type nitrogen atoms as in (b) are nonbasic because the lone pair electrons are delocalized into the aromatic π system. Thus, pyrrole (b) is by far the least basic compound in the series. Nitrogen bound to hydrogen or sp^3-hybridized carbon is generally more basic than nitrogen bound to sp^2-hybridized carbon (which is inductively more withdrawing). Thus, pyrrolidine (a) is a significantly stronger base than pyridine (c) or aniline (d). Pyridine is only a slightly stronger base than aniline.

Solution 5.4

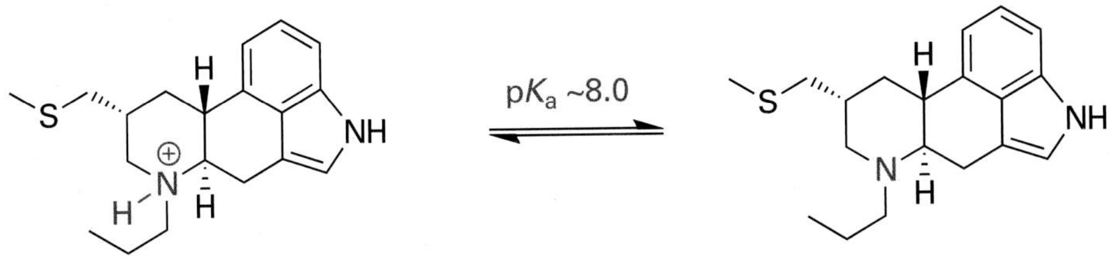

$pK_a \sim 8.0$

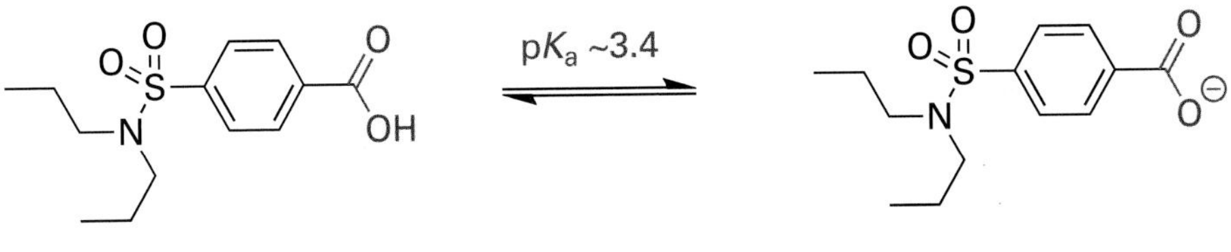

$pK_a \sim 3.4$

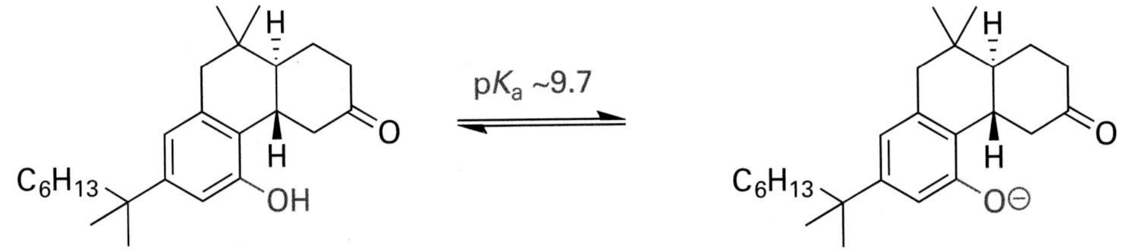

$pK_a \sim 9.7$

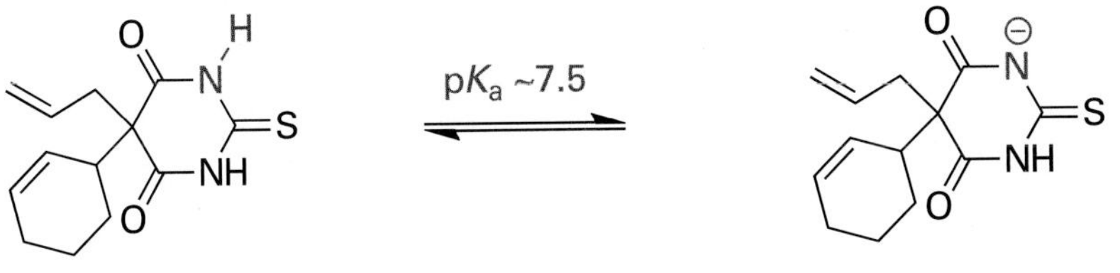

$pK_a \sim 7.5$

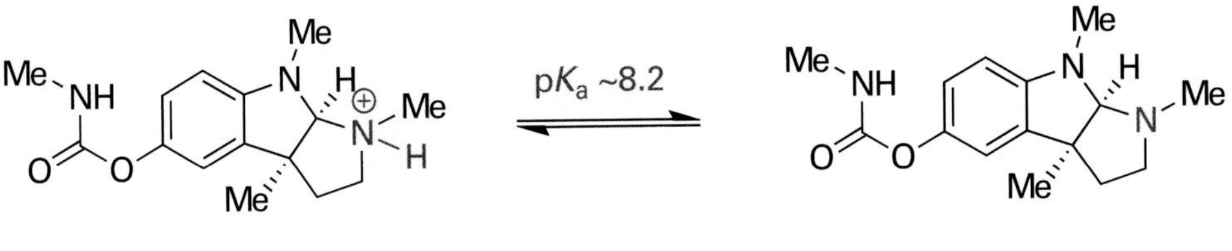

$pK_a \sim 8.2$

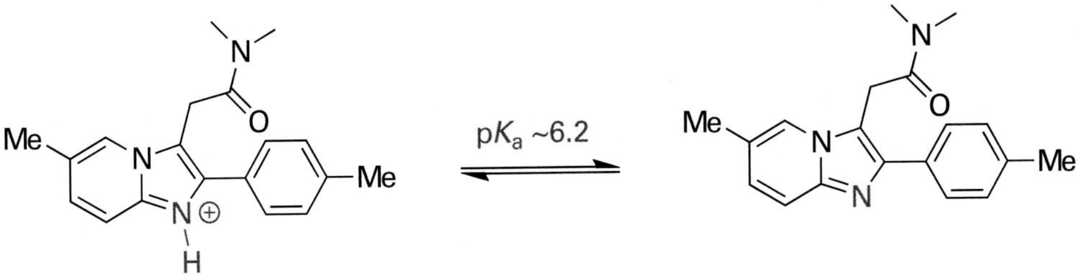

$pK_a \sim 6.2$

Solution 5.5

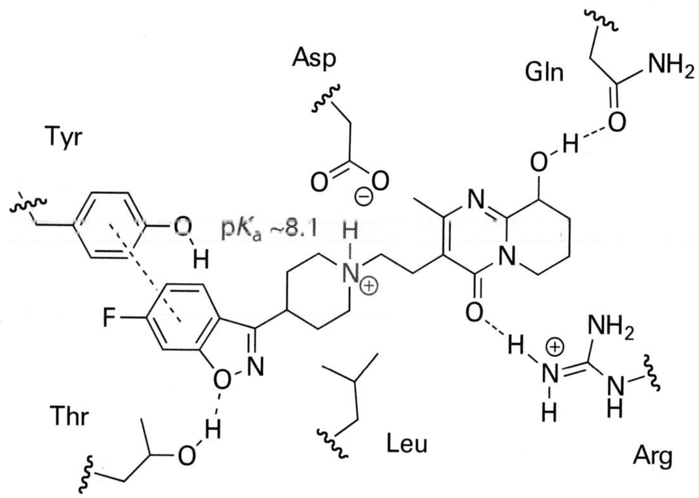

Solution 5.6

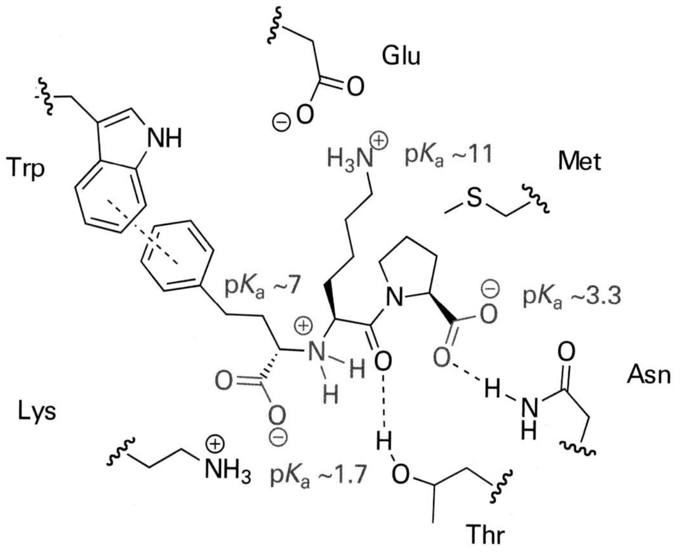

Solution 5.7

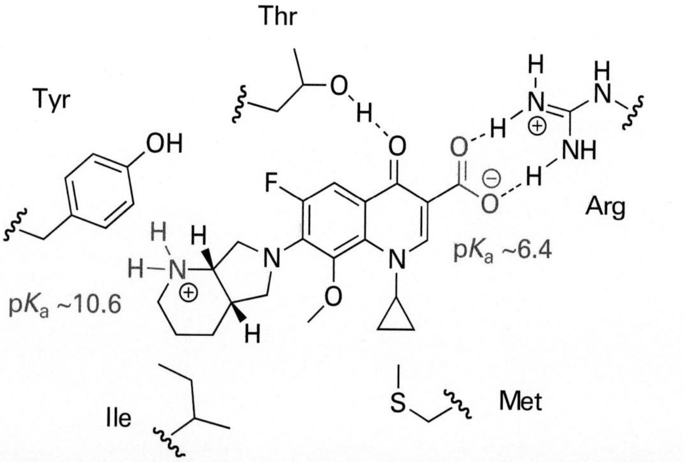

Solution 5.8

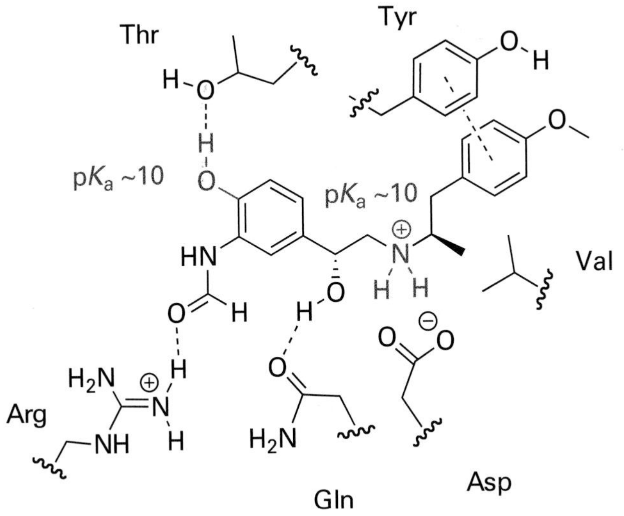

Thr — Tyr — Val — Arg — Gln — Asp

Solution 5.9

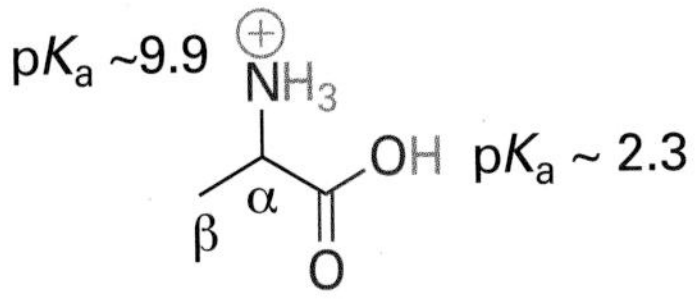

alanine 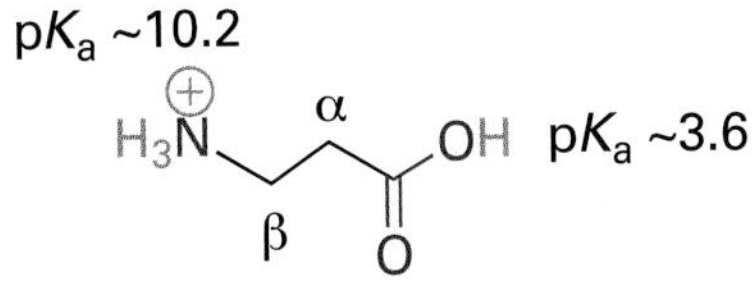   β-alanine

Explanation: The effects of the ammonium group is electron-withdrawing via an inductive effect. The carboxylic acid pK_a is therefore lower for alanine since the ammonium group is only two bonds away (compared to three bonds in β-alanine).

Solution 5.10

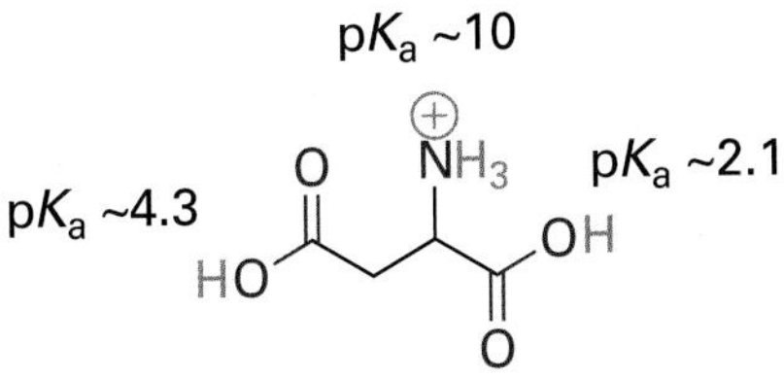

aspartic acid 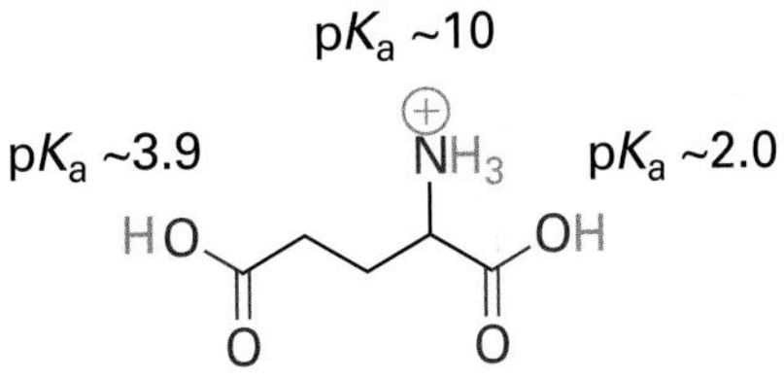   glutamic acid

Explanation: The inductive withdrawing effect of the ammonium function will make the proximal carboxylic acid more acidic than the distal one in both molecules. Once the first H−A deprotonation has occurred, the resulting carboxylate becomes a mildly electron-donating function. This inductive donating effect is modest but will be more strongly felt in aspartic acid, where fewer bonds separate the carboxylate and carboxylic acid groups. Thus, the second H−A type acid pK_a is higher for aspartic acid than glutamic acid. Unfavorable through space charge–charge interactions may also contribute, making the pK_a difference greater in aspartic acid, where the interacting negative charges are closer in space.

Chapter 6

Solution 6.1

Slower

Solution 6.2

No change

Solution 6.3

(a)

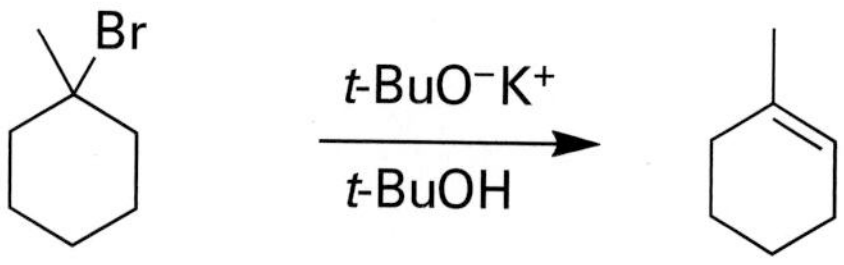

(b)

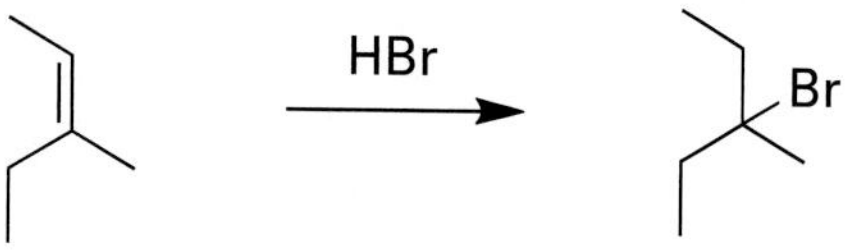

(c)

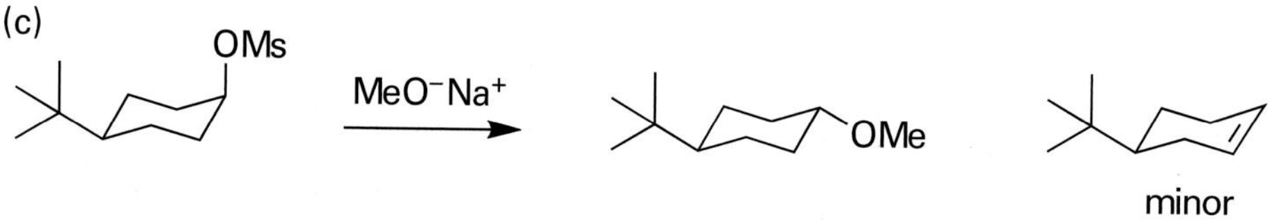

minor

Solution 6.4

(i)

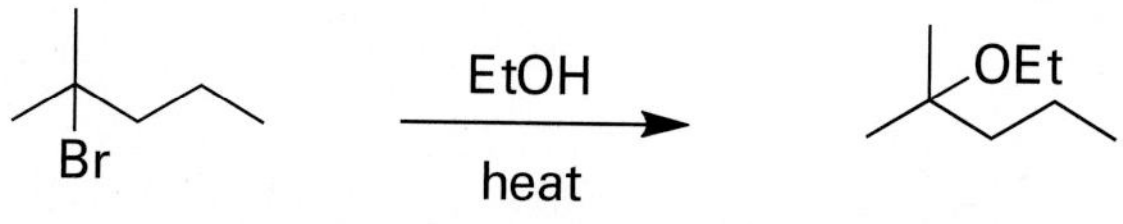

Explanation: These conditions suggest an S$_N$1 reaction since the nucleophile is weak and a tertiary carbocation can be formed by dissociation of the C–Br bond.

(ii)

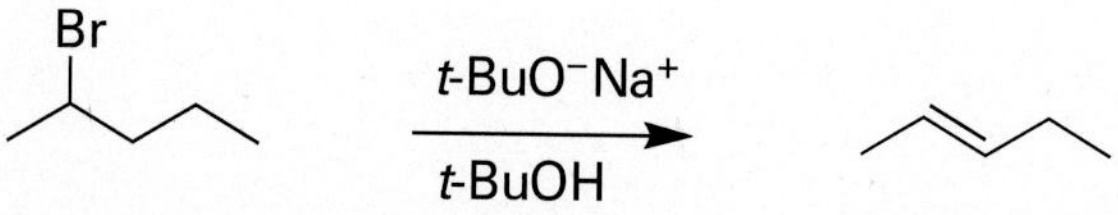

The use of a sterically hindered and strong base suggests that this reaction will proceed via the E2 mechanism. The more highly substituted alkene product is expected to predominate.

Solution 6.5

(a)

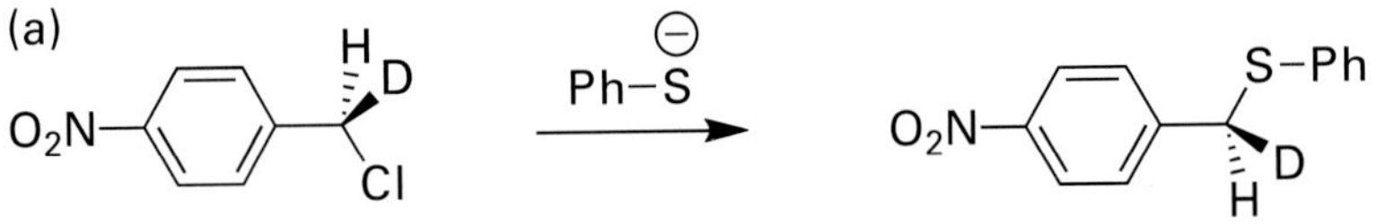

Predicted mechanism is S_N2 leading to product with inversion of configuration at the reacting carbon atom.

(b)

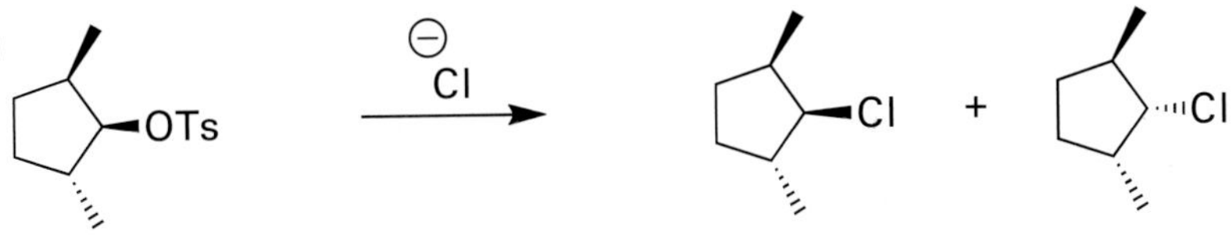

The nucleophile is a weak one and the C–OTs bond is in a crowded steric environment. Therefore, substitution by the S_N1 mechanism is more likely and would result in scrambling of stereochemical configuration at the reacting center, producing two diastereomeric products.

(c)

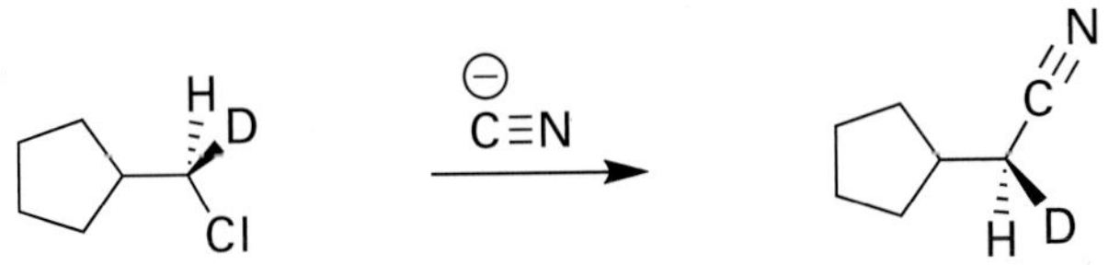

The nucleophile is a good one and the leaving group is good, so S_N2 reaction with inversion of configuration is expected.

Solution 6.6

(a)

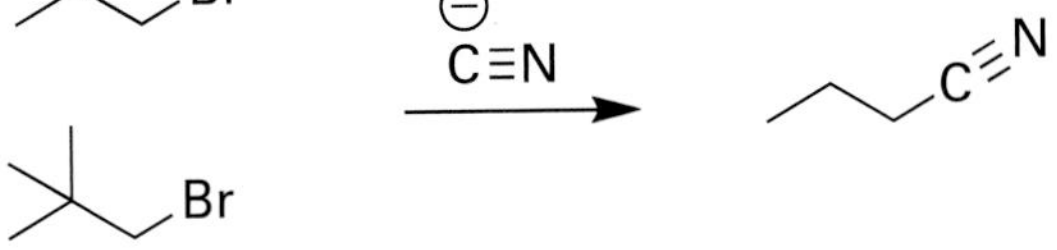

The reaction proceeds by an S_N2 mechansim since the formation of a primary carbocation is disfavored. The less hindered C–Br bond in the compound at top will react more rapidly.

(b)

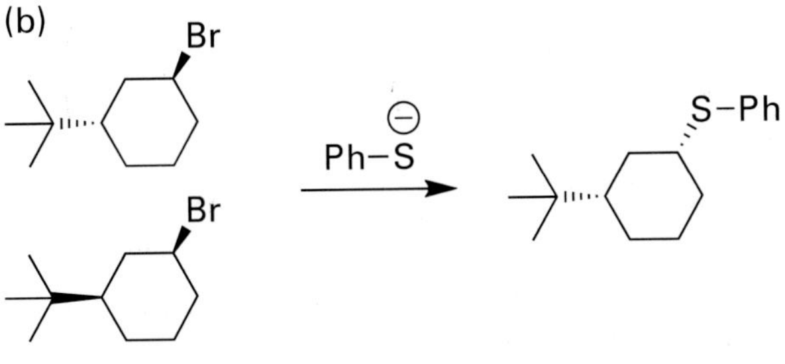

In both molecules, the *tert*-butyl group conformationally locks the cyclohexane ring into a single chair conformer with the *tert*-butyl substituent in an equatorial position. For the molecule at top this places the bromine in an axial position that permits S_N2 reaction with the nucleophile (with inversion of configuration). In the substrate at bottom the bromine is locked in an equatorial position and backside attack is blocked.

(c)

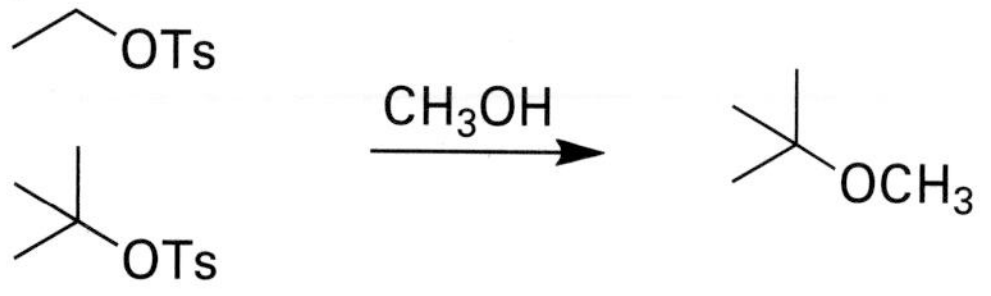

The nucleophile (methanol) is weak so the most likely reaction is an S_N1 type reaction. The starting material at bottom that can form a tertiary carbocation will react more rapidly under these conditions.

(d)

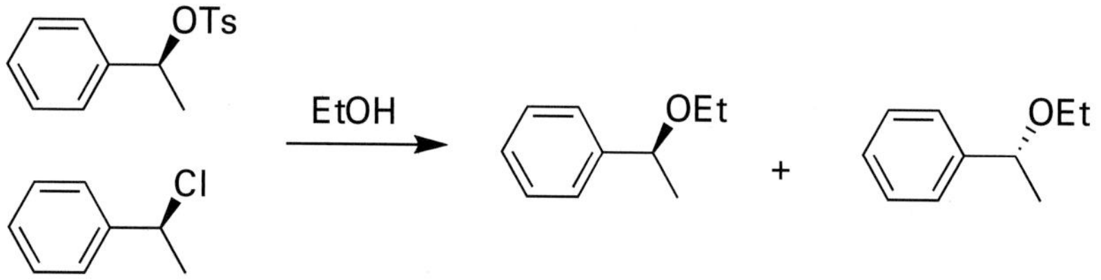

The nucleophile is weak, suggesting an S_N1 mechanism with formation of a stabilized benzylic carbocation as the reaction intermediate. Addition of the nucleophile can occur from either side of the carbocation resulting in a racemic product.

(e)

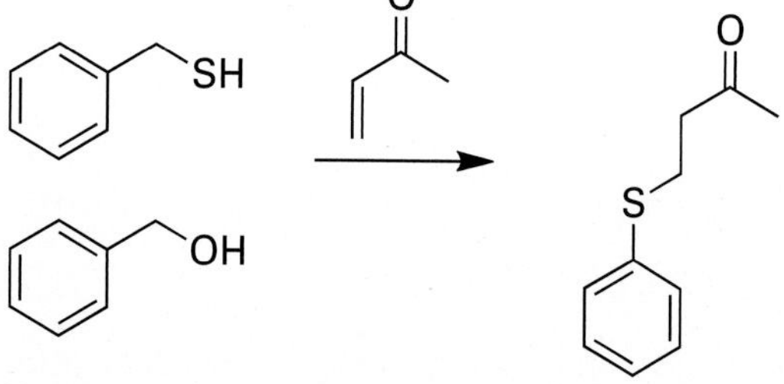

The thiol is a better nucleophile, so it will react more rapidly in a Michael addition reaction with the enone substrate.

Solution 6.7

Ans (a)

> **A** – retention
> **B** – inversion
> **D** - inversion

Ans (b)

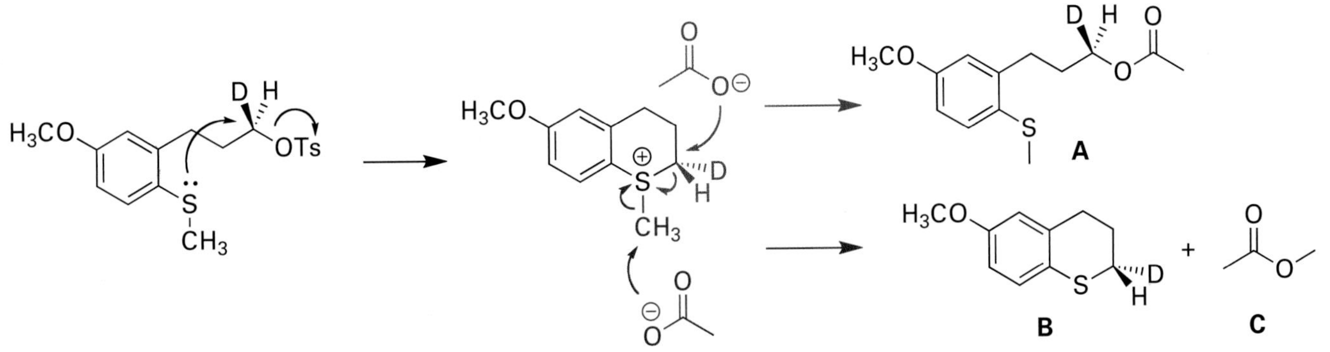

Ans (c)

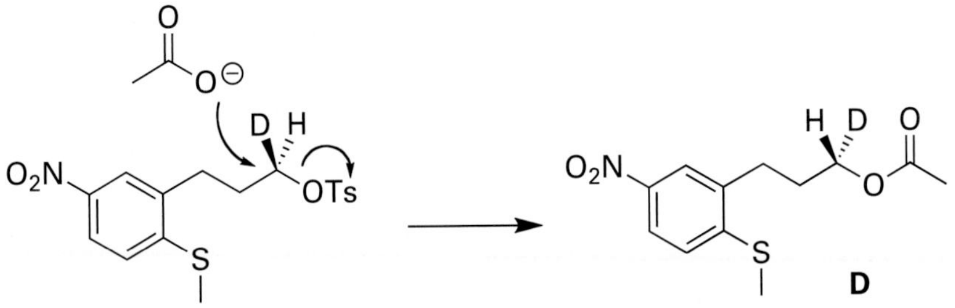

Ans (d)

The *para*-methoxy group is electron-donating by resonance through the aromatic ring and makes the sulfur
atom of the thioether more electron rich and nucleophilic. This more reactive thioether then participates
in the intramolecular S_N2 reaction that is the first step
in the reaction mechanism leading to products A–C. In
the second substrate, the thioether is deactivated by the
para-nitro group and does not act as a nucleophile. In
this case the S_N2 reaction occurs directly between acetate and the C–OTs center.

Chapter 7

Solution 7.1

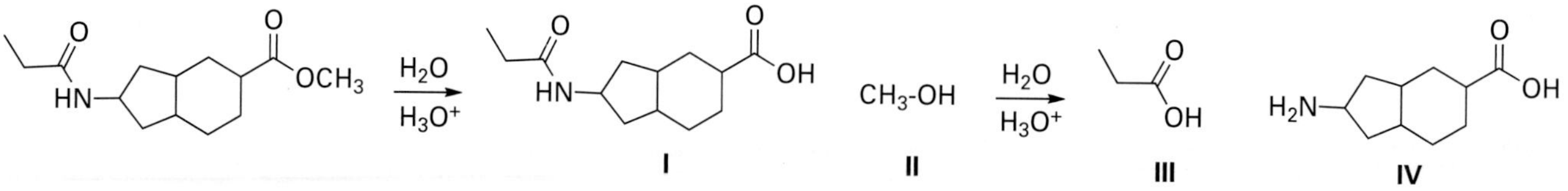

Solution 7.2

(a)

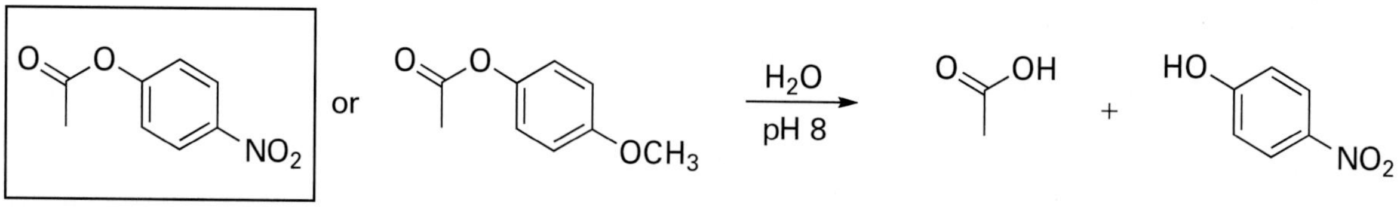

Explanation: Under neutral or basic conditions, it is the reactivity of the neutral (unprotonated) carbonyl species that is relevant. The *para*-nitro group makes the carbonyl more electrophilic and also makes the resulting phenoxide a better leaving group (weaker base).

(b)

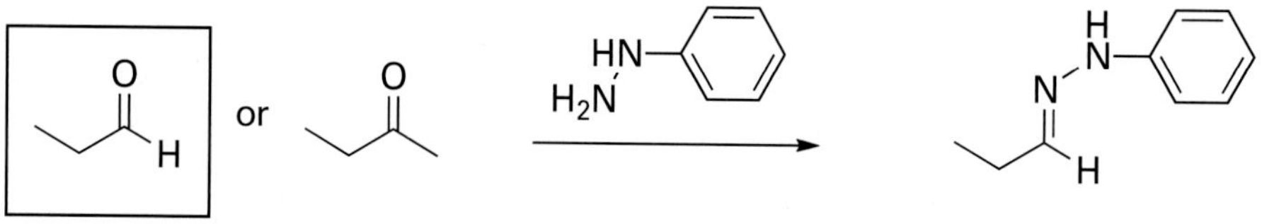

(c)

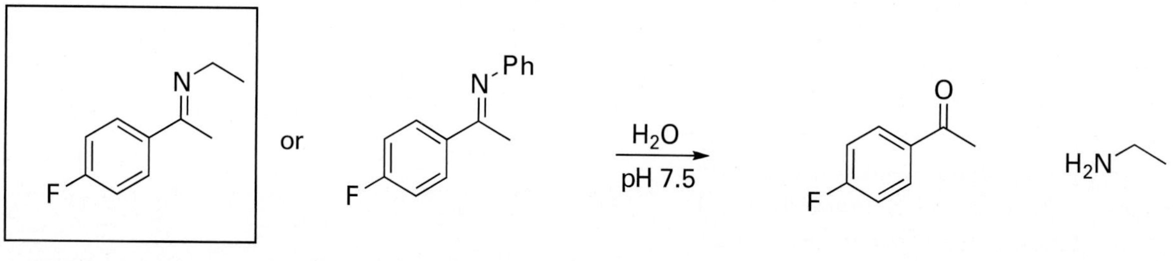

Explanation: The imine derived from aniline is less basic and thus less likely to become protonated at physiological pH. Since protonation is the first step in the hydrolysis reaction, the imine derived from ethylamine with its more basic nitrogen atom is more reactive.

(d)

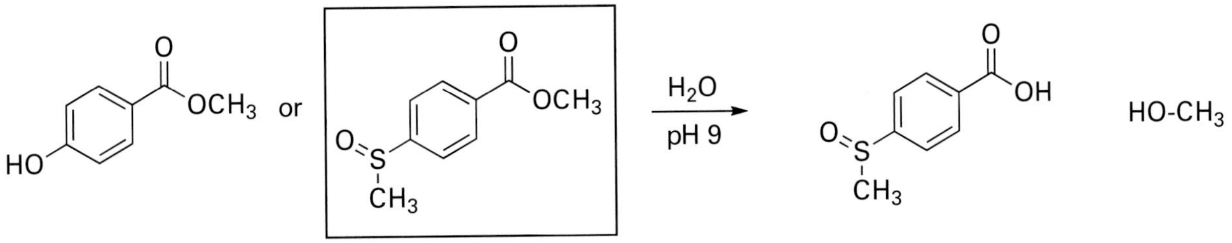

Solution 7.3

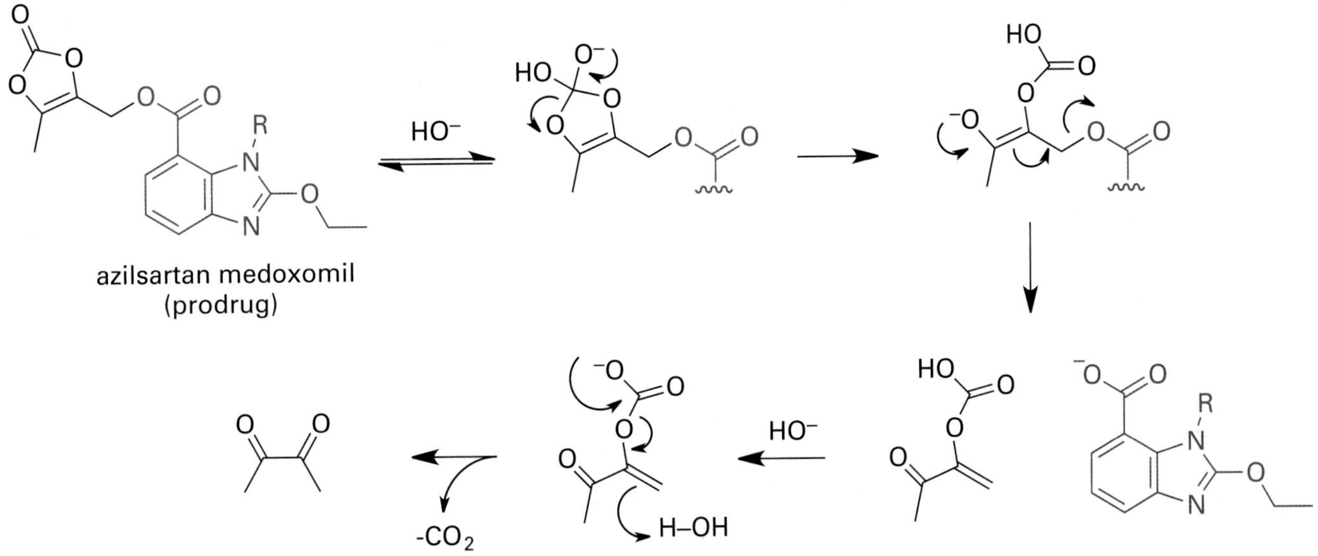

azilsartan medoxomil
(prodrug)

Note that at basic pH the relevant reaction is of hydroxide with the neutral, unprotonated carbonyl species.

Solution 7.4

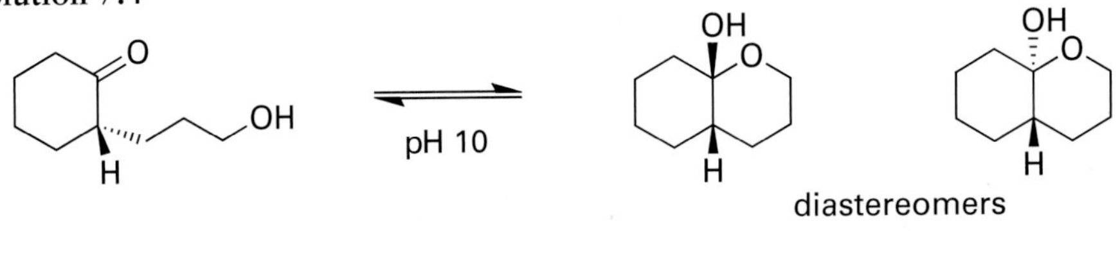

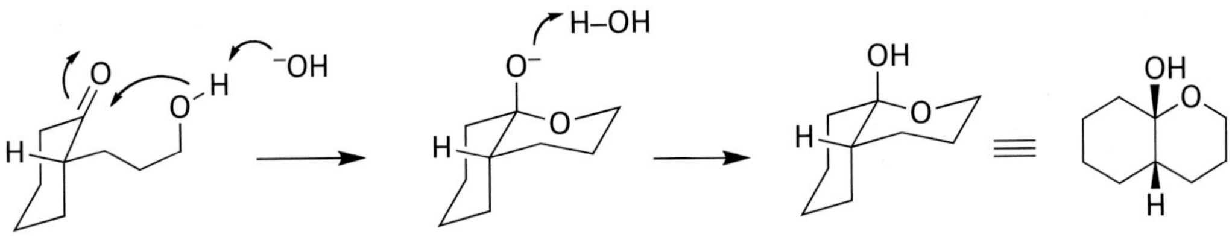

diastereomers

Explanation: The two products result from attack of the OH group from either side of the carbonyl function. The resulting products are diastereomers since they have a different configuration at one of the two stereocenters. A reaction mechanism using conformational drawings is shown above for formation of the diastereomer with a *cis* ring fusion.

Solution 7.5

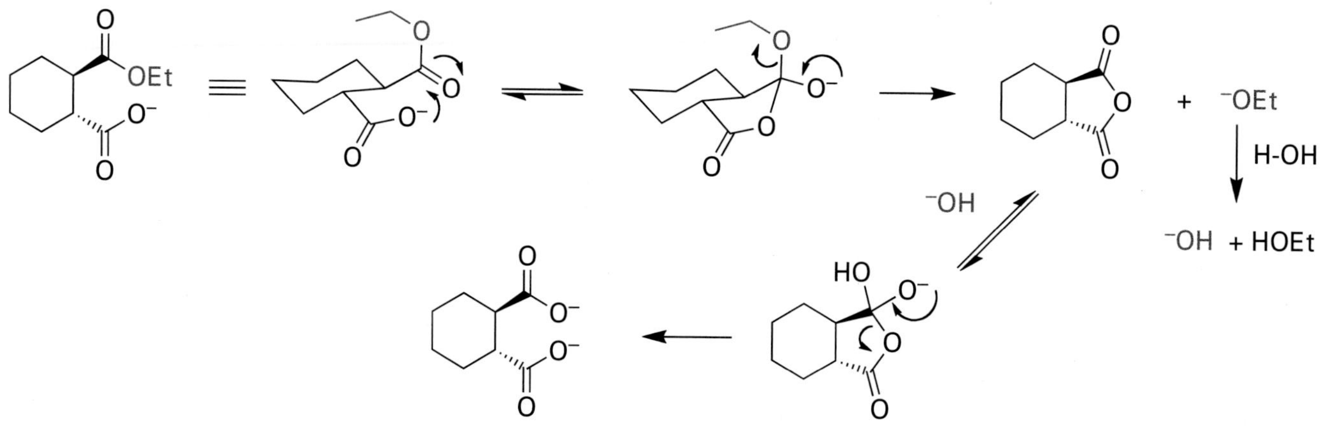

Explanation: The faster-reacting *trans* diastereomer exists with both ester and carboxylate in equitorial positions. This places the carboxylate in close proximity to the ester and enables the carboxylate to serve as a nucleophile and accelerate the reaction via initial formation of a cyclic anhydride intermediate, as shown. The slower-reacting *cis* diastereomer will always have one substituent in an axial position and one in an equatorial position. Because of this, the carboxylate is never close enough to provide neighboring group assistance and the reaction proceeds slowly at neutral pH.

Solution 7.6

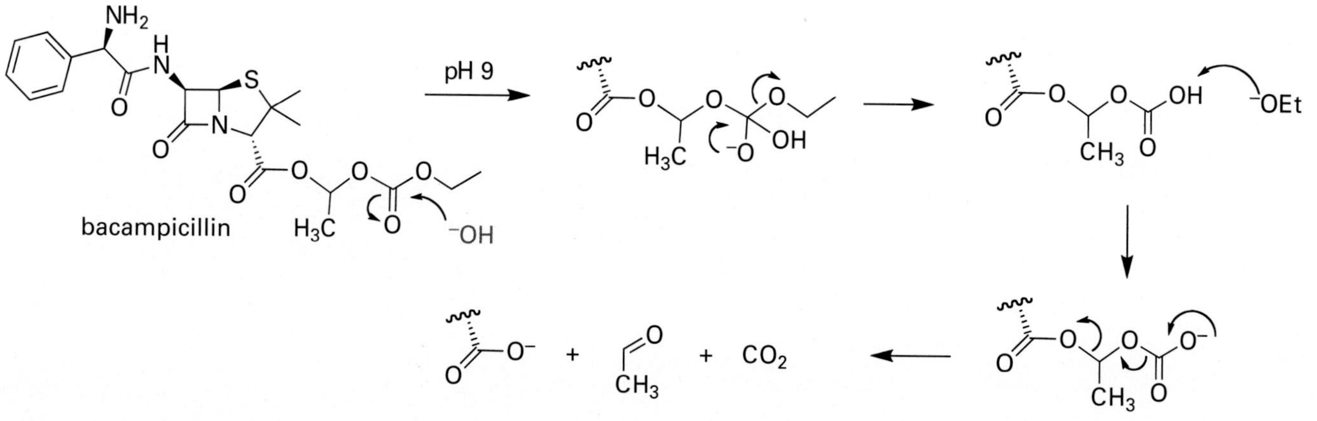

Solution 7.7

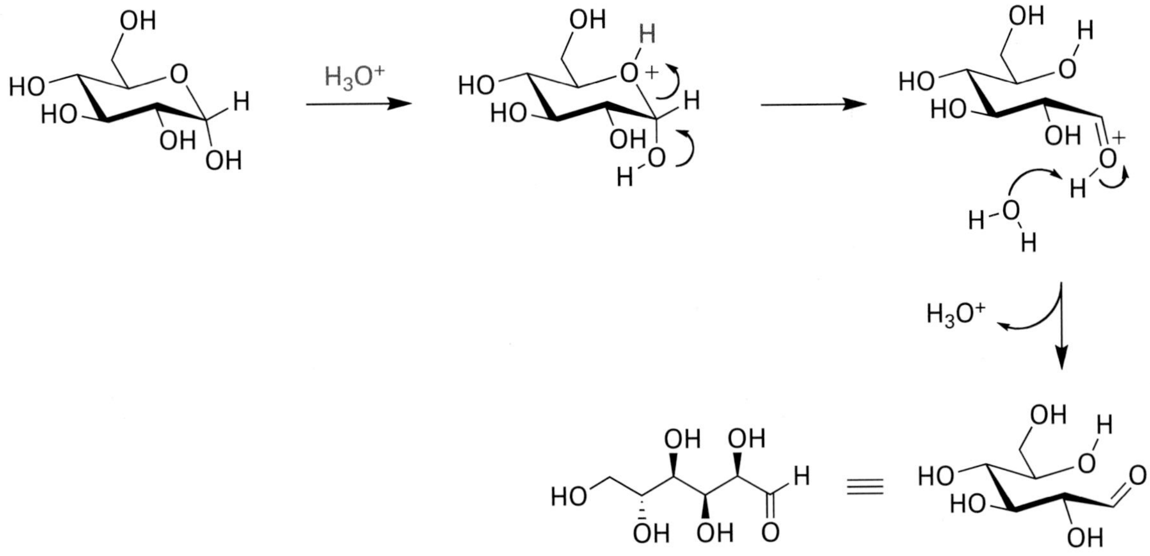

Solution 7.8

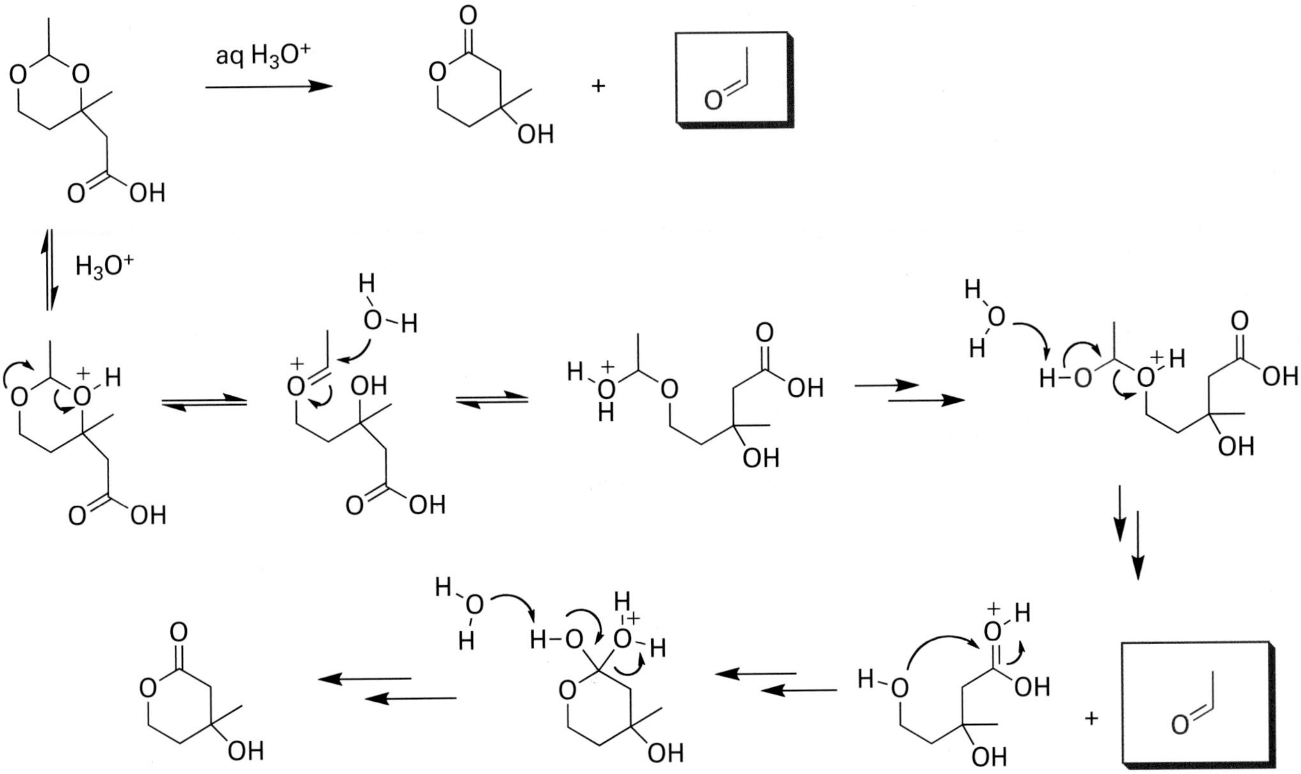

Explanation: The starting material is an acetal that reacts with water under the acidic reaction conditions to produce acetaldehyde (in orange in box) and an acyclic carboxylic acid with two free hydroxyl functions. One of the hydroxyls can react with the carboxylic acid in an acid catalyzed reaction to produce the observed lactone product, as shown above. Note that some steps (proton transfers) are omitted in the mechanism above.

Chapter 8

Solution 8.1

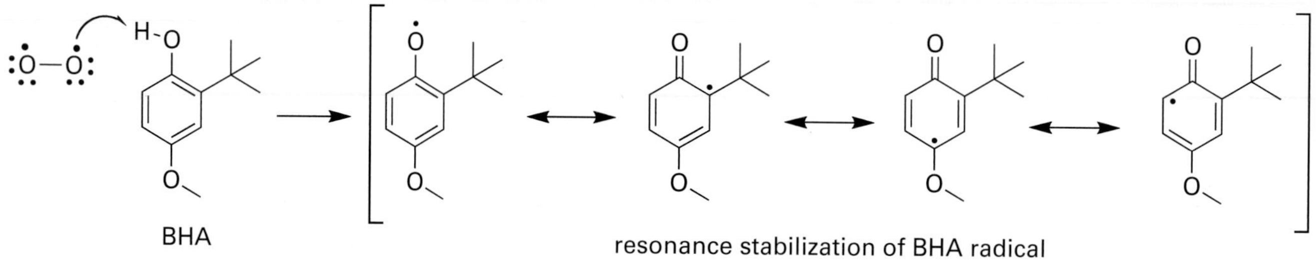

BHA

resonance stabilization of BHA radical

Solution 8.2

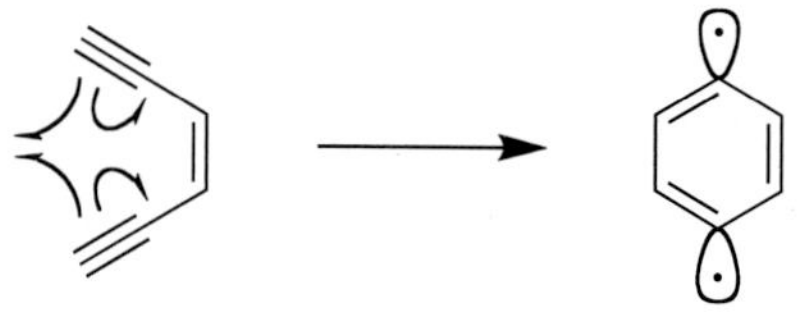

Solution 8.3

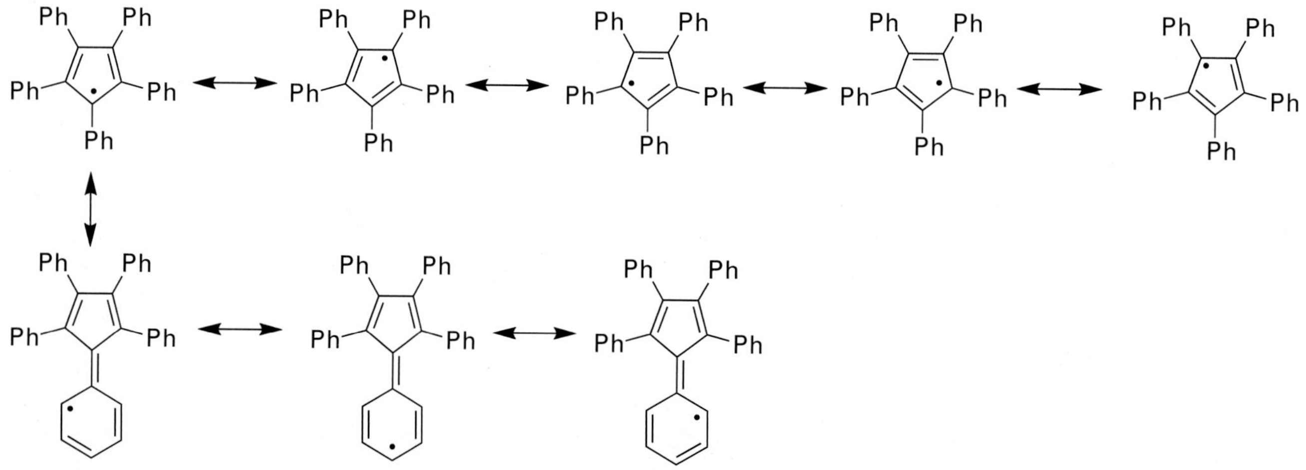

Explanation: This is a highly delocalized radical and thus relatively stable and unreactive. The radical is delocalized not only throughout the five-membered ring, as illustrated (top row of structures), but also into the pendant phenyl rings (as illustrated at bottom for one of the phenyl rings).

Solution 8.4

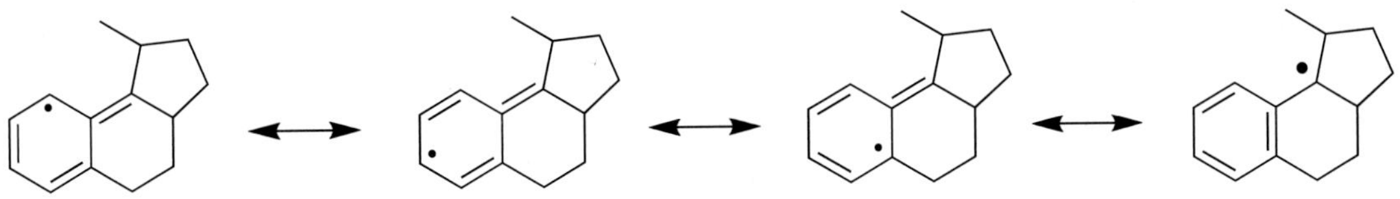

Explanation: Radical D is the most stable since it is a tertiary radical and is conjugated to the aromatic ring. Thus, radical D is delocalized throughout the aromatic ring, as illustrated above. While C is also a teriary radical, it does not benefit from the additional resonance stabilization of the aromatic ring. Radicals A and B are secondary and primary radicals, respectively, and thus less stable than either C or D.

Solution 8.5

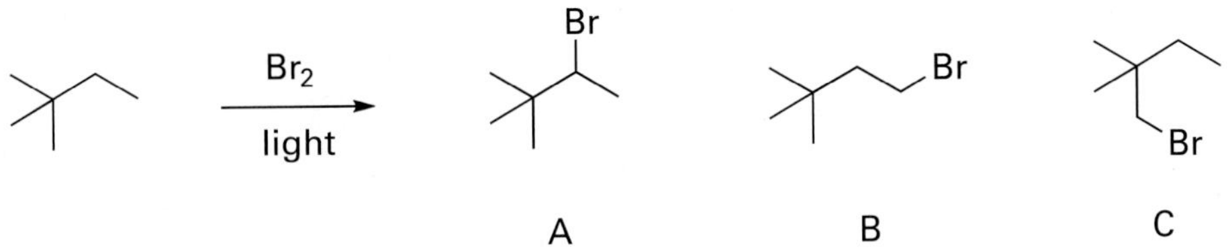

Product A is predicted to be the major product since it results from initial formation of the more stable secondary radical.

Solution 8.6

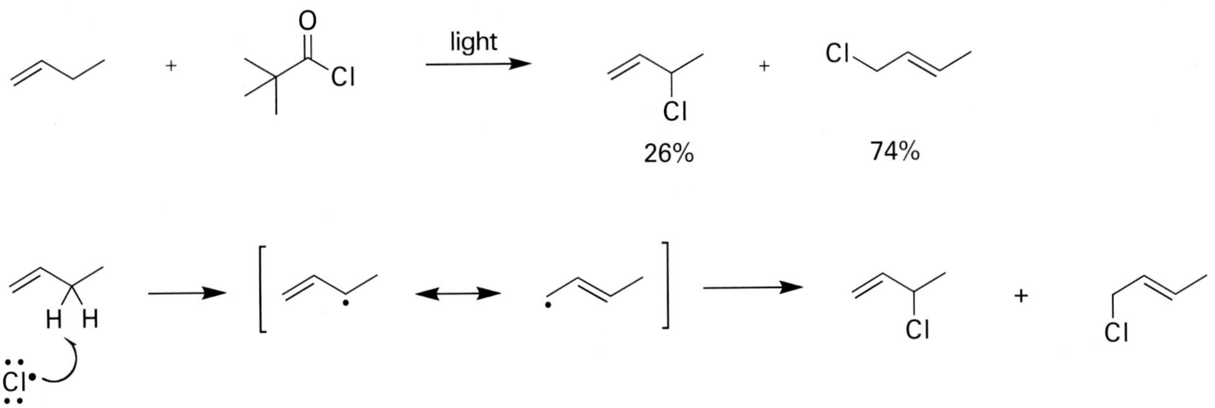

The chlorine radical produced in the initiation step abstracts a hydrogen atom from the substrate to produce a secondary radical that is conjugated to the double bond (forming an allylic radical). A resonance hybrid of the allylic radical is shown above and illustrates that two of the carbon atoms will have radical character. Either carbon can react further in a propagation or termination step to produce the observed products.

Solution 8.7

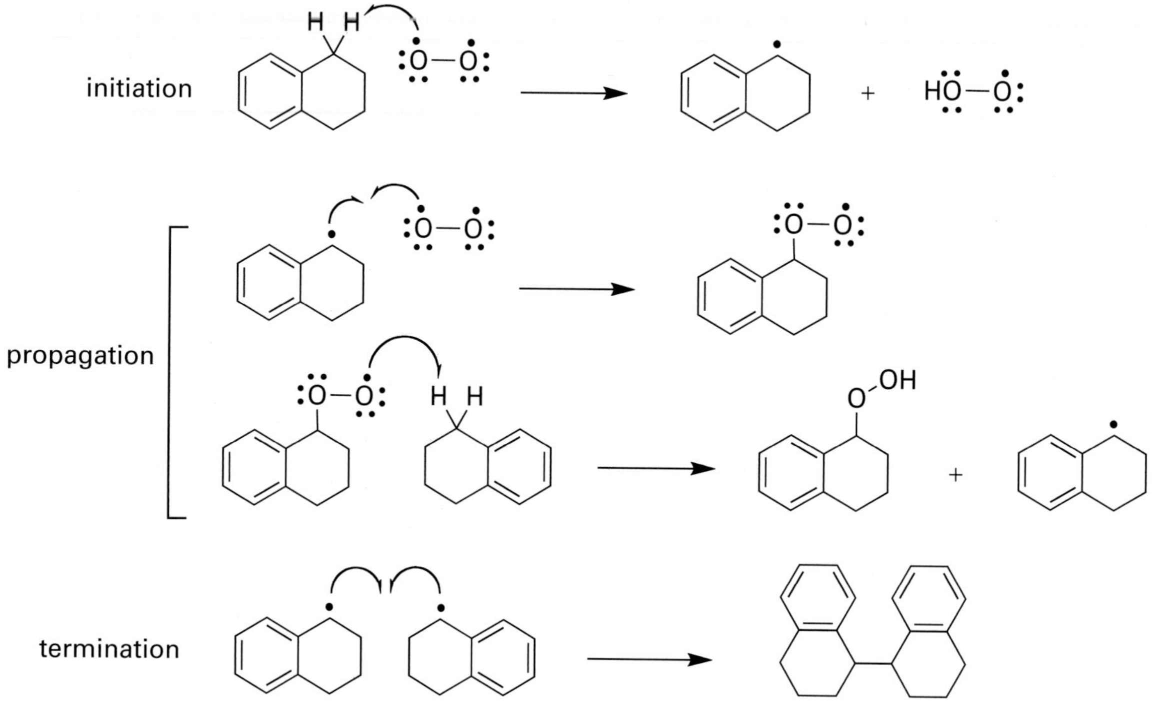

Solution 8.8

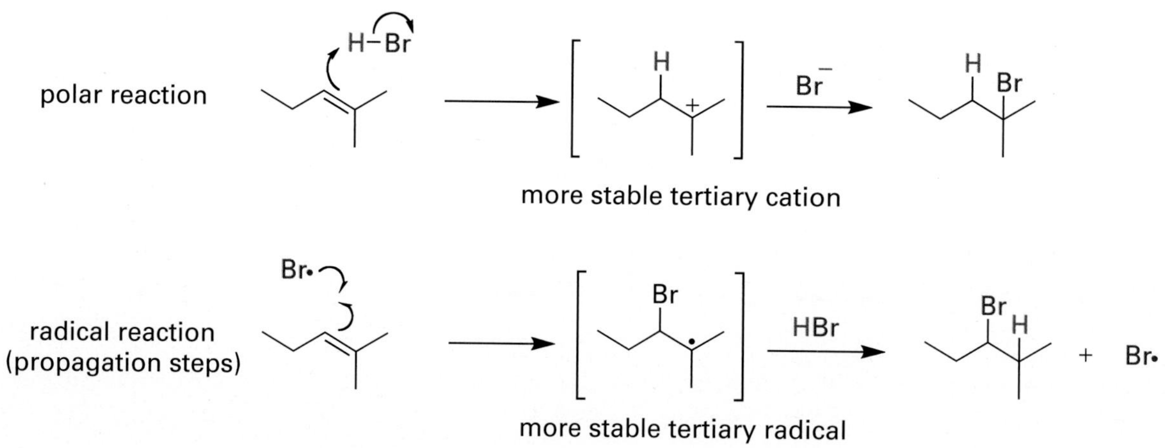

Explanation: The polar reaction involves reaction of HBr with the alkene, which proceeds with Markovnikov regioselectivity, placing hydrogen on the secondary carbon and producing the more stable tertiary carbocation intermediate. This reacts with bromide anion to form the observed product.

In the radical process, the regiochemistry-determining step is during propagation, when the bromine radical adds to the alkene. This addition proceeds with anti-Markovnikov regioselectivity, with bromine adding preferentially at the secondary carbon atom so as to produce the more stable tertiary radical intermediate. The radical then reacts with HBr to form the product and regenerate a bromine radical.

Index

Page numbers followed by *f* and *t* indicate figures and tables, respectively.

Acetal, 136
Acetal formation, 136, 137f
Acetaldehyde, 132f, 133
Acetamide, 81t
Acetate, 110f
Acetate anion, 86–87, 87f
Acetic acid, 82t, 86, 89–90, 90f, 91f
Acetone, 132f
Acetylcholine, 35b
Acetylcholine esterase, 35b
Acetylene, 3f, 81t
Acetylsalicylic acid, 96
Achiral objects/molecules, 42, 43
Achiral diastereomer, 44, 50
Acid, 78, 79
Acid anhydride, 134, 134f
Acid-base chemistry, 77–104
    acidic/basic, 79–80
    acidity/basicity, 80
    acidity constants, 80, 81–82t, 83–84t
    Arrhenius acid/base, 77–78, 79
    atom hybridization, 85–86, 86f
    atomic size, 85
    Brønsted-Lowry acid/base, 78, 79
    combined inductive and resonance effects, 92–95
    electronegativity, 82–85
    Henderson-Hasselbach equation, 96–97
    inductive electronic effects, 89–92
    Lewis acid/base, 78, 79
    pH scale, 79
    proximity and through-space effects, 95–96
    relative solubility, 77
    resonance electronic effects, 86–89
    self-ionization of water, 79
Acid-catalyzed amide hydrolysis, 147, 147f
Acid-catalyzed ester hydrolysis, 144, 144–145f
Acid chloride, 134, 134f
Acid dissociation constant (K_a), 80
Acidic solution, 79–80
Acidity, 80
Acidity constants, 80, 81–82t, 83–84t
Activation energy, 136
Active site, 148
Acyclic hydroxy aldehyde, 141b
Acyl-enzyme intermediate, 148
Acyl glucuronides, 141b
Acyl hydrazides, 142
ADC therapy. *See* Antibody-drug conjugate (ADC) therapy
Addition reactions, 119–121

Afatinib, 124–125, 125f
Alanine, 24t
Alcohol, 81t
Aldehyde, 13, 133t, 134–139
Aldimine, 139
Alendronate sodium, 12b
Alkoxyl radical, 163
Alkyl groups, 98
Alkylammonium ion, 95
Allylic radical, 160, 161f, 162
α-helix, 28
Alzheimer's therapies, 100
Amantadine, 29b, 72
Amide, 14, 134, 134f
Amide hydrolysis, 146–148
Amino acids, 23, 24–25t
Amino groups, 94, 95
Amphoteric molecules, 78
Angle strain, 62–63, 63b
Aniline, 81t, 88, 139
Anilinium, 83t
Anilinium ion, 88
Anion, 3, 7, 16, 17, 33, 78, 86, 87, 90, 96, 106, 107, 119, 164
Antacids, 99
Anti-aromatic, 16
Anti conformation, 60, 60f, 122
Antibiotic of last resort (vancomycin), 49b
Antibody-drug conjugate (ADC) therapy, 171
Anticoagulants, 38–39
Antimalarial therapy, 167b
Antiperiplanar orientation, 122
AO. *See* Atomic orbital (AO)
Apixaban, 38, 38f
Ar–NH$_2$, 81t
Ar–NH$_3$+, 83t
Ar–SH, 82t
Arginine, 25t
Aromatic amines, 139
Aromatic amino acids, 23
Aromatic compounds, 15
Aromatic heterocyclic ring systems, 17–18
Aromatic rings, 33
Aromaticity, 14–16
Arrhenius acid, 77–78, 79
Arrhenius base, 77–78, 79
Artemisinin, 167b
Artemisinin combination therapy, 167b
Aryl ammonium, 83t
Aryl diradical, 170

Aryl hydrazines, 142
Aryl thiol, 82t
Aryl-aryl interactions, 34
Aryl-aryl stacking interactions, 23, 26f, 34
Ascorbic acid, 164
Asparagine, 24t
Aspartic acid, 24t
Aspartyl proteases, 149–150
Aspirin, 124
Atom hybridization, 85–86, 86f
Atomic number, 7t
Atomic orbital (AO), 6
   1s orbital, 6
   2s orbital, 6
   p orbital, 6
   2p orbital, 6
   2p_x orbital, 6f
   2p_y orbital, 6f
   2p_z orbital, 6f
Atomic size, 85
Atropisomerism, 49b
Axial position, 64
Axid, 100

Backside attack, 112
Base, 78, 79. *See also* Acid-base chemistry
Basic solution, 79–80
Basicity, 80
Benzaldehyde, 134
Benzene, 15, 81t
Benzimidazole, 18f
Benzoic acid, 94
Benzylic radical, 160, 161f
Bergman cyclization, 170
Beryllium, 7t
β-secretase, 100
Betrixaban, 38, 38f
Bird flu (H5N1), 72
Bisphosphonates, 12b
Black, James, 100
Boat conformation, 64, 65, 65f
Bond dissociation energy, 160, 161f
Boron, 7t
Bridged ring system, 69, 69f
Bromine addition to cyclopentane, 120
Brønsted-Lowry acid, 78, 79
Brønsted-Lowry base, 78, 79
Bruton's tyrosine kinase (BTK), 125
BTK. *See* Bruton's tyrosine kinase (BTK)
Buried hydrophobic surface area, 28
Burimamide, 100
Buspirone, 69, 69f
n-butane conformers, 61

C–F bond, 36b
C–H–aryl interactions, 33
C–H hydrogen bond donor, 32
C–I bond, 36
C–X bond, 35, 36
Cahn-Ingold-Prelog (CIP) rules, 45–46, 46b
Calicheamicin γ₁, 169–171

Cancer drugs, 109b
Carbocation, 72, 114, 115, 116, 117, 119,
   120, 122, 138
Carbon, 1, 3, 7t
Carbon radical, 160, 161f
Carbonyl, 13
Carbonyl bonds, 152
Carbonyl-containing functional groups, 131–158
   aldehydes and ketones, 133t, 134–139
   amide hydrolysis, 146–148
   carbonyl group, 131–133
   enzyme-catalyzed hydrolysis, 148–151
   ester hydrolysis, 144–146
   imines and enamines, 139–142
   oximes and hydrazones, 142–143
   proteases, 148–151
   relative reactivity, 133–134, 134f
   steric effects, 132
Carbonyl group, 131–133
Carboxamide, 81t
Carboxylate anion, 90
Carboxylic acid, 82t
Carboxylic acid functional group, 90
Case studies
   calicheamicin γ₁, 169–171
   factor Xa inhibitors, 38–39
   kinase inhibitors, 124–125
   neuraminidase inhibitors and influenza virus, 74–75
   odanacatib, 153–154
   racemic and non-racemic drugs, 51–53
   Tagamet, 99–100
Catalytic triad, 149
Cathepsin K, 151b, 153
Cation, 3, 16, 17, 21, 34–35, 78, 114
Cation-π interactions, 34–35
Chair conformation, 64, 64f, 68–69
Chair-to-chair interconversion, 64
Chantix, 35b, 119, 119f
Chiral objects/molecules, 42
Chirality, 42
Chirality axis, 48, 48f
Chirality center, 44, 48
Chloroacetic acid, 90, 90f
Chronic lymphocytic leukemia (CLL), 125
Chymotrypsin, 149, 149f
Cimetidine, 99–100
CIP rules. *See* Cahn-Ingold-Prelog (CIP) rules
CLL. *See* Chronic lymphocytic leukemia (CLL)
Close proximity, 95, 99
Combined inductive and resonance effects, 92–95
Concerted process, 111
Configuration, 57
Configurational assignment, 44–46
Conformational constraint
   defined, 69
   drug molecules, 69f
   opiate analgesics, 70b
Conformational preferences of substituted cyclohexanes, 66–67
Conformations of organic molecules, 57–75
   angle strain, 62–63, 63b
   boat confirmation, 64, 65f

chair conformation, 64, 64f, 68–69
configuration/confirmation, distinguished, 57
conformational preferences of substituted cyclohexanes, 66–67
conformationally constrained ring systems, 69–70
cyclohexane and related six-membered rings, 64–66
dihedral angle, 58
eclipsed conformation, 57, 58f, 59
Newman projection, 58, 58f
staggered conformation, 57, 58f, 59
steric strain, 60–62, 63b
torsional strain, 58–60, 63b
twist-boat conformation, 64, 65f
wedge-hash type drawing, 66, 67f
Conformer, 57
Conjugate acid, 78
Conjugate base, 78
Constitutional isomers, 42
Cortisol, 70f
Covalent bond, 2
Covalent drugs, 124
COX enzyme, 52
Cyclobutadiene, 16
Cyclobutane, 62, 62t, 63
Cycloheptane, 62t
Cyclohexane, 62, 62t, 64f
Cyclohexane and related six-membered rings, 64–66
Cyclohexane substituents, 66t
Cyclooctane, 62t
Cyclooxygenase (COX), 52
Cyclopentadienyl anion, 17f
Cyclopentane, 62, 62t, 63, 63f
Cyclophosphamide, 109b
Cyclopropane, 62, 62t
Cyclotetradecane, 62t
CYP enzymes, 166, 167
Cys797, 125f
Cys805, 124
Cysteine, 24t
Cysteine protease inhibitors, 153–154
Cysteine proteases, 148, 149
Cytochrome P450 (CYP) enzymes, 166, 167
Cytoxan, 109b

Decalin, 69
cis-decalin, 70, 70f
trans-decalin, 69–70, 70f
Delocalization, 14, 19
Desolvation, 27–29
Desolvation penalty, 31
Dexketoprofen, 53
Dextrorphan, 42f
Diacetylimide, 81t
1,2-diaminoethane, 91f
1,3-diaminoethane, 91, 91f
Diastereomer, 43, 46, 49
Dielectric (medium), 27
Dihedral angle, 58
1,3-diketone, 82t
1,3-dimethylcyclohexane, 41, 41f, 42f, 43–44
cis-1,3-dimethylcyclohexane, 43
trans-1,3-dimethylcyclohexane, 43

Dimethyloxonium ion, 83t
Dipeptidyl peptidase-4 (DPP-4), 36b
Dipole, 34
Direct hydrogen bonding interaction, 95
Disproportionation, 166
Distomer, 51
DNA double helix, 26f
DNA intercalation, 34
Doxorubicin, 34
DPP-4, 36b
Drawing chair conformations, 68–69
Drawing organic molecules, 4b
Duocarmycins, 34

E1 elimination reaction, 122
E2 elimination reaction, 122
Eclipsed conformation, 57, 58f, 59
Edge-to-face, 34, 34f
Effective charge, 5
EGFR, 124
Electron, 2
Electron configuration, 7t
Electron donating, 89, 91, 98
Electron withdrawing, 89, 91, 98
Electronegative, 5
Electronegativity, 82–85, 87
Electrophiles, 105, 106, 108–109
Electrophilic chemotherapeutic drugs, 109f
Elimination reactions, 121–122
Eliquis, 38
Enamine, 139–142
Enamine formation, 141f
Enantiomer, 42, 42f, 46
End-on overlap, 10
Enthalpy-driven interactions, 26
Entropically driven interactions, 26
Entropy-driven hydrophobic effect, 28
Entropy-enthalpy compensation, 26
Envelope conformation, 63f
Enzyme-catalyzed hydrolysis, 148–151
Epoxidation reaction, 167, 168f
Epoxides, 109
Equatorial position, 64
Esomeprazole, 48, 48f, 52
Ester, 134, 134f, 144
Ester α-C–H, 81t
Ester hydrolysis, 144–146
Ethane, 3f, 58f, 59f
Ethyl acetate, 81t
Ethylamine, 91f
Ethylene, 3f, 10, 81t, 132f
Eutomer, 51

Face-to-face, 34, 34f
Factor Xa (fXa), 38
Factor Xa inhibitors, 38–39
Famotidine, 100
Faraday, Michael, 15
Fentanyl, 70b
Fenton chemistry, 166, 167b
Fenton reaction, 166, 166f

Fluorine, 5, 7f, 7t
Fluoroacetic acid, 90, 90f
Formaldehyde, 132f, 133
Formamide, 14f
Formic acid, 90, 90f
Fosamax, 12b
Frost circles, 16, 17f
Fructose, 138
D-fructose, 138f
Functional groups, 11, 12b
Furan, 17, 18f
Fused ring system, 69, 69f
fXa, 38
fXa inhibitors, 38–39

Gastric acid, 99
Gastroesophageal reflux disease (GERD), 99
Gauche conformation, 60, 60f
General acid, 148
General base, 148
GERD. *See* Gastroesophageal reflux disease (GERD)
Gilotrif, 124
Gleevec, 124
Glu, 151
D-glucose, 138f
Glucuronic acid, 137b
Glucuronidation reaction, 137b
Glucuronide, 137b, 167
Glutamic acid, 24t
Glutamine, 24t
Glutathione, 108
Glutathione S-transferase, 33b, 108
Glycine, 24t
Glycosidic bonds, 138
Guanidine, 100
Guanidinium ion, 83t, 88, 88f
Guanylhistamine, 100

H–C hydrogen bond donor, 32
H5N1 flu, 72
Half-chair conformation, 63f
Halides, 94, 110
Halogen bond, 35–36
Handedness of chirality centers, 44
Hands and gloves, 42
Hard acid or base, 107
Hard-soft acid base (HSAB) theory, 107
HDAC. *See* Histone deacetylase (HDAC)
Helium, 7t
Hemagglutinin, 72
Heme, 168f
Hemi-acetal, 136–138
Hemi-animal, 139
Hemi-ketal, 136–138
Henderson-Hasselbach equation, 96–97
HER2, 124
Heteratom, 19
Heteroaromatic ring systems, 17–18, 19
HI. *See* Hydroiodic acid (HI)
High-dielectric medium, 27
His 57, 149f

Histamine-2 receptor antagonists, 99
Histidine, 25t
Histone deacetylase (HDAC), 151b
Homolysis, 159, 160, 169
Homolytic cleavage, 160f
HSAB theory. *See* Hard-soft acid base (HSAB) theory
Hückel, Erich, 15
Hückel's rule, 15–16
Hybrid orbital, 9
   sp-hybridized carbon, 9f, 11
   *sp*²-hybridized carbon, 9f, 10
   *sp*³-hybridized carbon, 9f, 10
   sp-hybridized nitrogen, 13f
   *sp*²-hybridized nitrogen, 13, 13f
   *sp*³-hybridized nitrogen, 13, 13f
   *sp*²-hybridized oxygen, 13f
   *sp*³-hybridized oxygen, 13f
Hybridization, 85
Hybridization of carbon, 9, 9f
Hybridization of orbitals, 11–14
Hydration (aldehydes/ketones), 133t, 134–136
Hydrazide, 142
Hydrazine, 142
Hydrazone, 142–143
Hydrogen, 7t
Hydrogen atom radicals, 160f
Hydrogen bond, 27, 29–32
Hydrogen bond acceptor, 30, 32
Hydrogen bond donor, 30, 32
Hydrogen bond strength, 31
Hydrogen bromide, 82t
Hydrogen chloride, 82t
Hydrogen cyanide, 3
Hydrogen fluoride, 82t
Hydrogen iodide, 82t
Hydrogen sulfate, 82t
Hydrogen sulfate ion, 82t
Hydroiodic acid (HI), 107
Hydrolysis, 144
Hydronium, 83t
Hydrophilic/charged amino acids, 23
Hydrophilic/uncharged amino acids, 23
Hydrophobic amino acids, 23
Hydrophobic effect, 27–29
Hydrophobic substituents, 99
Hydroxide, 112
Hydroxylamine, 142
Hydroxylation reaction, 167, 168f
Hyperconjugation, 160

Ibrutinib, 125
Ibuprofen, 52
(R)-ibuprofen, 52, 52f
(S)-ibuprofen, 52f, 53
Imatinib, 124
Imbruvica, 124
Imidazole, 18f
Imidazolium ion, 83t, 89, 89f
Imine, 139–142
Imine formation, 140f
Iminium ion, 88, 88f, 139

In-phase combination, 8
Indazole, 18f
Indinavir, 151b
Indole, 18f
Inductive and resonance effects, 92–95
Inductive electronic effects, 89–92
Inductive withdrawing effect, 91
Influenza virus, 29–30b, 74–75
Initiation, 162, 164f
Intermolecular process, 117
Intramolecular hydrogen bond, 32
Intramolecular process, 117
Iodide, 110
Iodine, 61
Ionic bond, 2
Ionic interactions, 27, 29
Ionization state, 90
Iron-mediated radical reactions, 165–167
Isoleucine, 24t
Isopropyl ammonium ion, 83t
Isopropyl iminium ion, 83t
Isothiazole, 18f
Isoxazole, 18f

Januvia, 36b

K_a, 80
Kekulé benzene, 15, 15f
Kekulé naphthalene, 15
Kekulé structure, 15
Ketal, 136
Ketimine, 139
Ketones, 133t, 134–139
Ketoprofen, 52
(R)-ketoprofen, 52f, 53
(S)-ketoprofen, 52f
Kinase inhibitors, 124–125

Leaving group, 109–110
Left handed molecule, 45
Leucine, 24t
Leucine zipper, 28f
Levorphanol, 42f
Lewis, Gilbert N., 3, 78, 106
Lewis acid, 78, 79
Lewis base, 78, 79
Lewis structure, 3, 3f
Ligand/drug binding, 25–26
Linoleic acid, 163, 164f
Lipid oxidation, 163
Lithium, 5, 7t
Lone pair, 11
Lower energy conformers, 63
Lyrica, 121, 121f
Lysine, 25t

M2 proton channel, 29–30b
Maalox, 99
Magnesium, 7t
Malonic acid, 91f
Markovnikov's rule, 119

Mechlorethamine, 109b, 117f
Meisenheimer complex, 118
Meso compounds, 46–48
Mesylate, 110, 110f
Metalloprotease, 149, 150
Metalloprotease carboxypeptidase A, 150, 150f
Methane, 10, 81t
Methane sulfonate anion (mesylate), 110, 110f
Methanesulfonic acid, 82t
Methanethiol, 81t
Methanol, 62, 81t, 86
Methionine, 24t
Methoxide anion, 86
Methoxy group, 93
Methyl bromide, 109, 112
Methyl groups, 94
4-methyl-histamine, 100
Methyl radical, 160, 160f
Methylamine, 62, 81t
Methylammonium ion, 83t
Methylcyclohexane, 66
Methylsulfonate anion, 87f
Metiamide, 100
Michael acceptor, 119
Michael addition, 119, 121f, 170
Microsomal CYPs, 166, 167
Mirror-image molecules, 42
Mirror-image stereoisomer
        (enantiomer), 42, 42f
Molecular orbital (MO), 7
    π bond, 11
    sigma (σ) bond, 8, 10
    sigma (σ) orbital, 8, 8f
    sigma star (σ*) orbital, 8, 8f
Molecular oxygen (O_2), 163–165
Mono-chlorobutanoic acids, 91
Morphine, 70b
Mustard gas, 109b
Mylanta, 99
Mylotarg, 171

$n \rightarrow \pi^*$ interaction, 36b
Naproxen, 52, 53
(S)-naproxen, 52f, 53
Neighboring group assistance, 116–118
Neon, 6, 7f, 7t
Neuraminidase, 72
Neuraminidase inhibitors and
        influenza virus, 74–75
Neutron, 2
Newman projection, 58, 58f
Nexium, 48, 52
Nicotine, 35b
Nitrile functional group, 11
Nitro (NO_2) group, 92
Nitrogen, 7t
Nitrogen mustard, 109b
Nizatidine, 100
NO_2 group, 92
Noble gases, 2
Non-carbon chirality center, 50

Non-covalent interactions, 23–40
   amino acids, 23, 24–25t
   aryl-aryl interactions, 34
   aryl rings as hydrogen bond acceptors, 33
   cation-π interactions, 34–35
   desolvation, 27–29
   enthalpy-driven interactions, 26
   entropically driven interactions, 26
   C–H as hydrogen bond donor, 32
   halogen bond, 35 36
   hydrogen bond, 29–32
   hydrophobic effect, 27–29
   ionic interactions, 29
   π-hydrogen bond, 33
   strength of, 27
Non-mirror image stereoisomer (diastereomer), 43, 49
Nonclassical hydrophobic effect, 28
Nonsteroidal anti-inflammatory drugs (NSAIDs), 52–53
NSAIDs. *See* Nonsteroidal anti-inflammatory drugs (NSAIDs)
Nucleophiles, 105, 106–108
Nucleophilic aliphatic substitution
   neighboring group assistance, 116–118
   S_N1 reactions, 114–118
   S_N2 reactions, 110–113
Nucleophilic aromatic substitution, 118–119
Nucleophilic catalysis, 148
Nucleophilic reactions. *See* Substitution, addition, and elimination
   reactions
Nucleophilicity, 106, 107, 107t

O–H–aryl interactions, 33
Odanacatib, 151b, 153–154
Omeprazole, 48, 51–52, 124
(S)-omeprazole, 52
One-electron redox chemistry, 169
Opiate analgesics, 70b
Orbital overlap, 8
Organic molecules, 1, 4b
Oseltamivir, 72–73, 72f, 73f
Osteoporosis, 12b, 154
Out-of-phase combination, 8
1,3,4-oxadizole, 18f
Oxazole, 18f
Oxidation of linoleic acid, 163, 164f
Oxidative phosphorylation, 169
Oxime, 142–143
Oxy-anion hole, 149
Oxygen, 7t, 13
Oxygen-mediated lipid oxidation, 163

p orbital, 6
2*p* orbital, 6
2p_x orbital, 6f
2p_y orbital, 6f
2p_z orbital, 6f
Parallel-displaced, 34, 34f
Partial antagonists, 100
Pauli exclusion principle, 6
Pauling, Linus, 5, 9
Pauling electronegativity scale, 5, 5f
Pentane-2,4-dione, 82t

Pepcid, 100
Periodic table, 2, 2f
Peroxy radical, 163
pH scale, 79
Phenol, 81t, 86, 108f
Phenolic acid, 94
Phenoxide, 108f
Phenoxide anion, 86, 87f
Phenylalanine, 25t
Phosphate, 12b
Phosphate group, 12b
Phosphonate group, 12b
Phosphorus, 12b
π bond, 11
π-hydrogen bond, 33
pK_a, 80
Planar conformation, 63f
Polarizability, 107
Polarization, 4–5
Potential energy diagram, 61f, 65f
Pregabalin, 121, 121f
Prilosec, 48, 51
"Profen" class, 52
Proline, 25t
Propagation, 162, 164f
Prostaglandins, 52
Protease, 38, 148–151
Protease inhibitors, 38, 151b
Prothrombin, 38
Proton, 2
Protonate acetone, 84t
Protonate amide, 83t
Protonated isopropyl alcohol, 83t
Protonated methanethiol, 84t
Protonated methanol, 83t
Protonated methyl acetate, 84t
Proximity and through-space effects, 95–96
Pyrazine, 17, 17f
Pyrazole, 18f
Pyridazine, 17, 17f
Pyridine, 17f
Pyridine ring, 107
Pyridinium ion, 83t, 89, 89f
Pyrimidine, 17, 17f
Pyrrole, 18, 18f

Qinghaosu, 167b
Quadrupole, 34
Quantum mechanics, 5–6
Quetiapine, 118
Quinoline, 18f

R configuration, 45, 45f
Racemic and non-racemic drugs, 51–53
Radical chemistry, 159–173
   Fenton chemistry, 166
   homolysis, 159, 160, 169
   hydroxylation and epoxidation reactions, 167, 168f
   hyperconjugation, 160
   iron-mediated radical reactions, 165–167
   molecular oxygen (O_2), 163–165

radical, defined, 169
  radical reactions, 161–163
  steric crowding, 160
  vitamin C, 159f, 164–165
  vitamin E, 159f, 163–164
Radical reactions, 161–163
Ranitidine, 100
Regioselective reaction, 119
Relative solubility, 77
Resonance delocalization, 86–89, 160
Resonance effects, 92
Resonance electron donating, 86, 92, 94, 98
Resonance electron donor, 98
Resonance electron withdrawer, 98
Resonance electron withdrawing, 86, 92, 94, 98
Resonance electronic effects, 86–89
Resonance form, 14
Resonance hybrid, 12b, 14
Resonance stabilization, 14
Retro-Michael reaction, 122
Ring flip, 64
Ring fusion, 69
Ring systems, 17
Rivaroxaban, 38–39
Rolaids, 99

1s orbital, 6
2s orbital, 6
S-adenosyl methionine (SAM), 112
S configuration, 45f, 46
Salicylamide, 96, 96f
Salicylic acid, 96
Salt bridge, 29
SAM. See S-adenosyl methionine (SAM)
Sawhorse, 58f, 59f
Schiff base, 139
Schrödinger equation, 5, 6
Self-ionization of water, 79
Serine, 24t
Serine proteases, 148, 149
Sialic acid, 72–73, 72f
Side-on overlap, 11
sigma (σ) bond, 8, 10
sigma (σ) orbital, 8, 8f
sigma star (σ*) orbital, 8, 8f
Singlet oxygen, 163, 163f
Sitagliptin, 36b
S_N1 reactions, 114–118
S_N2 reactions, 110–113
S_NAr reactions, 118–119
Sodium, 6, 7f, 7t
Sodium chloride, 2
Soft acid or base, 107
Solvolysis reaction, 110f
sp-hybridized carbon, 9f, 11
sp²-hybridized carbon, 9f, 10
sp³-hybridized carbon, 9f, 10
sp-hybridized nitrogen, 13f
sp²-hybridized nitrogen, 13, 13f
sp³-hybridized nitrogen, 13, 13f
sp²-hybridized oxygen, 13f

sp³-hybridized oxygen, 13f
Spirocyclic ring system, 69, 69f
Staggered conformation, 57, 58f, 59
Stereochemistry, 41–56
  atropisomerism, 49b
  chirality, 42
  chirality axis, 48, 48f
  chirality center, 44, 48
  CIP rules, 45–46, 46b
  configurational assignment, 44–46
  constitutional isomers, 42
  determining isomeric/stereochemical
    relationships, 43b
  diastereomer, 43, 46, 49
  enantiomer, 42, 42f, 46
  meso compounds, 46–48
  stereoisomer, 41, 42
Stereoisomer, 41, 42
Stereospecific reaction, 112
Steric crowding, 160
Steric effects, 132
Steric strain, 60–62, 63b
Stern (boat), 65
Structural scaffolding, 17
Substituted cyclohexanes, 66–67
Substitution, addition, and elimination reactions, 105–129
  addition reactions, 119–121
  electrophiles, 108–109
  elimination reactions, 121–122
  leaving group, 109–110
  neighboring group assistance, 116–118
  nucleophiles, 106–108
  nucleophilic aliphatic substitution, 110–118
  nucleophilic aromatic substitution, 118–119
  S_N1 reactions, 114–118
  S_N2 reactions, 110–113
  S_NAr reactions, 118–119
Succinic acid, 91f
Sucrose, 137f
Sulfide group, 12b
Sulfonamide, 81t
Sulfonamide group, 12b
Sulfonate anion, 87
Sulfone group, 12b
Sulfonic group, 12b
Sulfoxide group, 12b
Sulfur functional groups, 12b
Sulfuric acid, 82t
Sulphenamide intermediate, 51f, 52
Syn conformation, 60, 60f

Table salt, 2
Tagamet, 99–100
Tamiflu, 72
Termination, 162–163
Tetrahedral oxygen, 48
Tetrahedral sulfur, 50
Thiazole, 18f
Thiele benzene, 15f
Thiele naphthalene, 15
Thiele-type drawings, 15

Thioester, 134, 134f
Thioether, 12b
Thiol group, 12b
Thiophene, 18f
Thiophenol, 82t
Threonine, 24t
Thrombin, 38
Through-bond electronic effects, 95
Through-space hydrophobic effect, 95
Thyroxine, 36
Torsional strain, 58–60, 63b
Transition-state intermediate, 73f
Transthyretin, 36
1,2,4-triazole, 18f
Triflate, 110, 110f
Trifluoroacetaldehyde, 133
Trifluoroacetate, 110, 110f
Trifluoromethyl group, 133
Trifluoromethylsulfonate anion (triflate), 110, 110f
Trigonal-planar arrangement, 10
Triplet oxygen, 163, 163f
Trovafloxacin, 69, 69f
Tryptophan, 25t
Tums, 99

Twist-boat conformation, 64, 65f
Tyrosine, 24t, 25t
Valence, 3
Valence bond theory, 5–8
Valence shell electrons, 85
Valine, 24t
van der Waals interactions, 27, 37
Vancomycin, 49b
Varenicline, 35b, 69, 69f, 119, 119f
Vitamin C, 159f, 164–165
Vitamin E, 159f, 163–164
Vorinostat, 151b

Water, 81t
Wedge-and-dash, 58f, 59f, 66, 67f

Xarelto, 38

Zaitsev's rule, 122
Zanamivir, 72–73, 72f
Zantac, 100
Zomepirac, 137b, 141b
Zomepirac acylglucuronide, 141b
Zomepirac glucuronide, 137b, 141b